THE

HEART

AND

HYPERTENSION

THE
HEART
AND
HYPERTENSION

Franz H. Messerli, MD
Editor

Associate Head, Division of Hypertension, Ochsner Clinic

Director of Hemodynamic Laboratory,
Alton Ochsner Medical Foundation, New Orleans

Professor of Medicine, Department of Medicine,
Tulane University, New Orleans

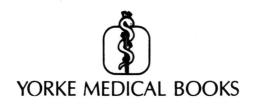

YORKE MEDICAL BOOKS

NOTICE

While every effort has been made to ensure the accuracy of the drug dosage and administration data, the reader is advised to check the package insert of each drug he/she plans to administer for possible changes in information resulting from new research or clinical experience after publication of this work.

Printed in the United States of America.

THE HEART AND HYPERTENSION
First Edition

Library of Congress Cataloging in Publication Data

The Heart and hypertension.

   Includes index.
   1. Heart—Hypertrophy.   2. Hypertension—Complications and sequelae. I. Messerli, Franz H. [DNLM: 1. Heart—drug effects. 2. Heart—
physiopathology.   3. Hypertension—drug   therapy.   4. Hypertension—
physiopathology. WG 340 H4357]
 RC685.H9H4   1987   616.1′29   87-13316
 ISBN 0-914316-45-1

Contents

PART IV
PATHOPHYSIOLOGY OF LEFT VENTRICULAR HYPERTROPHY

PART V
CLINICAL ASPECTS

**PART VII
SPECIAL CONSIDERATIONS**

Dedication

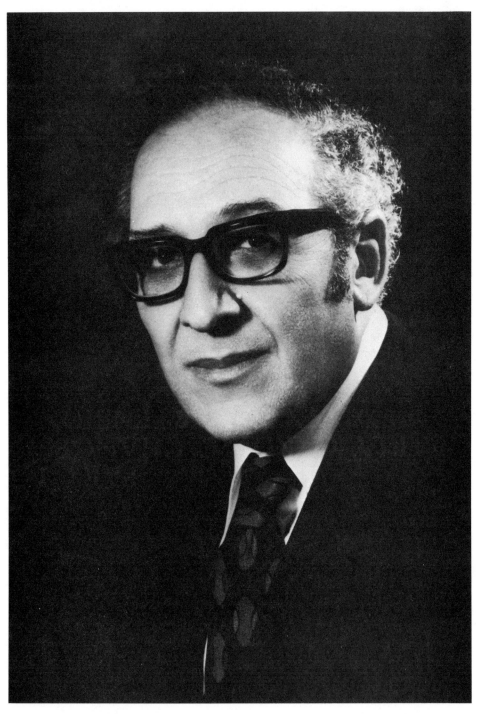

This book is dedicated to the late Robert C. Tarazi, M.D., who for many years led the way in this field.

Franz Messerli

Contributors

FREDDY ABI-SAMRA, MD, Research Division, Cleveland Clinic Foundation, Cleveland, Ohio

JAMES K. ALEXANDER, MD, Department of Cardiology, Baylor College of Medicine, Houston, Texas

CELSO AMODEO, MD, Department of Internal Medicine, Section on Hypertensive Diseases, Ochsner Clinic and Alton Ochsner Medical Foundation, New Orleans, Louisiana

STEPHEN L. BACHARACH, PhD, Department of Nuclear Medicine, Clinical Center, National Institutes of Health, Bethesda, Maryland

ROBERT BARNDT, MD, Department of Medicine, Section of Hypertension, USC School of Medicine, Los Angeles, California

EDWARD BLANCHARD, PhD, Department of Cardiology, State University of New York at Albany, Albany, New York

PETER BOLLI, Division of Cardiology, University Hospital, Basel, Switzerland

JEFFREY S. BORER, MD, Cardiology Division, The New York Hospital-Cornell Medical Center, New York, New York

ARCHER BROUGHTON, Baker Medical Research Institute, Melbourne, Australia

FRITZ R. BÜHLER, Division of Cardiology, University Hospital, Basel, Switzerland

JOSEPH M. CAPASSO, PhD, Cardiovascular Research Laboratories, Department of Medicine, Division of Cardiology, Albert Einstein College of Medicine, Bronx, New York

ANNE COULL, MRC/University Circulation Research Unit, University of the Witwatersrand Medical School, Johannesburg, South Africa

WALTER S. CULPEPPER III, MD, Department of Pediatric Cardiology, Ochsner Clinic and Alton Ochsner Medical Foundation, New Orleans, Louisiana

ANDREW L. DANNENBERG, MD, MPH, National Heart, Lung, and Blood Institute, Bethesda, Maryland

VINCENT DeQUATTRO, MD, Hypertension Service, Department of Medicine, University of Southern California School of Medicine, Los Angeles, California

RICHARD B. DEVEREUX, MD, Cardiology Division, Department of Medicine, The New York Hospital-Cornell Medical Center, New York, New York

V. M. DIMITRIU, Diagnosis Center and the Hypertension Research Center, Broussais Hospital, Paris, France

DONALD B. DOTY, MD, Department of Cardiac Surgery, Latter Day Saints Hospital, Salt Lake City, Utah

JAN I. M. DRAYER, MD, Hypertension Center, Section of Cardiology, Veterans Administration Medical Center, Long Beach, California

ELENA G. DYAKONOVA, MD, Myasnikov Institute of Clinical Cardiology, USSR Cardiology Research Center, Moscow, USSR

CHARLES L. EASTHAM, BA, Cardiovascular Center, University of Iowa Hospitals, Iowa City, Iowa

BRENT M. EGAN, MD, Division of Hypertension, Department of Internal Medicine, University of Michigan Medical Center, Ann Arbor, Michigan

PAUL ERNE, Division of Cardiology, University Hospital, Basel, Switzerland

MURRAY D. ESLER, Baker Medical Research Institute, Melbourne, Australia

BONITA FALKNER, MD, Department of Pediatrics, Hahnemann University, Philadelphia, Pennsylvania

VICTOR J. FERRANS, MD, PhD, Chief, Ultrastructural Section, Pathology Branch, National Heart, Lung and Blood Institute, National Institutes of Health, Bethesda, Maryland

JEFFREY FISHER, MD, Cardiology Division, The New York Hospital-Cornell Medical Center, New York, New York

ANDRAS G. FOTI, PhD, Department of Medicine, Section of Hypertension, USC School of Medicine, Los Angeles, California

FETNAT M. FOUAD, MD, Research Division, Cleveland Clinic Foundation, Cleveland, Ohio

JOSEPH A. FRANCIOSA, MD, Cardiovascular Division, Veterans Administration Medical Center and University of Arkansas for Medical Sciences, Little Rock, Arkansas

EDWARD D. FREIS, MD, Senior Medical Investigator, Veterans Administration Medical Center, Professor of Medicine, Georgetown University, Washington, D.C.

PETER FRIBERG, PhD, Department of Physiology, University of Goteborg, Goteborg, Sweden

EDWARD D. FROHLICH, MD, Vice President, Academic Affairs, Alton Ochsner Medical Foundation, Staff Member, Division on Hypertensive Diseases, Ochsner Clinic, New Orleans, Louisiana

JULIUS M. GARDIN, MD, Hypertension Center, Section of Cardiology, Veterans Administration Medical Center, Long Beach, California and the University of California, Irvine, California

CARMEL GOODMAN, MRC/University Circulation Research Unit, University of the Witwatersrand Medical School, Johannesburg, South Africa

MICHAEL V. GREEN, MS, Department of Nuclear Medicine, Clinical Center, National Institutes of Health, Bethesda, Maryland

MAURIZIO D. GUAZZI, MD, Institute of Cardiology, Milan, Italy

DAVID G. HARRISON, MD, Department of Medicine, University of Iowa Hospitals, Iowa City, Iowa

LOREN F. HIRATZKA, MD, Department of Surgery, Division of Thoracic & Cardiovascular Surgery, University of Iowa Hospitals, Iowa City, Iowa

ALAN T. HIRSCH, MD, Cardiovascular Division, Harvard Medical School, Beth Israel Hospital, Boston, Massachusetts

U. LENNART HULTHÉN, Division of Cardiology, University Hospital, Basel, Switzerland

ISAO K. INOUYE, MD, Department of Medicine, Baylor College of Medicine, Houston, Texas

MICHAEL JASON, MD, Cardiology Division, The New York Hospital-Cornell Medical Center, New York, New York

GARRY L. JENNINGS, Baker Medical Research Institute, Melbourne, Australia

STEVO JULIUS, MD, Division of Hypertension, Department of Internal Medicine, University of Michigan Medical Center, Ann Arbor, Michigan

WILLIAM B. KANNEL, MD, MPH, Boston University School of Medicine, Boston, Massachusetts

NORMAN M. KAPLAN, Professor of Internal Medicine, University of Texas Health Science Center at Dallas, Southwestern Medical School, Dallas, Texas

ARNOLD M. KATZ, MD, Division of Cardiology, Department of Medicine, University of Connecticut, Farmington, Connecticut

VIKTOR V. KHRAMELASHVILI, MD, Myasnikov Institute of Clinical Cardiology, USSR Cardiology Research Center, Moscow, USSR

WOLFGANG KIOWSKI, Division of Cardiology, University Hospital, Basel, Switzerland

PAUL I. KORNER, Baker Medical Research Institute, Melbourne, Australia

SAMON KOYANAGI, MD, Research Institute of Angiocardiography and Cardiovascular Clinic, Kyushu University Medical School, Fukuoka, Japan

EDWARD G. LAKATTA, MD, Cardiovascular Section, Gerontology Research Center, National Institute on Aging, National Institutes of Health, Baltimore, Maryland

JOHN H. LARAGH, MD, Cardiology Division, Department of Medicine, The New York Hospital-Cornell Medical Center, New York, New York

VLADIMIR B. LEBEDEV, PhD, Myasnikov Institute of Clinical Cardiology, USSR Cardiology Research Center, Moscow, USSR

J. F. LIARD, MD, Professor of Physiology, Department of Physiology, Medical College of Wisconsin, Milwaukee, Wisconsin

IRINA A. LICHITEL, MD, Myasnikov Institute of Clinical Cardiology, USSR Cardiology Research Center, Moscow, USSR

PER LUND-JOHANSEN, MD, Medical Department, Haukeland Hospital, Professor of Medicine, University of Bergen School of Medicine, Bergen, Norway

ELIZABETH M. LUTAS, MD, Cardiology Division, Department of Medicine, The New York Hospital-Cornell Medical Center, New York, New York

MELVIN L. MARCUS, MD, Professor of Medicine, University of Iowa Hospitals, Iowa City, Iowa

BARRY M. MASSIE, MD, Cardiology Division, Veterans Administration Medical Center, San Francisco, California

FRANZ H. MESSERLI, MD, Department of Internal Medicine, Section on Hypertensive Diseases, Ochsner Clinic and Alton Ochsner Medical Foundation, New Orleans, Louisiana

MARGARETA NORDLANDER, PhD, Department of Cardiovascular Pharmacology, A. B. Hassle, Molndal, Sweden

ELENA V. PARFENOVA, MD, Myasnikov Institute of Clinical Cardiology, USSR Cardiology Research Center, Moscow, USSR

BARBARA L. PEGRAM, PhD, Section on Research, Alton Ochsner Medical Foundation, New Orleans, Louisiana

THOMAS PICKERING, MD, Cardiology Division, The New York Hospital-Cornell Medical Center, New York, New York

NATHANIEL REICHEK, MD, Noninvasive Laboratory, Hospital of the University of Pennsylvania, Philadelphia, Pennsylvania

E. RENÉ RODRÍGUEZ, MD, Ultrastructure Section, Pathology Branch, National Heart, Lung and Blood Institute, National Institutes of Health, Bethesda, Maryland

CLIVE ROSENDORFF, MRC/University Circulation Research Unit, University of the Witwatersrand Medical School, Johannesburg, South Africa

M. E. SAFAR, Diagnosis Center and the Hypertension Research Center, Broussais Hospital, Paris, France

BORIS B. SALENKO, MD, Myasnikov Institute of Clinical Cardiology, USSR Cardiology Research Center, Moscow, USSR

DANIEL D. SAVAGE, MD, PhD, National Center of Health Statistics, U.S. Department of Health and Human Services, Bethesda, Maryland

SUBHA SEN, PhD, DSc, Research Division, Department of Cardiovascular Research, Cleveland Clinic Foundation, Cleveland, Ohio

IGOR K. SHKHVATSABAYA, MD, Myasnikov Institute of Clinical Cardiology, USSR Cardiology Research Center, Moscow, USSR

B. SILKE, University Department of Cardiovascular Studies, The General Infirmary, Leeds, England

VIVIENNE-ELIZABETH SMITH, MD, Division of Cardiology, Department of Medicine, University of Connecticut, Farmington, Connecticut

B. E. STRAUER, Department of Medicine, University of Munich, Munich, West Germany

JAY M. SULLIVAN, MD, Professor of Medicine, Chief, Division of Cardiovascular Diseases, University of Tennessee Center for the Health Sciences, Memphis, Tennessee

ROBERT C. TARAZI, MD, Research Division, Cleveland Clinic Foundation, Cleveland, Ohio

S. H. TAYLOR, Department of Medical Cardiology, The General Infirmary, Leeds, England

JULIO F. TUBAU, MD, Cardiology Division and Clinical Pharmacology Division, Veterans Administration Medical Center, San Francisco, California

SVETLANA E. USTINOVA, MD, Myasnikov Institute of Clinical Cardiology, USSR Cardiology Research Center, Moscow, USSR

HECTOR O. VENTURA, MD, Department of Internal Medicine, Section on Hypertensive Diseases, Ochsner Clinic and Alton Ochsner Medical Foundation, New Orleans, Louisiana

MICHAEL A. WEBER, MD, Hypertension Center, Section of Cardiology, Veterans Administration Medical Center, Long Beach, California and the University of California, Irvine, California

SAXON W. WHITE, Faculty of Medicine, Discipline of Human Physiology, University of Newcastle, New South Wales, Australia

JOHN WIKSTRAND, MD, PhD, Associate Professor, Department of Clinical Physiology, Sahlgrenska Hospital, University of Goteborg, Goteborg, Sweden

YUKIO YAMORI, MD, Department of Pathology, Shimane Medical University, Izumo, Japan

ALEXEI P. YURENEV, MD, Myasnikov Institute of Clinical Cardiology, USSR Cardiology Research Center, Moscow, USSR

Preface

"The course of any case of cardiac hypertrophy may be divided into three stages: (a) the period of development which varies with the nature of the primary lesion, (b) the period of full compensation—the latent stage—during which the heart's vigor meets the requirement of the circulation, (c) the period of broken compensation." Little remains to be added to these sentences written by Sir William Osler in the first edition of his textbook, *Principles and Practice of Medicine*, almost a century ago. Osler's three stages of left ventricular adaptation to an increased afterload were substantiated in 1962 by the lucid observation of Meerson. An elegant experimental design allowed him to identify: (1) a stage of increased cardiac function that was followed by (2) a stage of adaptation (hypertrophy) of the myocardium, which represented a compensation for the increased afterload bringing the wall stress back to normal; and (3) a stage of the failing left ventricle that leads to venous congestion and pulmonary edema. A similar sequence of pathophysiologic events was subsequently described in patients with essential hypertension.

However, although it is still fashionable to consider the heart as a hollow viscus that provides mechanical energy to propel blood through the vascular tree, it is not a muscular pump only. It can be considered a sophisticated biologic apparatus that contains a complex of control and effective mechanisms that are involved in electric excitation, contraction coupling, contraction, and possibly endocrine function. Like the kidney and the brain, the heart plays a threefold role in essential hypertension: first, it is directly involved in the pathogenesis of arterial hypertension. Its contractile force generates the energy needed to increase blood pressure. Recent evidence indicates that a natriuretic factor generated in the atrium of the heart may directly participate in the pathogenesis of essential hypertension. Second, the heart suffers as a target organ of long-standing hypertension. Long-standing blood pressure elevation leads to left ventricular hypertrophy and hypertensive heart disease with their grave outlook. Third, cardiac function and structure are directly and indirectly affected by a variety of antihypertensive agents.

This volume provides a critical review of recent research into these three areas that connect the heart to arterial hypertension. Our book is intended to provide a synoptic view of our present knowledge in this rapidly expanding area. The text is written for physicians, cardiologists, or investigators who would like to deepen their understanding of cardiac involvement in hypertension and of progression as well as regression of left ventricular hypertrophy, and the heart's structural and functional response to various blood pressure lowering agents.

I would like to express my gratitude to the authors of the chapters, all experts in their field, who have given willingly of their talents and efforts so that this needed critique could be compiled. In addition, my deep appreciation goes to Marion Stafford, Medical Editor of Alton Ochsner Medical Foundation, for her invaluable support, and her able and efficient handling of the manuscript material. To the staff of Yorke Medical Books, and in particular to Herb Paureiss, I owe many thanks for the personal care and attention I received.

Franz H. Messerli, M.D.

New Orleans, Louisiana
January 1987

PART I
EARLY CARDIAC CHANGES
IN HYPERTENSION

1

Cardiogenic Hypertension: Experimental Findings

J. F. LIARD, MD

Cardiogenic hypertension is defined here as a sustained elevation of mean arterial pressure (MAP) initiated (but not necessarily maintained) by an increase in cardiac output (CO) due to enhanced myocardial contractility. Other definitions have been proposed, notably to include a potential role of the heart as a source of pressor or deinhibitory reflexes,[1,2] but the more restrictive definition adopted allows one to focus on a few specific pathogenetic considerations. First, does a primary increase in myocardial contractility ever increase CO? Second, if it does, can the increased output be sustained? Finally, what is the effect, if any, of a sustained increase in CO on the peripheral vasculature when it is not determined by increased tissular needs? These questions have been addressed in detail previously[3] and will be briefly dealt with after summarizing the few experimental attempts that have been made to create cardiogenic hypertension.

Stellate Ganglion Stimulation

Stimulation of the cardiac sympathetic innervation was shown a long time ago to increase arterial pressure and CO.[4–6] This pressor response could be maintained for several hours in the anesthetized dog,[7] but the possibility that prolonged electrical stimulation of cardiac nerves might produce hypertension was not tested until Liard et al[8] studied the hemodynamic changes resulting from a continuous, 7-day stimulation of the left stellate ganglion in conscious dogs. These changes are summarized in Figure 1. Hypertension of a moderate degree developed and was maintained as long as the stimulation lasted. During the first hours of stimulation, CO was increased and calculated peripheral resistance did not change. Later, CO decreased back to its control value and resistance was increased above control levels. Measurements of circulating catecholamines, blood volume, sodium balance, and plasma renin activity suggested that none of these factors could explain the development of hypertension. When the stimulation was ended, arterial pressure decreased rapidly, and this decrease was accounted for by a decrease in CO. Total peripheral resistance (TPR) returned toward control only later. Thus, both at the onset and at the offset of hypertension elicited by

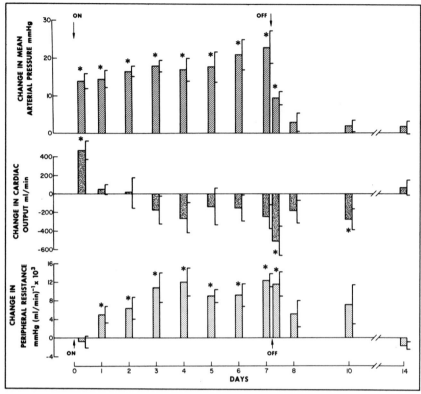

Figure 1. *Hemodynamic changes ± SE in 6 dogs between 6 hours and 7 days of continuous left stellate ganglion stimulation (between arrows ON and OFF), as well as following discontinuation of the stimulation. Asterisk indicates a significant change from the prestimulation value.*

stellate ganglion stimulation, changes in cardiac output preceded the peripheral resistance modifications. This experimental model seemed to support the concept of cardiogenic hypertension. However, we could not exclude the fact that high blood pressure developed as a result of stimulation of afferent fibers from the heart, which are known to induce pressor reflexes.[9] A more selective enhancement of myocardial contractility was therefore necessary.

Intracoronary Infusion of Dobutamine

Figure 2 illustrates the hemodynamic changes measured over a 7-day period of continuous administration of dobutamine, a powerful stimulant of cardiac inotropism, through a catheter implanted in the left coronary artery in conscious dogs.[10] Mean arterial pressure increased rapidly and was elevated during the whole infusion period. Cardiac output was significantly

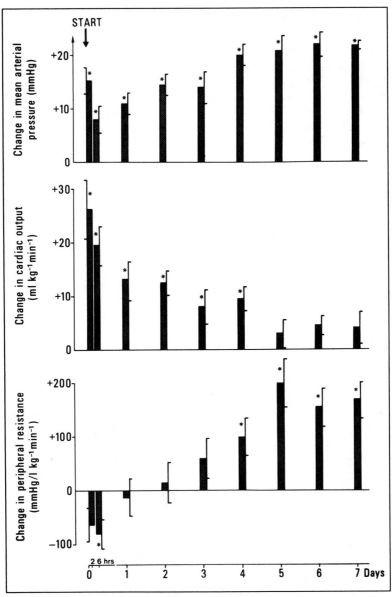

Figure 2. *Hemodynamic changes ± SE in 7 dogs between 2 hours and 7 days of continuous infusion of dobutamine into the left coronary artery started at arrow at a rate of 4.5 ± 0.2 µ/kg/min. Asterisk indicates a significant change from the preinfusion value.*

increased during the first few days, then decreased back toward control as TPR increased progressively. When the infusion was stopped, MAP decreased rapidly because of a decrease in CO. Only later did the elevated TPR return to its control value. In this model again, there was no expansion of blood volume nor of extracellular fluid volume that could have explained the development of hypertension, and plasma renin activity decreased. In a subsequent study[11] it was shown that the intravenous infusion of dobutamine at the same rate as that administered into the coronary circulation produced no increase in arterial pressure. Thus, systemic effects of the drug could not explain the development of hypertension observed on intracoronary administration. Furthermore, preventing the increase in CO elicited by intracoronary administration of dobutamine with propranolol eliminated any increase in arterial pressure.[11] It was therefore concluded that hypertension characterized by increased peripheral resistance could develop as a consequence of an increase in systemic flow of cardiac origin.

The experimental evidence summarized indicates that both prolonged stellate ganglion stimulation and intracoronary administration of dobutamine produced moderate levels of hypertension that seem to fit the definition of "cardiogenic." How, then, should we answer the following questions?

Can an Increase in Myocardial Contractility Increase Cardiac Output? The prevalent concept is that CO is normally determined by peripheral factors and not by the heart itself,[12] which is certainly verified under most circumstances. Thus, the heart pumps whatever amount of blood is returned to the right atrium, and increased pumping ability of the heart should not increase CO. Indeed, even the normal heart has a large excess pumping ability, which obviously does not lead to hypertension.[13] However, increasing pumping ability of the heart does, in fact, increase CO because the steady state venous return increases as a result of both increased mean systemic pressure (caused by a shift of blood volume out of the thoracic region) and decreased right atrial pressure.[14] To that extent, the heart may therefore control CO, which has been verified repeatedly. Liedtke et al[15] were able to increase CO by infusing calcium chloride into the left coronary artery in anesthetized dogs. Liard et al[16] demonstrated that left stellate ganglion stimulation increased left CO transiently when venous return was kept constant with a pump, indicating that blood was transferred from the cardiopulmonary area to the systemic circulation.

Can an Increased Cardiac Output due to Increased Cardiac Pumping Ability be Maintained Despite the Renal-Body Fluid Mechanism for Arterial Pressure Control? Raising arterial pressure without modification of the renal function curve should promote urinary output of salt and water in excess of intake and consequently return blood pressure to its control value.[13] Therefore, the argument has been made that any increase in cardiac output induced by increased pumping ability would be rapidly corrected by progressive fluid loss and hypertension could not develop.[13] We have suggested that the renal function curve can actually be shifted as a consequence of increased arterial pressure through the following mechanism.[3]

As the renal-body fluid volume mechanism attempts to correct for an arterial pressure increase, it depletes extracellular and plasma volumes, which in turn modifies renal function to prevent further losses of salt and water. Thus, the renal function curve changes as a result of the operation of the mechanism that controls blood pressure, limiting its ability to correct the disturbance completely. Possible mechanisms for such a change in renal function as a consequence of volume depletion include an increase in plasma protein concentration or in efferent renal nerve activity. Omvik et al[17] have shown in hypertensive subjects that the slope of the pressure natriuresis curve appears to be decreased by volume contraction. They also suggested that a shift of renal function curve may be a consequence rather than a cause of hypertension. We conclude that hypertension may result from extrarenal causes because of a secondary shift of the renal function curve.

What are the Consequences of an Increased Cardiac Output due to Increased Pumping Ability of the Heart on the Vascular System? As shown in Figures 1 and 2, TPR increased progressively in both models of cardiogenic hypertension. Although the time course differed between the two studies, the hemodynamic changes were sufficiently similar to warrant the suggestion that resistance increased as a result of augmented CO. One possible interpretation of the findings in Figures 1 and 2 is based on the theory widely known as whole-body autoregulation,[18,19] which postulates that peripheral tissues exposed to an unwarranted increase in flow would respond locally by an increase in vascular resistance. However, the evidence supporting a role of autoregulation of blood flow in hypertension is only indirect. Actually, it has been difficult to detect any autoregulation of systemic blood flow when a perfusion pump was used to vary mean aortic flow for periods up to 20 minutes in dogs,[20] and the existence of whole-body autoregulation of blood flow seems to be linked to a high arteriovenous oxygen difference.[21] Furthermore, studies of regional circulation in dogs developing hypertension because of salt and water loading have indicated that most tissues did not receive an excess perfusion when CO was elevated.[22] The only vascular beds exposed to an increased blood flow were the skeletal muscle and the heart. Even though this pattern is modified by baroreceptor denervation,[23] these findings do not support the concept that tissue overperfusion is necessary for the development of increased vascular resistance in a model of hypertension in which CO increase precedes modifications of TPR.

Yet there is no easy alternative explanation for the increased vascular resistance found in the two models of cardiogenic hypertension described. The stellate ganglion stimulation might have induced a generalized increase in sympathetic tone through activation of afferent nerves, but this possibility has not been tested experimentally. Such an explanation would certainly not apply to intracoronary dobutamine administration. Increased plasma levels of angiotensin II as well as decreased activity of the sodium-potassium adenosine triphosphatase (ATPase) of vascular smooth muscle as a result of body fluid expansion can be excluded. Therefore, an increase in systemic flow appears to trigger an increase in peripheral resistance, but the mechanisms involved have not been established.

In conclusion, the few experiments that have been conducted to test the concept of cardiogenic hypertension indicate that increased arterial pressure characterized by high peripheral resistance may develop as a consequence of an increase in systemic flow of cardiac origin.

Acknowledgments

Supported by a grant from Fondation Suisse de Cardiologie and NIH Program Project PO1 HL 29587.

References

1. TARAZI RC, FOUAD FM, FERRARIO CM: Can the heart initiate some forms of hypertension? Fed Proc 1983; 42: 2691–2697.
2. DUSTAN HP, TARAZI RC: Cardiogenic hypertension. Annu Rev Med 1978; 29: 485–493.
3. LIARD JF: Cardiogenic hypertension. In: Guyton AC, Young DB, eds. Cardiovascular physiology III, Vol. 18. Baltimore: University Park Press, 1979.
4. SHIPLEY RE, GREGG DE: Cardiac response to stimulation of the stellate ganglia and cardiac nerves. Am J Physiol 1945; 143: 396–401.
5. ANZOLA J, RUSHMER RF: Cardiac responses to sympathetic stimulation. Circ Res 1956; 4: 302–307.
6. SARNOFF SJ, BROCKMAN SK, GILMORE JP, LINDEN RJ, MITCHELL JH: Regulation of ventricular contraction: influence of cardiac sympathetic and vagal nerve stimulation on atrial and ventricular dynamics. Circ Res 1960; 8: 1108–1122.
7. ROHSE WG, KAYE M, RANDALL WC: Prolonged pressor effects of selective stimulation of the stellate ganglion. Circ Res 1957; 5: 144–148.
8. LIARD JF, TARAZI RC, FERRARIO CM, MANGER WM: Hemodynamic and humoral characteristics of hypertension induced by prolonged stellate ganglion stimulation in conscious dogs. Circ Res 1975; 36: 455–464.
9. MALLIANI A: Cardiovascular sympathetic afferent fibers. Rev Physiol Biochem Pharmacol 1982; 94: 11–74.
10. LIARD JF: Hypertension induced by prolonged intracoronary administration of dobutamine in conscious dogs. Clin Sci 1978; 54: 153–160.
11. LIARD JF: Cardiogenic hypertension: experimental evidence from a comparison between intravenous and intracoronary administration of dobutamine in conscious dogs. Clin Sci 1980; 58: 271–277.
12. GUYTON AC, JONES CE, COLEMAN TG: Circulatory physiology: cardiac output and its regulation. 2nd ed. Philadelphia: W.B. Saunders, 1973.
13. GUYTON AC: Arterial pressure and hypertension. Circulatory physiology III. Philadelphia: W.B. Saunders, 1980.
14. MITZNER W, GOLDBERG H, LICHTENSTEIN S: Effect of thoracic blood volume changes on steady-state cardiac output. Circ Res 1976; 38: 255–261.

15. LIEDTKE JA, URSCHEL CW, KIRK ES: Total systemic autoregulation in the dog and its inhibition by baroreceptor reflexes. Circ Res 1973; 32: 673–677.

16. LIARD JF, TARAZI RC, FERRARIO CM: Hemodynamic effects of stellate ganglion stimulation in conscious dogs. In: Julius S, Esler MD, eds: The nervous system in arterial hypertension. Springfield, IL: Charles C Thomas, 1976; 151–160.

17. OMVIK P, TARAZI RC, BRAVO EL: Regulation of sodium balance in hypertension. Hypertension 1980; 2: 515–523.

18. COLEMAN TG, SAMAR RE, MURPHY WR: Autoregulation versus other vasoconstrictors in hypertension. Hypertension 1979; 1: 324–330.

19. COWLEY AW: The concept of autoregulation of total blood flow and its role in hypertension. Am J Med 1980; 68: 906–916.

20. SAGAWA K, EISNER A: Static pressure-flow relation in the total systemic vascular bed of the dog and its modification by the baroreceptor reflex. Circ Res 1975; 36: 406–413.

21. SHEPHERD AP, GRANGER HJ, SMITH EE, GUYTON AC: Local control of tissue oxygen delivery and its contribution to the regulation of cardiac output. Am J Physiol 1973; 225: 547–755.

22. LIARD JF: Regional blood flows in salt loading hypertension in the dog. Am J Physiol 1981; 240: H361–H367.

23. LIARD JF, SILENZIO R: Baroreceptor reflex influence on peripheral circulations in salt-loading hypertension in dogs. Hypertension 1982; 4: 597–603.

2

Cardiac Reflexes and Blood Pressure Elevation

BRENT M. EGAN, M.D.
STEVO JULIUS, M.D.

Interest in cardiac baroreflexes was first stimulated by von Bezold and Hirt[1] in the 19th century. The interest was rekindled some 30 years ago by such investigators as Jarisch and Zotterman,[2] Henry and associates,[3] and Roddie et al.[4] Much of the physiologic data on reflexes originating from receptors in the "low-pressure" or capacitance side of the circulation are derived from complex animal studies. However, an impressive and growing volume of human research suggests that these reflexes may be important in man. This chapter will focus on the positive studies and their potential importance to human hypertension.

The human heart is a four-chambered pump with the "prime" goal of sending and receiving blood to and from the pulmonary and systemic circulations. It is, for all practical purposes, centrally located—the focal point of the cardiovascular system. Therefore, one could postulate that the heart, as the center of such a vital system, should have some capacity for monitoring and influencing variables crucial to its role. These variables would include blood volume or preload, chronotropic and inotropic state, and vascular resistance, an important component of afterload. Before reviewing studies that lend substance to this hypothesis, we will first review some basic principles and methods important to the study of cardiopulmonary reflexes.

Background Information and Methodology

The healthy heart, particularly the atria, is a compliant structure in which relatively small changes in pressure produce large changes in volume. Thus, the cardiac receptors respond predominantly to changes in volume. Changes in the blood volume within the central circulation elicit altered activity from these receptors.[5] For example, increasing central blood volume increases afferent vagal nerve traffic from a subset of these cardiopulmonary receptors to regions in the brainstem important in cardiovascular control. This, in turn, elicits increased vagal and decreased sympathetic outflow. Decreasing central blood volume reduces the stretch of the cardiopulmonary receptors and decreases the inhibitory traffic converging on the central regulatory centers manifested as decreased vagal and increased sympathetic efferent outflow.

In human studies, maneuvers are utilized that change the volume of blood in the cardiopulmonary circulation. It is important to avoid maneuvers that also cause significant changes in mean arterial pressure or pulse pressure, since reflexes from arterial baroreceptors in the aorta, carotid, renal, and mesenteric vessels could cause interpretative problems. Interventions in humans that preferentially decrease central blood volume and right atrial pressure without significantly affecting mean arterial or pulse pressure include nonhypotensive hemorrhage, lower body negative pressure at levels of 20 to 30 mmHg or less, and thigh cuff inflation. Interventions that predominantly increase central blood volume and right atrial pressure (or prevent gravity-induced decreases) include water immersion, lower body water suit, lower body positive pressure, tight bandaging of the abdomen and lower extremities, and elevation of the lower extremities.

Cardiac Reflexes and the Neurohumoral Control of the Circulation

As stated earlier, the heart as the center of the cardiovascular system should have some capacity to regulate important variables, such as preload, inotropic and chronotropic state, and afterload. Some of the earliest human studies on cardiac reflexes demonstrated that elevation of the extremities induced reflex vasodilation of the forearm vessels.[4] Subsequent studies with lower body negative pressure showed, conversely, that reduction of right atrial pressure induced vasoconstriction in the forearm and to a lesser degree in the mesenteric circulation.[6] Thus, the heart has some capacity to rapidly change afterload.

The next area of cardiac reflexes in humans to generate considerable interest was the neural regulation of renin release. The first study showed that tightly bandaging the abdomen and lower extremities prevented the increase in plasma renin, which occurs with upright posture.[7] Subsequent studies utilizing more sophisticated antigravity suits confirmed the ability of these devices to prevent both the gravitationally mediated decreases in central blood volume and increases in renin.[8,9] Taken together, these studies suggest that decreases in central blood volume are an important controlling influence on renin response to upright posture. However, these studies did not prove that the renin response to upright posture was a neural reflex originating in the heart, as opposed to gravity-mediated decreases in arterial pulse pressure, renal blood flow, glomerular filtration rate, and sodium excretion.[8]

Some of these uncertainties were addressed in a series of experiments to determine if the cardiopulmonary receptors could effect a neurally mediated increase of plasma renin activity in man.[9–11] Thigh cuff inflation to

70 mmHg in healthy volunteers reduced right atrial pressure and central blood volume without altering mean arterial or pulse pressure. This maneuver caused approximately a doubling of plasma renin activity. However, thigh cuff inflation to this level also reduced the cardiac output (CO) slightly so that it was possible that changes in intrarenal hemodynamics caused the increase in renin. The neurogenic origin of this reflex has been confirmed in three ways: First, the increase in renin was abolished by propranolol, which suggests but does not prove a neurogenic basis. Second, the increase in renin did not occur in subjects with bilateral nephrectomies who had a recent (presumably denervated) well-functioning renal transplant, although these kidneys released renin normally in response to isoproterenol infusion. Third, renin activity increased significantly in sodium replete subjects after thigh cuff inflation to lower pressures that produced decreases in right atrial pressure and central blood volume without changing MAP, pulse pressure, or CO. These studies demonstrated further the capacity of the heart to influence an enzyme important in regulating the peripheral resistance (angiotensin) and volume (aldosterone).

The next area of human investigation in neurohumoral regulation of the circulation by cardiopulmonary receptors, which followed very closely in time the renin studies, was vasopressin or antidiuretic hormone (ADH). Several investigators showed that water immersion reduced urinary and plasma ADH levels.[12–14] Water immersion obviously increases central blood volume and right atrial pressure, which may have been responsible for the reduction in plasma and urinary ADH.[15] However, interpretation of these studies is complicated by reported decreases in plasma osmolality with water immersion, which may also contribute to the decrease in ADH.[14,16] Furthermore, although arterial pressure does not appear to change, major changes in CO and peripheral resistance are elicited and may affect ADH levels.[15,17] Despite the complexities, these studies strongly implicate a role for the cardiopulmonary receptors in the regulation of plasma vasopressin levels.

The role of cardiopulmonary receptors in ADH regulation was furthered by the observation that 30 mmHg lower body negative pressure, which did not alter noninvasively measured mean arterial or pulse-pressure induced increases in plasma ADH.[18] However, no invasively obtained hemodynamic data were produced to confirm the stimulus selectivity. Clearly, 20 mmHg lower body negative pressure predominantly affects cardiopulmonary receptors, whereas 40 mmHg lower body negative pressure affects cardiopulmonary and arterial baroreceptors.[19] In studies utilizing modest levels of thigh cuff inflation (30 to 40 mmHg), which decreased right atrial pressure and central blood volume without altering MAP or pulse pressure, CO, or plasma osmolality, the plasma ADH levels increased significantly.[20] Although, as with renin, studies utilizing various methods obtain results to the contrary,[21,22] we interpret the overall evidence as favoring the conclusion that cardiopulmonary receptors in man influence plasma ADH levels. Once again, evidence suggests that the heart modulates a hormone involved in volume and pressure homeostasis.

Cardiopulmonary Receptors and Regulation of Sympathetic Activity

Plasma norepinephrine serves as an indirect but nevertheless useful index of efferent sympathetic activity.[23,24] Upright posture (standing and head-up tilt) in man elicits substantial increases in plasma norepinephrine.[8,9,11] Application of antigravity measures that restore central blood volume without correcting the hydrostatic unloading of the carotid baroreceptor, which occurs with upright posture, largely reverses the increase in norepinephrine.[8,9] In addition, thigh cuff inflation to 70 mmHg in supine healthy subjects, which induces a relatively selective unloading of low-pressure receptors, elicits increases in plasma norepinephrine.[10] These studies support a role for cardiopulmonary receptors in regulation of sympathetic activity in man. Thus, the heart may modulate the activity of a system capable of altering preload, inotropic and chronotropic state, and afterload.

Evidence for Physiologic Importance of the Cardiopulmonary Receptors in Human Essential Hypertension

Several lines of evidence indicate that some pathophysiologic abnormalities in hypertensive patients involve low-pressure receptors. First, abnormal renin responses to upright posture are observed in a subset of patients.[25] A group of patients with low renin and with either borderline[26] or established hypertension[27] have an increased central blood volume without an expanded total blood volume. The redistribution of the blood volume through an effect on low-pressure receptors may explain the suppressed renin values. Furthermore, these patients with low renin also have low values for plasma norepinephrine[27] and vasopressin.[28] All of these abnormalities, the low values for renin, norepinephrine, and vasopressin, could be explained by an increased tonic inhibition originating in the low-pressure receptors.

The arterial and cardiopulmonary baroreceptors interact in regulating many of the variables previously discussed.[29,30] However, because the arterial baroreceptors are often impaired in the hypertensive process,[31,32] the cardiopulmonary receptors may assume a more dominant role in neurohumoral control of the circulation. For example, lower body negative pressure causes larger increases in forearm vascular resistance in patients with borderline hypertension compared with normotensive control subjects.[33] This observation is consistent with the view that the low-pressure receptors play a greater regulatory role in hypertension.

Summary

An impressive and growing number of studies in humans confirm a physiologic role for the cardiopulmonary low-pressure receptors in the acute regulation of renin release, sympathetic activity (Fig. 1) and plasma vasopressin

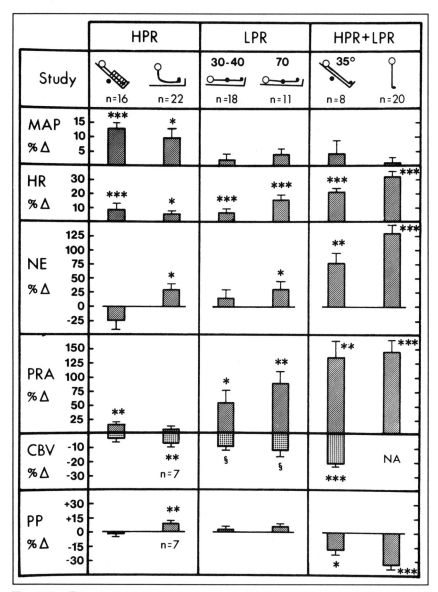

Figure 1. The interventions that cause a hydrostatic unloading of the high-pressure baroreceptor (HPR), or carotid baroreceptor (when the patient is sitting with legs horizontal and tilt with water suit) are at the left. Maneuvers that predominantly unload the low-pressure baroreceptors (LPR; thigh cuff inflation) are in the center. Stimuli that unload both HPR and LPR (standing and head-up tilt) are at the right. Please observe the overall trend between changes in LPR load (central blood volume [CBV]), HPR load (mean arterial pressure [MAP] and pulse pressure [PP]) and the responses in heart rate (HR), plasma renin activity (PRA) and plasma norepinephrine (NE). The trends suggest that relatively selective unloading of HPR causes a small increase in heart rate without consistent changes in PRA or NE. Unloading of LPR causes a small increase in heart rate, plasma renin activity, and plasma NE. Unloading both HPR and LPR elicits large increases in HR, PRA, and NE, which suggests an interaction between the HPR and LPR in regulating these variables. P values were obtained from either the Student t-test (*) or Wilcoxon's rank sum test (§) of paired differences from baseline. * or § p <0.05; ** p <0.01; *** p <0.001. NA = not available.

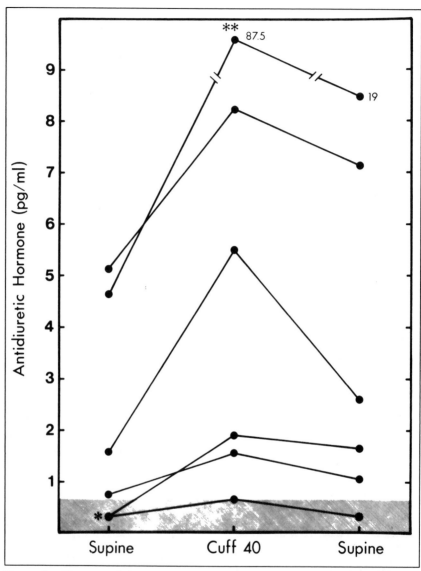

Figure 2. *Plasma antidiuretic hormone (ADH) response to selective unloading of low-pressure receptors. Following a 30-minute supine baseline, thigh cuffs were inflated to 40 mmHg for 30 minutes. Thigh cuffs were then deflated and subjects remained supine for an additional 45 minutes. Plasma ADH increased during thigh cuff inflation and returned partially toward baseline following deflation. * = Plasma ADH less than 0.63 pg/ml, which is below assay limits. ** = The subject whose ADH increased to 87.5 pg/ml did not differ hemodynamically from the others. Specifically, there were no hypotensive episodes during continuous intra-arterial monitoring.*

levels (Fig. 2). Chronically altered levels of these values may be explained in part by abnormalities in blood volume distribution, perhaps reflecting altered venous tone,[34,35] with consequent effects on low-pressure receptor activity. The relative importance of the low-pressure receptors in hypertensive patients may be further enhanced by impaired arterial baroreflexes and contribute to the observed abnormalities. It is not yet clear if primary abnormalities in low-pressure receptors could account for observed abnormalities in renin, vasopressin, and norepinephrine or if the abnormal blood volume distribution or impaired arterial baroreceptors are altering the activity of otherwise normal cardiopulmonary reflexes. Future investigations will, it is hoped, resolve these questions and address the role of the heart in regulating various natriuretic factors.

References

1. VON BEZOLD A, HIRT L: Uber die physiologischen Wirkungen des essigsauren veratrins. Untersuchungen aus dem physiologischen Laboratorium in Wurzburg 1867; 1: 75–156.

2. JARISCH A, ZOTTERMAN Y: Depressor reflexes from the heart. Acta Physiol Scand 1948; 16: 31–51.

3. HENRY JP, GAUER OH, REEVES JL: Evidence of the atrial location of receptors influencing urine flow. Circ Res 1956; 4: 85–90.

4. RODDIE IC, SHEPHERD JT, WHELAN RF: Reflex changes in vasoconstrictor tone in human skeletal muscle in response to stimulation of receptors in a low-pressure area of the intrathoracic vascular bed. J Physiol (Lond) 1957; 139: 369–376.

5. GUPTA PD, HENRY JP, SINCLAIR R, VON BAUMGARTEN R: Responses of atrial and aortic baroreceptors to nonhypotensive hemorrhage and to transfusion. Am J Physiol 1966; 211: 1429–1437.

6. ABBOUD FM, ECKBERG DL, JOHANNSEN UJ, MARK AL: Carotid and cardiopulmonary baroreceptor control of splanchnic and forearm vascular resistance during venous pooling in man. J Physiol (Lond) 1979; 286: 173–184.

7. BROWN E, GOEI JS, GREENFIELD ADM, PLASSARAS GC: Circulatory responses to simulated gravitational shifts of blood in man induced by exposure of the body below the iliac crests to sub-atmospheric pressure. J Physiol (Lond) 1966; 183: 607–627.

8. HESSE B, RING-LARSEN H, NIELSEN I, CHRISTENSEN NJ: Renin stimulation by passive tilting: the influence of an anti-gravity suit on postural changes in plasma renin activity, plasma noradrenaline concentration and kidney function in normal man. Scand J Clin Lab Invest 1978; 38: 163–169.

9. JULIUS S, COTTIER C, EGAN B, IBSEN H, KIOWSKI W: Cardiopulmonary mechanoreceptors and renin release in humans. Fed Proc 1983; 42: 2703–2708.

10. KIOWSKI W, JULIUS S: Renin response to stimulation of cardiopulmonary mechanoreceptors in man. J Clin Invest 1978; 62: 656–663.

11. EGAN BM, JULIUS S, COTTIER C, OSTERZIEL KJ, IBSEN H: Role of cardiovascular receptors on the neural regulation of renin release in normal men. Hypertension 1983; 5: 779–786.

12. EPSTEIN M, PINS DS, MILLER M: Suppression of ADH during water immersion in normal man. J Appl Physiol 1975; 38: 1038–1044.

13. EPSTEIN M, PRESTON S, WEITZMAN RE: Isoosmotic central blood volume expansion suppresses plasma arginine vasopressin in normal man. J Clin Endocrinol Metab 1981; 52: 256–262.

14. GREENLEAF JE, SHVARTZ E, KEIL LC: Hemodilution, vasopressin suppression, and diuresis during water immersion in man. Aviat Space Environ Med 1981; 52: 329–336.

15. ARBORELIUS M JR, BALLDIN UI, LILJA B, LUNDGREN CEG: Hemodynamic changes in man during immersion with the head above water. Aerospace Med 1972; 43: 592–598.

16. KHOSLA SS, DuBOIS AB: Fluid shifts during initial phase of immersion diuresis in man. J Appl Physiol 1979; 46: 703–708.

17. BEGIN R, EPSTEIN M, SACKNER MA, LEVINSON R, DOUGHERTY R, DUNCAN D: Effects of water immersion to the neck on pulmonary circulation and tissue volume in man. J Appl Physiol 1976; 40: 293–299.

18. ROGGE JD, MOORE WW: Influence of lower body negative pressure on peripheral venous ADH levels in man. J Appl Physiol 1968; 25: 134–138.

19. MARK AL, ABBOUD FM, FITZ AE: Influence of low and high pressure baroreceptors on plasma renin activity in humans. Am J Physiol 1978; 235: H29–H33.

20. EGAN B, JULIUS S, GREKIN R, OSTERZIEL K, IBSEN H: The role of cardiopulmonary mechanoreceptors in the ADH release in normal man. Hypertension 1984; 6: 832–836.

21. GOETZ KL, BOND GC, SMITH WE: Effect of moderate hemorrhage in humans on plasma ADH and renin. Proc Soc Exp Biol Med 1974; 145: 277–280.

22. GOLDSMITH SR, FRANCIS GS, COWLEY AW, COHN JN: Response of vasopressin and norepinephrine to lower body negative pressure in humans. Am J Physiol 1982; 243: H970–H973.

23. GOLDSTEIN DS, McCARTY R, POLINSKY RJ, KOPIN IJ: Relationship between plasma norepinephrine and sympathetic neural activity. Hypertension 1983; 5: 552–559.

24. WALLIN BG, SUNDLOF G: A quantitative study of muscle nerve sympathetic activity in resting normotensive and hypertensive subjects. Hypertension 1979; 1: 67–77.

25. ESLER M, ZWEIFLER A, RANDALL O, JULIUS S, DeQUATTRO V: The determinants of plasma-renin activity in essential hypertension. Ann Intern Med 1978; 88: 746–752.

26. ESLER M, JULIUS S, RANDALL O: Relationship of volume factors, renin and neurogenic vascular resistance in borderline hypertension. In: Rorive G, Van Cauwenberge H, eds. The arterial hypertension disease. A symposium. New York: Masson USA, 1976; 231–249.

27. ESLER M, ZWEIFLER A, RANDALL O, JULIUS S, BENNETT J, RYDELEK P: Suppression of sympathetic nervous function in low-renin essential hypertension. Lancet 1976; 2: 115–118.

28. ANDO T, SHIMAMOTO K, NAKAHASHI Y, et al: Plasma antidiuretic hormone levels in patients with normal and low renin essential hypertension, and secondary hypertension. Endocrinol Jpn 1983; 30: 567–570.

29. KOIKE H, MARK AL, HEISTAD DD, SCHMID PG: Influence of cardiopulmonary vagal afferent activity on carotid chemoreceptor and baroreceptor reflexes in the dog. Circ Res 1975; 37: 422–429.

30. THAMES MD, JARECKI M, DONALD DE: Neural control of renin secretion in anesthetized dogs. Interaction of cardiopulmonary and carotid baroreceptors. Circ Res 1978; 42: 237–245.

31. ECKBERG DL: Carotid baroreflex function in young men with borderline blood pressure elevation. Circulation 1979; 59: 632–636.

32. BRISTOW JD, HONOUR AJ, PICKERING GW, SLEIGHT P, SMYTH HS: Diminished baroreflex sensitivity in high blood pressure. Circulation 1969; 39: 48–54.

33. MARK AL, KERBER RE: Augmentation of cardiopulmonary baroreflex control of forearm vascular resistance in borderline hypertension. Hypertension 1982; 4: 39–46.

34. WALSH JA, HYMAN C, MARONDE RF: Venous distensibility in essential hypertension. Cardiovasc Res 1969; 3: 338–349.

35. TAKESHITA A, MARK AL: Decreased venous distensibility in borderline hypertension. Hypertension 1979; 1: 202–206.

3

Sodium and the Heart

JAY M. SULLIVAN, M.D.

The cardiovascular system is profoundly influenced by sodium. Dietary intake of sodium has been proposed to be a major influence in the development of high blood pressure,[1] which, if untreated, affects the heart by predisposing to the development of left ventricular hypertrophy (LVH), congestive heart failure, coronary artery disease, and other cardiovascular disorders. The prevalence of hypertension has been shown to vary directly with sodium intake in a number of populations. However, even in populations consuming enormous quantities of sodium, such as the northern Japanese, who ingest 25 g of salt daily, the majority of individuals do not become hypertensive, that is, only 35% to 40% in northern Japan.[2] Although it has been shown that stringent sodium restriction sometimes lowers blood pressure[3] and reduces extracellular fluid (ECF)[4] and that moderate salt restriction reduces average blood pressure by about 8/4 mmHg,[5] all individuals do not respond to sodium restriction with a decrease in blood pressure.[6] These observations suggest that certain individuals are more sensitive to sodium than others. However, at present, we cannot prospectively and reliably distinguish between the two.

The manner by which sodium chloride ingestion results in blood pressure elevation has not been clearly defined. One proposal, derived from a number of lines of experimental evidence, suggests that excessive intake of sodium chloride leads to sodium and water retention, expansion of ECF and intravascular volume, increased venous return, and elevated cardiac index (CI). As elevated blood flow to the tissues continues, whole body autoregulation takes place, with subsequent increase in total peripheral resistance (TPR) and the ultimate development of hypertension.[7] The elevated blood pressure leads to increased urine output and restoration of ECF and CI to normal, whereas hypertension is sustained because of the elevated TPR. Guyton and coworkers[8] have applied systems analysis to the problem and have derived data that support this general outline. In studies of the relative effects of the various feedback loops involved in blood pressure control, they have concluded that chronic blood pressure elevation will not occur unless the kidney fails to increase salt and water excretion appropriately and therefore does not reduce ECF or arterial blood pressure back to normal.

Certain animal experiments have supported this proposal. Coleman and Guyton[9] have shown that sodium and water loading of dogs with reduced renal mass causes a chronic expansion of ECF, followed by a series of events similar to those observed in rats with renovascular hypertension by Ledingham, with sequential elevation of CI, TPR, and blood pressure and with increased urine output ultimately lowering ECF. Dahl[10] has selectively inbred strains of rats to produce groups that invariably develop hypertension when fed salt and others that never develop hypertension despite salt loading, a circumstance similar to the human experience. Bianchi et al[11] and Dahl et al[12] have transplanted the kidneys of salt-resistant rats into hypertensive salt-sensitive rats who subsequently become normotensive. Transplantation of kidneys from hypertensive rats has succeeded in making salt-resistant rats salt sensitive, thus suggesting that the genetic predisposition resides in the kidney. In parabiotic experiments, Dahl et al[13] and coworkers have demonstrated transmittal of a humoral factor from the plasma of salt-sensitive animals that increases the blood pressure of salt-resistant rats. Tobian et al[14] have produced chronic hypertension in rats fed 8% sodium for 4 months and have observed that the kidneys of rats with persistent hypertension require a higher level of perfusion pressure for a given amount of sodium excretion. Ganguli et al[15] have studied the hemodynamic effects of sodium loading in Dahl "S" and "R" rats, observing that the salt-resistant rats responded with vasodilation that allowed blood pressure to remain normal despite an increased CI. In contrast, the salt-sensitive rats responded with an increase in blood pressure, CI, and TPR, the latter increasing with time as the CI decreased to control levels, and the elevated blood pressure was maintained.

Cardiac function and sodium homeostasis are interrelated in a number of fascinating ways that might influence the way that an individual responds to sodium. One of the most interesting recent findings in this area has been the discovery of atrial natriuretic factor (ANF). Granular structures in the atria, interposed among myocytes, were described by Kisch[16] in 1956. DE Bold[17] later observed that these granules were altered by changes in water and electrolyte balance and, with his coworkers, that atrial extracts caused a rapid and potent natriuretic response.[18] Subsequent studies have shown that ANF has a molecular weight of 5,000 to 30,000 daltons, contains one or more peptide fragments, relaxes vascular and intestinal smooth muscle, lowers blood pressure, and does not inhibit sodium-potassium adenosine triphosphatase (Na-K ATPase) nor change glomerular filtration rate. Natriuresis takes place because ANF inhibits resorption of sodium, potassium, chloride, and water in the renal tubule, probably distal to the loop of Henle.[19] A deficiency of this factor could underlie sodium sensitivity.

In addition to their hormonal function, the left atrium and posterior left ventricle also contain stretch receptors[20] that respond to sodium-induced changes in heart size. As left atrial size increases, the receptors are activated, vagal afferent nerve traffic increases, and heart rate, TPR, and blood pressure decrease. Furthermore, the release of ADH is inhibited and water excretion increases, thus reducing heart size. Concomitantly, renal blood flow, glomerular filtration rate, and sodium excretion increase because stimulation of the stretch receptors also results in decreased efferent nerve traffic to the kidney, which in turn reduces renin release, angiotensin II formation, and aldosterone secretion. With chronic increases in heart size, the sensitivity of atrial and ventricular receptors decreases, thereby reducing the capacity to

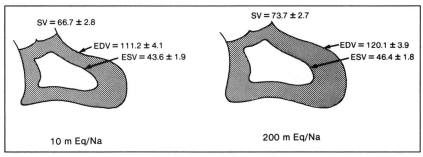

Figure 1. *Alterations of heart size measured by echo with variations of sodium intake in 109 normal and borderline hypertensive subjects. The responsiveness of the borderline hypertensive patients did not differ significantly from that of the normal subjects. The increase in diastolic size and stroke volume (SV) were statistically significant (P <0.0001). EDV = end-diastolic volume; ESV = end-systolic volume.*

restore fluid components to normal levels. Impaired receptor function could explain why TPR does not decrease appropriately in salt-sensitive persons when heart size is increased by a high sodium intake.

Expansion of intravascular volume by sodium loading in volume-dependent forms of experimental hypertension leads to the appearance in plasma of a digoxin-like substance, endoxin.[21] This nonpeptide compound, of less than 500 dalton molecular weight, inhibits Na-K ATPase, thus preventing resorption of sodium throughout the renal tubule and causing natriuresis. However, by inhibiting Na-K ATPase throughout the body, particularly in vascular smooth muscle, endoxin leads to intracellular accumulation of sodium, then of calcium in cells, thus causing vasoconstriction and elevation of blood pressure.[22] Hamlyn et al[23] have observed that plasma levels of an Na-K ATPase inhibitor are proportional to the level of blood pressure in patients with essential hypertension. Such a substance could have an important influence on the way in which an individual responds to dietary sodium.

In studies of normotensive volunteers, Kirkendall et al[24] have found that salt loading is followed by increased forearm blood flow without an increase in blood pressure or in right atrial pressure, thus suggesting that local vasodilation took place. Mark et al[25] found that patients with borderline hypertension decreased forearm blood flow when salt loaded, suggesting that sodium acts to cause vasoconstriction in such patients. Studies of patients with labile[26] or mild essential hypertension[27] have shown normal ECF and plasma volumes but have demonstrated elevated CI and normal vascular resistance, suggesting that these patients are in a phase of hypertension development and will later develop elevated vascular resistance if their tissues undergo autoregulation. Whether sodium intake contributes to this elevation of CI in man is not known.

Sullivan et al,[28] using echo techniques to study each subject as their own control during states of high and low sodium intake, have made serial measurements of CI. First, they observed that a high sodium diet increased heart size[28] (Fig. 1). They subsequently found that a 200 mEq sodium diet, given

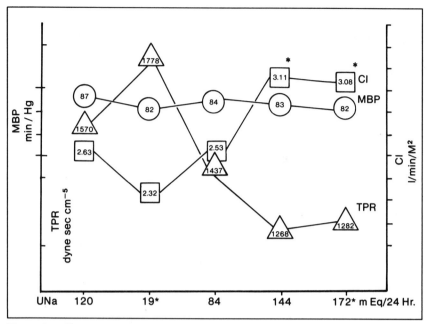

Figure 2. *Chronic hemodynamic effects of a relatively high sodium intake in 7 normal subjects. The first measurements were made during an ad libitum diet, the second after 4 days of sodium depletion, the third after 4 to 6 days of sodium repletion, the fourth after a liberal sodium intake for 6 months, and the fifth after 1 year of high sodium intake.*

after a period of sodium restriction, result in a 5% or greater increase in mean blood pressure in about 40% of borderline hypertensive subjects but in only 22% of normal subjects.[29] The normal subjects responded to sodium repletion with an increase in CI and a decrease in TPR. The response in the hypertensive subjects was more varied; of those showing an increase in blood pressure, 50% did so because of an increase in CI without an adequate decrease in TPR, and 50% on the basis of an increase in TPR, suggesting that the human population of North America is far less genetically homogenous than the Dahl salt-sensitive rat. Whether these changes persist and which, if any, are associated with the eventual development of hypertension are important, unanswered questions. Sullivan and Ratts[30] have found that the increased CI and decreased TPR persist more than 12 months in sodium- resistant subjects (Fig. 2) and have made unpublished observations that blood pressure remained elevated at 6 months in sodium-sensitive subjects because of an inadequate decrease in resistance.

This heterogeneity of response has been found by other investigators under different circumstances. In patients receiving hemodialysis, Onesti et al[31] found that expansion of ECF did not cause an increase in TPR or blood pressure in previously normotensive subjects, whereas blood pressure increased along with TPR in 60% or with CI in 20% of the hypertensive patients. Similarly, Bravo et al[32] have found that mineralocorticoid-induced hypertension in the dog was, in some cases, associated with an increased TPR and in other cases with an increased CI. Berecek and Bohr[33] have made similar observations in the pig. Luft et al[34] have studied the hemodynamic and metabolic response of normal subjects to extremes of sodium intake, 10 to 1,500 mEq daily. They found that an intake of 800 mEq or more was associated with a significant increase in blood pressure and in CI.

Epidemiologic studies also suggest a link between potassium deficiency and hypertension.[35] Direct infusion of potassium chloride and slight increases in serum potassium concentration have been found to have a vasodilatory effect in several vascular beds in man and in experimental animals.[36,37] Evidence has been presented to suggest that this vasodilator effect is attenuated in hypertensive humans.[38] Potassium has natriuretic effects, due to a decreased tubular absorption of sodium. Luft et al[39] have found that potassium replacement promotes saluresis and reduces the blood pressure elevating effects of sodium in normal subjects, and MacGregor et al[40] found that potassium supplementation lowered blood pressure in hypertension. Thus, potassium might be an important modifier of the effects of sodium on the cardiovascular system.

Impaired left ventricular (LV) diastolic function has been found in patients with cardiac hypertrophy.[41] Al-Aouar et al[42] observed that the maximum LV filling rates in young, borderline hypertensive patients without LVH did not vary as heart size was altered by variations in sodium intake, as did normal subjects. Recently, Ratts et al[43] reported that of a group of patients presenting with chronic hypertension and heart failure of recent onset, only 39% had echo evidence of impaired LV contraction, and of these, 91% had a history of alcoholism, prior myocardial infarction, or other illness that could explain abnormal LV function. Fully 61% had normal systolic shortening despite hypertrophied ventricles, suggesting that sodium-induced volume overload, plus a stiff left ventricle with abnormal diastolic relaxation, explained the development of pulmonary congestion.

Thus, in normal, sodium-resistant individuals, a high sodium diet results in an increase in LV end-diastolic and end-systolic size and an increase in stroke volume and in CI that is accommodated by a decrease in TPR, which in turn maintains arterial blood pressure at usual levels. The sodium-sensitive person usually shows the same cardiac response but does not lower vascular resistance to the same degree, or even vasoconstricts; therefore, blood pressure increases. The reason for this abnormal interplay between flow and resistance has intrigued investigators for decades and remains an exciting area of investigation.

Acknowledgment

Supported in part by Grant HL-21523 from the National Heart, Lung, and Blood Institute and Grant RR-0211 from the General Clinical Research Center.

References

1. AMBARD L, BEAUJARD E: Causes de l'hypertension arterielle. Arch Gen Med 1904; 1: 530.
2. SASAKI N: The relationship of salt intake to hypertension in the Japanese. Geriatrics 1964; 19: 735–744.
3. KEMPNER W: Treatment of kidney disease and hypertensive vascular disease with rice diet. NC Med J 1944; 5: 125–133.
4. MURPHY RJF: The effect of "rice diet" on plasma volume and extracellular fluid space in hypertensive subjects. J Clin Invest 1950; 29: 912–917.
5. PARIJS J, JOOSENS JV, VAN DER LINDEN L, VERSTREKEN G, AMERY AKPC: Moderate sodium restriction and diuretics in the treatment of hypertension. Am Heart J 1973; 85: 22–34.
6. LUFT FC, WEINBERGER MH, GRIM CE, FINEBERG NS, MILLERY JZ: Sodium sensitivity in normotensive human subjects. Ann Intern Med 1983; 98: 758–762.
7. LEDINGHAM JM, COHEN RD: The role of the heart in the pathogenesis of renal hypertension. Lancet 1963; 2: 979–981.
8. GUYTON AC, COLEMAN TG, COWLEY AW, MANNING RD, NORMAN A, FERGUSON JD: A systems analysis approach to understanding long-range arterial blood pressure control and hypertension. Circ Res 1974; 35: 159.
9. COLEMAN TG, GUYTON AC: Hypertension caused by salt loading in the dog. III. Onset transients of cardiac output and other variables. Circ Res 1969; 25: 153–160.
10. DAHL LK: Salt and hypertension. Am J Clin Nutr 1972; 25: 231–244.
11. BIANCHI G, DiFRANCESCO GF, et al: Blood pressure changes produced by kidney cross-transplantation between spontaneously hypertensive rats (SHR) and normotensive rats (NR). Clin Sci Mol Med 1974; 47: 435–448.
12. DAHL LK, HEINE M, THOMPSON K: Genetic influence of the kidneys on blood pressure. Evidence from chronic renal homografts in rats with opposite predispositions to hypertension. Circ Res 1974; 40: 94–101.
13. DAHL LK, KNUDSEN KD, OWAI J: Humeral transmission of hypertension: evidence from parabiosis. Circ Res 1976; 24, 25 (suppl): 21.
14. TOBIAN L, ISHII M, DUKE M: Relationship of cytoplasmic granules in renal papillary interstitial cells to "post-salt" hypertension. J Lab Clin Med 1969; 73: 309–319.
15. GANGULI M, TOBIAN L, IWAI J: Cardiac output and peripheral resistance in strains of rats sensitive and resistant to NaCl hypertension. Hypertension 1974; 1: 3.
16. KISCH B: Electron microscopy of the atrium of the heart. Exp Med Surg 1956; 15: 99–112.
17. DEBOLD AJ: Heart atria granularity effects changes in water-electrolyte balance. Proc Soc Exp Biol Med 1979; 161: 508–511.
18. DEBOLD AJ, BORENSTEIN HB, VERESS AT, SONNENBERG H: A rapid and potent natriuretic response to intravenous injection of atrial myocardial extract in rats. Life Sci 1981; 28: 89–94.
19. SONNENBERG H, CUPPLES WA, DEBOLD AJ, VERESS AT: Intrarenal localization of the natriuretic effect of cardiac atrial extract. Can J Physiol Pharmacol 1982; 60: 1149–1152.

20. MARK AL: The Bezold-Jarisch reflex revisited: clinical implications of inhibitory reflexes originating in the heart. J Am Coll Cardiol 1983; 1: 90–102.

21. DE WARDENER HE, CLARKSON EM: The natriuretic hormone: recent developments. Clin Sci 1982; 63: 415–420.

22. BLAUSTEIN MP: Sodium ions, calcium ions, blood pressure regulation, and hypertension: a reassessment and a hypothesis. Am J Physiol 1977; 232: 165–173.

23. HAMLYN JM, RINGEL R, SCHAEFFER J, LEVINSON PD, HAMILTON BP, KOWARSKI AA, BLAUSTEIN MP: A circulating inhibitor of (Na + K) ATPase associated with essential hypertension. Nature 1982; 300: 650–652.

24. KIRKENDALL WM, CONNOR WE, ABBOUD F, RASTOGI SP, ANDERSON TA, FRY M: The effect of dietary sodium on the blood pressure of normal man. In: Genest J, Koiw E, eds. Hypertension '72. Berlin: Springer-Verlag, 1972; 360–374.

25. MARK AL, LAWTON WJ, ABBOUD FM, FITZ AE, CONNOR WE, HEISTAD DD: Effects of high and low sodium intake on arterial pressure and forearm vascular resistance in borderline hypertension. A preliminary report. Circ Res 1975; 36 (suppl 1): 194–198.

26. FROHLICH ED, TARAZI RC, DUSTAN HP: Re-examination of the hemodynamics of hypertension. Am J Med Sci 1969; 257: 9–23.

27. JULIUS S, PASCUAL AV, REILLY K, et al: Abnormalities of plasma volume in borderline hypertension. Arch Intern Med 1971; 127: 116–119.

28. SULLIVAN JM, RATTS TE, SCHOENEBERGER AA, SAMAHA JK, PALMER ET: The effect of diet on echocardiographic left ventricular dimensions in normal man. Am J Clin Nutr 1979; 32: 2410–2415.

29. SULLIVAN JM, RATTS TE, TAYLOR JC, KRAUS DH, BARTON BR, PATRICK DR, REED SW: Hemodynamic effects of dietary sodium in man. A preliminary report. Hypertension 1980; 2: 506–514.

30. SULLIVAN JM, RATTS TE: Hemodynamic mechanisms of adaptation to chronic high sodium intake in normal humans. Hypertension 1983; 5: 814–820.

31. ONESTI G, KIM KE, GRECO JA, DEL GUERICIO E, FERNANDES J, SWARTZ C: Blood pressure regulation in end-stage renal disease and anephric man. Circ Res 1975; 36 (Suppl 1): 145–152.

32. BRAVO EL, TARAZI R, DUSTAN H: Multifactorial analysis of chronic hypertension induced by electrolyte-active steroids in trained unanesthetized dogs. Circ Res 1977; 40 (Suppl 1): I–140–145.

33. BERECEK KH, BOHR DF: Whole body vascular reactivity during the development of deoxycorticosterone acetate hypertension in the pig. Circ Res 1978; 42: 764–771.

34. LUFT FC, WEINBERGER MH, GRIM CE: Sodium sensitivity and resistance in normotensive humans. Am J Med 1982; 72: 726–736.

35. LANGFORD HG: Dietary potassium and hypertension: epidemiologic data. Ann Intern Med 1983; 98: 770–772.

36. EMANUEL DA, SCOTT JB, HADDY FJ: Effect of potassium on small and large blood vessels of the dog forelimb. Am J Physiol 1959; 197: 637–642.

37. LOWE RD, THOMPSON JW: The effect of intra-arterial potassium chloride infusion upon forearm blood flow in man. J Physiol (Lond) 1962; 162.

38. OVERBECK HW, DERIFIELD RS, PAMNANI NB: Attenuated vasodilator responses to K in essential hypertensive men. J Clin Invest 1964; 53: 678.

39. LUFT FC, RANKIN LI, BLOCH R, WEYMAN AE, WILLIS LR, MURRAY RH, GRIM CE, WEINBERGER MH: Cardiovascular and humoral responses to extremes of sodium intake in normal black and white men. Circulation 1979; 60: 697–706.

40. MACGREGOR GA, SMITH SJ, MARHANDU ND, BANKS RA, SAGNELLA GA: Moderate potassium supplementation in essential hypertension. Lancet 1982; 2: 567–570.

41. GIBSON DG, TRAIL TA, HALL RJC, BROWN DJ: Echocardiographic features of secondary left ventricular hypertrophy. Br Heart J 1979; 41: 54–59.

42. AL-AOUAR ZR, RATTS TE, CUNNINGHAM BR, SULLIVAN JM: Altered ventricular diastolic properties in borderline hypertension: effect of sodium intake. Circulation 1981; 64: IV–322.

43. RATTS TE, ADDINGTON B, GERLACH P, CONWAY L, SULLIVAN JM: Echocardiographic-clinical correlation of heart failure in hypertension (abstr.). J Am Coll Cardiol 1984; 3: 592.

4

Cardiovascular Changes in Prehypertension

BONITA FALKNER, M.D.

It is currently recognized that the dysregulatory mechanisms that direct the pathogenesis of hypertension have their onset in the young.[1–3] The ability to identify with certainty young prehypertensive people would provide a population in which the evolving pathogenesis of hypertension could be delineated. However, the entity of hypertension is defined in terms of blood pressure determinations that exceed certain levels, with higher than normal levels related to vascular and target organ injury. Thus, prehypertensive juveniles cannot be concisely identified by similar criteria, that of blood pressure, since their blood pressures have not yet exceeded the normal range. Since definitive criteria to identify the prehypertensive individual are as yet nonexistent, the available parameters are limited to measures that assess risk for development of hypertension. The characteristics of those at high risk provide an approximation of those with prehypertension.

Epidemiologic investigations in the young have contributed a greater overall understanding of correlates and variations of blood pressure in juveniles.[4,5] These studies have characterized levels of blood pressure in the young and delineated related parameters, such as body weight, height, and maturation.[6–8] When race is considered as a parameter of blood pressure and hypertension risk, black children have been shown to have higher levels of blood pressure than white children in the Bogalusa Heart Study[9] and in the young of Evans County,[10] whereas other reports relate no racial difference in blood pressure. In another investigation of related parameters of black and white children, subgrouped according to the presence of parental hypertension or normotension, Hohn et al[11] demonstrated racial differences in heart rate, blood pressure, urinary electrolytes, urinary kallikrein, and plasma renin activity. These results indicate that black children of hypertensive parents not only have higher levels of blood pressure, but also may have identifiable biochemical characteristics that portray an increased risk status for essential hypertension.[11]

Longitudinal studies have provided data that indicate that blood pressure tracking occurs throughout childhood and adolescence.[8] Thus, children with blood pressure measurements in the upper quintiles of the blood pressure distribution tend to maintain this position during growth and maturation, as do those in lower levels of blood pressure distribution. A pertinent issue then is the relationship of these higher levels of blood pressure in the young to the disease of essential hypertension with its inherent vascular and target organ injury. Relevant to this issue are the reports by Zahka et al[12] and Schieken et al.[13] These investigators have demonstrated by echo that juveniles with blood pressure in the higher deciles have greater left ventricular (LV) mass and posterior wall thickness of the myocardium. These differences remain significant when subjects are matched for body mass indices. In another study by Schieken et al[14] it was demonstrated that juveniles with the higher levels of blood pressure have an increasing peripheral vascular resistance.[14] The relevance of these observations must be determined. On the one hand, these cardiovascular differences may only reflect one extreme of normal cardiovascular maturation processes. On the other hand, it is conceivable that a relatively greater LV mass and higher peripheral vascular resistance in juveniles with blood pressures in the higher normal range may reflect an early phase of a disease that is already effecting some degree of cardiovascular injury.

Further studies will be necessary to determine the correlation of these observations with the pathogenesis of essential hypertension. Of particular interest is the question of whether these differences in blood pressure, ventricular mass, or vascular resistance can be altered by some intervening treatment. Related to these issues is the report by Falkner et al[15] in a group of adolescents with fixed hypertension. These patients had blood pressures consistently above the 95th percentile. During exercise stress testing by multistage treadmill exercise, it was observed that the persons with hypertension did not demonstrate the normal reduction in R-wave amplitude with increasing workload and heart rate that was observed in the normotensive adolescents.[15] After blood pressure reduction with either diuretics or with a centrally acting drug (clonidine), the adolescents with hypertension then demonstrated a progressive reduction in R-wave amplitude similar to the normotensive subjects (Fig. 1). These observations indicate that there may be functional as well as structural changes in adolescents with mild hypertension, and these changes may be related to a relatively greater vascular resistance.[16]

Cardiovascular characteristics of early or borderline hypertension include an increased cardiac output with normal peripheral resistance. These changes are consistent with increased adrenergic systems activity. In adolescents, McCory et al[17] have demonstrated higher norepinephrine values in patients with both hypertension and borderline hypertension, with a blunted response in both blood pressure and norepinephrine to upright postural change.

A number of investigations have linked these neurogenic-mediated cardiovascular responses to hereditary risk for hypertension.[18,19] Studies in the young have also demonstrated that children with hypertensive parents respond to mental stress with greater heart rate and blood pressure responses.[20,21] We have studied adolescents from families with and without hypertension. When these juveniles were exposed to a standardized alerting stimulus of forced mental arithmetic, the offspring of hypertensive parents

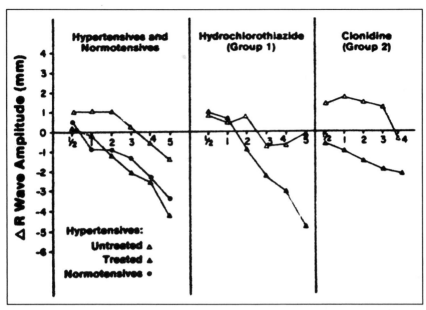

Figure 1. *The mean R-wave amplitude change at each stage of progressive exercise. Left panel, normotensive control subjects, all untreated hypertensive subjects as a group, and all hypertensive subjects after treatment. Middle panel, the R-wave response before and during hydrochlorothiazide therapy. Right panel, the R-wave response before and during clonidine therapy.*

showed higher basal heart rates as well as a heart rate and blood pressure response to stress that was both greater and more prolonged than the genetically normotensive control subjects. This increased responsiveness, expressed not only in blood pressure and heart rate, but also in higher catecholamine levels, was present among adolescents already displaying marginal hypertension and also in those who were still normotensive (Fig. 2).[20]

This study and others suggested that a stress-mediated hyperresponsivity of the cardiovascular system could be associated with an increased risk for subsequent essential hypertension. To evaluate the clinical relevance of a high stress response, stress testing data were obtained in a group of 50 adolescents with borderline hypertension. Over a follow-up period of 5 years more than 50% progressed to a phase of fixed hypertension defined as diastolic or systolic blood pressure above the 95th percentile for more than 3 months. This progression rate to fixed hypertension is considerably greater than that reported for other populations with borderline hypertension and indicates that the characteristics of marginally elevated blood pressure with a strong family history of hypertension and increased cardiovascular response to stress in the young place them at a greater risk for essential hypertension.[22]

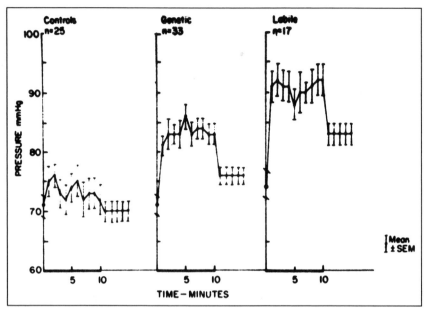

Figure 2. *The change in diastolic pressure during stress is plotted against time. Mean pressure ± SE of each group is presented at 1-minute intervals during stress and in the recovery phase. The mean of the pressure changes for all subjects of each group during the entire period of stress is: controls, 3.5 mmHg; genetic, 11.3 mmHg; labile, 16.2 mmHg. A significant difference exists between controls and labiles (p < 0.001) and controls and genetics (p < 0.001). There is also a difference between genetics and labiles (p < 0.05). (Reproduced with permission from Falkner et al.[20])*

Early cardiovascular changes in the young prehypertensive person may be due to factors other than enhanced sympathetic nervous system activity. In studies of sodium sensitivity, patients with borderline hypertension respond to a dietary load with an increase in blood pressure and a disproportionate increase in cardiac index, and some may also have an increase in peripheral vascular resistance.[23] In children we have found that sodium loading will increase blood pressure both under baseline conditions and during stress in offspring of persons with hypertension, but the heart rate is lower. In offspring of normotensive persons the sodium loading resulted in no change.[24] These studies indicate that manipulations of blood volume appear to unmask an aberrant relationship between sympathetic nervous system activity and vascular sensitivity, with resultant changes in cardiovascular response. Not only are these variations identifiable in borderline hypertension, but there is an indication that they are operative in the prehypertensive state.

Summary

The objective determination of cardiovascular changes in the prehypertensive phase requires a retrospective analysis of extended longitudinal studies. However, no such data are currently available. Prehypertension in the young may be approached by identifying those with blood pressures consistently in the higher range of distribution and having other risk factors. In these juveniles the available data indicate that some have increased adrenergic activity with greater cardiovascular reactivity. There is also evidence of slight but distinguishable increases in myocardial mass, with relatively greater peripheral vascular resistance than age- and size-matched children with lower blood pressure. The significance of these differences has not been determined, nor has it been determined whether these cardiovascular changes can be altered by any intervention maneuvers. Further studies in the young will be necessary to clarify these issues.

References

1. LONDE S, BOURGOIGNIE JJ, ROBSON AM, GOLDRING D: Hypertension in apparently normal children. J Pediatr 1971; 78: 569–577.
2. Report of the Task Force on Blood Pressure Control in Children. Pediatrics 1977; 59 (suppl): 797–820.
3. ZINNER SH, LEVY PS, KASS EH: Familial aggregation of blood pressure in childhood. N Engl J Med 1971; 284: 401–404.
4. HARLAN WR, CORNONI-HUNTLEY J, LEAVERTON PE: Blood pressure in childhood. The National Health Examination Survey. Hypertension 1979; 1 (suppl): 559–565.
5. CORNONI-HUNTLEY J, HARLAN WR, LEAVERTON PE: Blood pressure in adolescence, United States Health Examination Survey. Hypertension 1979; 1: 566–571.
6. PRINEAS RJ, GILLUM RF, HORIBE H, HANNAN PJ: The Minneapolis Children's Blood Pressure Study. Part 2: Multiple determinants of children's blood pressure. Hypertension 1980; 2 (suppl): I: 18–24.
7. KATZ SH, HEDIGER MC, SCHALL JI, et al: Blood pressure, growth, and maturation from childhood through adolescence. Hypertension 1980; 2 (suppl): I: 55–69.
8. VOORS AW, WEBBER LS, BERENSON GS: Time course study of blood pressure in children over a three-year period. Hypertension 1980; 2 (suppl): I: 102–108.
9. VOORS AW, FOSTER TA, FRERICHS RR, WEBBER LS, BERENSON GS: Studies of blood pressures in children ages 5–14 years in a total biracial community. Circulation 1976; 54: 319–327.
10. JOHNSON AL, CORNONI JC, CASSEL JC, TYROLER HA, HEYDEN S, HAMES CG: Influence of race, sex and weight on blood pressure behavior in young adults. Am J Cardiol 1975; 35: 523–530.
11. HOHN AR, RIOPEL DA, KEIL JE, et al: Childhood familial and racial differences in physiologic and biochemical factors related to hypertension. Hypertension 1983; 5: 56–70.
12. ZAHKA KG, NEILL CA, KIDD L, CUTILLETTA MA, CUTILLETTA AF: Cardiac involvement in adolescent hypertension. Echographic determination of myocardial hypertrophy. Hypertension 1981; 3: 664–668.
13. SCHIEKEN RM, CLARKE WR, LAUER RM: Left ventricular hypertrophy in children

in the upper quintile of the distribution: the Muscatine Study. Hypertension 1981; 3: 669–675.

14. SCHIEKEN RM, CLARKE WR, LAUER RM: The cardiovascular responses to exercise in children across the blood pressure distribution: the Muscatine Study. Hypertension 1983; 5: 71–78.

15. FALKNER B, LOWENTHAL DT, AFFRIME MB, HAMSTRA B: Changes in R-wave amplitude during aerobic exercise stress testing in hypertensive adolescents. Am J Cardiol 1982; 50: 152–156.

16. FALKNER B, LOWENTHAL DT, AFFRIME MB, HAMSTRA B: R-wave amplitude during aerobic exercise in hypertensive adolescents after treatment. Am J Cardiol 1983; 51: 459–463.

17. McCORY WW, KLEIN AA, ROSENTHAL RA: Blood pressure, heart rate, and plasma catecholamines in normal and hypertensive children and their siblings at rest and after standing. Hypertension 1982; 4: 507–513.

18. LIGHT KC, OBRIST PA: Cardiovascular reactivity to behavioral stress in young males with and without marginally elevated casual systolic pressure: a comparison of clinic, home, and laboratory measures. Hypertension 1980; 2: 802–808.

19. MANUCK SB, PROIETTI JM: Parental hypertension and cardiovascular response to cognitive and isometric challenge. Psychophysiology 1982; 19: 481–489.

20. FALKNER B, ONEST G, ANGELAKOS ET, FERNANDEZ M, LANGMAN C: Cardiovascular response to mental stress in normal adolescents with hypertensive parents. Hemodynamics and mental stress in adolescents. Hypertension 1979; 1: 23–30.

21. LAWLER KA, ALLEN NT: Risk factors for hypertension in children: their relationship to psychophysiologic responses. J Psychosom Res 1981; 25: 199–205.

22. FALKNER B, KUSHNER H, ONESTI G, ANGELAKOS ET: Cardiovascular characteristics in adolescents who develop essential hypertension. Hypertension 1981; 3: 521–527.

23. SULLIVAN JM, RATTS TE, TAYLOR JC, et al: Hemodynamic effects of dietary sodium in man: a preliminary report. Hypertension 1980; 2: 506–514.

24. FALKNER B, ONESTI G, ANGELAKOS ET: Effects of salt loading on the cardiovascular response to stress in adolescents. Hypertension 1981; 3 (suppl): II–195–199.

5

Cardiac Adaptation in Hypertensive Children

WALTER S. CULPEPPER III, M.D.

Study of the early developmental stages of hypertensive heart disease in man has been greatly enhanced by the introduction of echo and by intensive study of the origins of essential hypertension in children. Longitudinal studies of blood pressure in children suggest that adult essential hypertension has its origin in adolescence and possibly earlier.[1,2] Recently, several groups of investigators have found subtle cardiac changes very early in the development of primary hypertension: increased left ventricular (LV) mass has been demonstrated by echo in 10% to 15% of children with mild hypertension.[3-7] Early left ventricular hypertrophy (LVH) may also be present in some adolescents before blood pressure exceeds the 95th percentile for age and sex.[3,7] This chapter will summarize current information about cardiac adaptation during the incipient phases of essential hypertension.

Brief Comparison of Study Designs

Echo studies of American children with borderline hypertension in Chicago and New Orleans,[3] in St. Louis,[4] Dallas,[5] Baltimore,[6] and Muscatine, Iowa,[7] have been published since 1979. The cardiac status of young subjects with persistent borderline or mild hypertension was compared with that of cohorts with normal blood pressure. All studies involved relatively small numbers of total subjects, approximately 50 to 250, with the largest group of children studied by Schieken et al[7] in Muscatine, Iowa. The average age of all the subjects was about 14 years. Two of the studies included children under 12 years of age.[6,7] Males predominated in all studies, but only the Muscatine group was nearly all white. Conditions under which blood pressures were measured were roughly comparable: multiple sitting blood pressures were obtained with mercury sphygmomanometers in a school survey or outpatient department setting. Most of the investigators used the fifth Korotkoff sound for diastolic blood pressure levels. Three studies[4,5,7] used normal blood pressure values obtained from local population surveys. Each study defined their high blood pressure subject groups differently and somewhat arbitrarily. Specifically, Goldring et al[4] selected patients with blood pressures greater than 1.65 SD above the mean for their hypertensive group. Laird and Fixler[5] defined hypertension as systolic or diastolic pressures greater than 95th percentiles from their Dallas school survey normal data. Only the Baltimore study by Zahka et al[6] included subjects with moderately severe essential hypertension. (Their ranges for hypertensives were systolic pressures between 136 and 176 mmHg and diastolic pressures between 82 and 110 mmHg.) Our study and that of the Muscatine group[3,7] were limited exclusively to subjects whose blood pressures were within normal limits, although relative strata differed significantly for high and low blood pressure groups in both studies. For example, average systolic and diastolic pressures for our borderline hypertensive group were 137/89 mmHg compared with 110/68 mmHg for our normotensive controls.

All of the investigators followed the standard recommendations of the American Society of Echocardiography for obtaining and measuring the echo.[8] However, the formulas used to derive volumetric data and LV mass[9–11] differed in some studies. Also, different methods were used to normalize variables for group comparisons. Despite these methodologic differences between studies, many of their findings were qualitatively similar.

Anatomic Adaptations

Echo findings reported in the five studies are summarized in Table I. Left ventricular posterior wall thickness in our group[3] of borderline hypertensive teenagers was significantly greater than in control subjects ($p < 0.001$). The Dallas and Baltimore studies also found significantly greater indexed LV wall thickness for their hypertensive group.[5,6] All studies except that of Goldring et al[4] in St. Louis examined echo estimates of LV mass, and all four reported increased LV mass in teenagers with hypertension. The Muscatine study[7] also found significantly greater interventricular septal thickness when their teenagers with high normal blood pressure levels were compared

TABLE I   Echo Anatomy in Hypertensive Adolescents

	Culpepper et al[3]	Goldring et al[4]	Laird et al[5]	Schieken et al[7]	Zahka et al[6]
Increased LVWT	Yes ($p < 0.001$)	No	Yes ($p < 0.001$)	No	Yes ($p < 0.005$)
Increased IVST	ND	Yes ($p < 0.05$)	No	Yes ($p < 0.01$)	Yes ($p < 0.005$)
Increased LVM	Yes ($p < 0.001$)	ND	Yes ($p < 0.001$)	Yes ($p < 0.05$)	Yes ($p < 0.001$)
Increased T/R	Yes ($p < 0.001$)	ND	ND	ND	Yes ($p < 0.001$)
Increased LA	No	No	No	Yes ($p < 0.05$)	Yes ($p < 0.005$)
NL or decreased LVEDD	Yes	Yes	Yes	Yes	Yes
LVWT $> +2$ SD	2/27 (7%)	ND	9/50 (18%)	ND	ND
LVM $> +2$ SD	3/27 (11%)	ND	18/50 (16%)	ND	ND

LVWT = left ventricular posterior wall thickness in end-diastole; IVST = interventricular septal thickness in end-diastole; LVM = left ventricular mass; T/R = relative wall thickness; LA = maximal left atrial dimensions; LVEDD = left ventricular end-diastolic dimension; ND = not done; NL = normal; SD = standard deviation. p values are hypertensive group means compared with normotensive group means.

with groups in the low and middle quintiles of blood pressure. Only hypertensive male subjects in the study by Goldring et al[4] had significantly greater LV end-diastolic volumes when compared with control subjects. In all other studies LV chamber dimensions and volumes did not differ between the hypertensive groups and the control subjects.

Teenagers with borderline hypertension also had significantly increased relative wall thickness (thickness to radius ratio) compared with controls. Increased relative wall thickness is consistent with the concentric form of LVH. Previous echo studies by Dunn et al[12] and others[13,14] found concentric LVH in adults with primary hypertension. However, in a recent report by Safar and associates[15] a majority of young adults with borderline hypertension was found to exhibit disproportionate septal thickening. In the five studies reviewed here, only 1 hypertensive teenage girl in the Dallas group had asymmetric septal hypertrophy.

In two studies estimates of prevalence and degree of early LVH were presented, based on prediction intervals or confidence limits from their normal echo data. In our study, 2 of 27 (7%) of hypertensive subjects had indexed LV wall thicknesses greater than 2 SD above predicted normal. Three of 27 (11%) of hypertensives had indexed LV mass greater than 2 SD above predicted normals. None of the normotensive patients exceeded normal limits for either variable. In the Dallas study, 8 of 50 (16%) of the hypertensive teenagers had indexed LV mass above their 95th percentile, whereas 2 of 50 of the control subjects were above this level.

Some of the data suggest that early LVH in juvenile borderline hypertension is only partly related to modest elevations in blood pressure. Although LV mass correlated weakly but significantly with casual blood pressures in our subjects, the thickness to radius ratio (Fig. 1) showed moderate correlation with systolic and diastolic pressures ($r = 0.47$ and $r = 0.51$, respectively; $p < 0.01$ for both). There was a linear regression of relative wall thickness on systolic and diastolic pressures that was independent of ventricular cavity size. However, there was a large standard error for both regression lines, and the association only accounted for about 25% of the observed variability as predicted by the square of the correlation coefficients. Thus, it would appear that factors other than average pressure load or afterload may influence the development of LVH very early in the natural history of essential hypertension.

Functional Adaptations

In young subjects the net changes in ventricular mass and geometry are not only relatively mild but also apparently physiologically adaptive with regard to preservation of resting hemodynamics. No significant differences were found for heart rate and cardiac output (CO) between the high and low blood pressure groups in any of the studies. There were wide distributions for randomly measured heart rate and CO in teenagers that may have masked important subgroups within the small number of hypertensive sub-

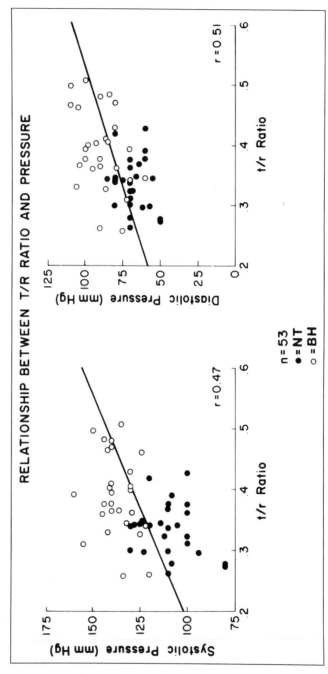

Figure 1. *Left ventricular wall thickness to radius (T/R) ratios versus systolic and diastolic blood pressures for 53 subjects. Closed circles represent normotensive subjects and open circles represent borderline hypertensive subjects. (Reproduced with permission from Culpepper WS III et al.[3])*

jects studied. The Muscatine Study found a tendency toward higher CO in the higher blood pressure quintiles, but again, they showed no statistical differences between strata.

Echo ejection phase indices of LV function (minor axis shortening, velocity of circumferential fiber shortening, ejection fraction, and systolic time intervals) were within normal limits for normal and high blood pressure groups for each study. Our borderline hypertensive subjects had statistically lower ejection fractions, minor axis shortening values, and velocities of circumferential fiber shortening than the controls. However, the practical clinical significance of these findings is difficult to interpret, particularly since ejection phase indices are afterload-dependent variables. Also, the absolute values for the borderline hypertensive group were still within normal limits for our laboratory.

Little is known about LV performance during exercise in hypertensive teenagers, but blood pressure and heart rate responses were evaluated in the St. Louis study. Goldring et al[4] found that peak exercise systolic and diastolic blood pressures during upright bicycle ergometry were significantly higher in their hypertensive men and women. Furthermore, they found that the relative change in diastolic blood pressure during exercise was significantly higher in hypertensive men than in normotensive men ($p < 0.0001$). Although normotensive and hypertensive subjects had similar baseline heart rates, the hypertensive male and female groups had significantly higher peak heart rates during bicycle exercise ($p < 0.05$ for both groups). Because both peak heart rates and peak systolic pressures were higher in the hypertensive subjects, rate-pressure product estimates of myocardial oxygen consumption would appear to be considerably higher for the hypertensive subjects. In experimental forms of pressure overload hypertrophy, decreased coronary reserve[16] and subendocardial ischemia during pacing tachycardia[17] have been documented. Part of the long-term "cost" of early LVH in hypertensive children may be subclinical abnormalities of myocardial perfusion during exercise stress.

Clinical Implications

Juvenile-onset essential hypertension and echo evidence for LVH are probably separate but interrelated long-term cardiovascular risk factors.[18] However, several decades will be required to assess accurately the predictive value of echo indices of LVH for cardiac morbidity and mortality. Meanwhile, the conscientious clinician who tries to individualize treatment of the juvenile hypertensive based not only on blood pressure level and trend but on the patient's total cardiovascular risk profile is faced with the following information: (1) routine electrocardiographic methods have very low specificity and sensitivity for identifying LVH[19]; and (2) as many as 10% to 15% of teenagers with mild persistent hypertension will have LVH. As a result, it is anticipated that increasing numbers of physicians will use M-mode echo to assess cardiac status and to help tailor therapy for hypertensive individuals.

Unfortunately, no comprehensive evaluation and treatment guidelines have been established for young patients with mild essential hypertension. At present, I suggest that physicians avoid needless and possibly harmful drug therapy in children with mild hypertension who have no echo evidence of LVH or coexistent risk factors.

References

1. VOORS AW, WEBBER LS, BERENSON GS: Time course study of blood pressure in children over a three-year period (Bogalusa Heart Study). Hypertension 1980; 2 (suppl I): 102–108.

2. LAUER RM, CLARKE WR, BEAGLEHOLE R: Level, trend and variability of blood pressure during childhood: The Muscatine Study. Circulation 1984; 69: 242–249.

3. CULPEPPER WS III, SODT PC, MESSERLI FH, RUSCHHAUPT DG, ARCILLA RA: Cardiac status in juvenile borderline hypertension. Ann Intern Med 1983; 98: 1–7.

4. GOLDRING D, HERNANDEZ A, CHOI S, et al: Blood pressure in a high school population. II. Clinical profile of the juvenile hypertensive. J Pediatr 1979; 95: 298–304.

5. LAIRD WP, FIXLER DE: Left ventricular hypertrophy in adolescents with elevated blood pressure: Assessment by chest roentgenography, electrocardiography, and echocardiography. Pediatrics 1981; 67: 255–259.

6. ZAHKA KG, NEILL CA, KIDD L, CUTILLETTA MA, CUTILLETTA AF: Cardiac involvement in adolescent hypertension. Hypertension 1981; 3: 664–668.

7. SCHIEKEN RM, CLARKE WR, LAUER RM: Left ventricular hypertrophy in children with blood pressures in the upper quintile of the distribution (the Muscatine Study). Hypertension 1981; 3: 669–675.

8. SAHN DJ, DEMARIA A, KISSLO J, WEYMAN A: Recommendations regarding quantitation in M-mode echocardiography: Results of a survey of echocardiographic measurements. Circulation 1978; 58: 1072–1083.

9. CAHILL N, SODT P, LESTER L, MATTHEW R, ARCILLA RA: Cardiac echo-angio correlation in children (abstr.). Am J Cardiol 1976; 37: 125.

10. TROY BL, POMBO J, RACKLEY CE: Measurement of left ventricular wall thickness and mass by echocardiography. Circulation 1972; 45: 602–611.

11. McFARLAND IN, ALAM M, GOLDSTEIN S, PICKARDS S, STEIN T: Echocardiographic diagnosis of left ventricular hypertrophy. Circulation 1978; 57: 1140–1144.

12. DUNN FG, CHANDRARATNA PN, BASTA LL, FROHLICH ED: Pathophysiologic assessment of hypertensive heart disease by echocardiography (abstr). Am J Cardiol 1976; 37: 133.

13. SCHLANT RC, FELNER JM, HEYMSFIELD SB, et al: Echocardiographic studies of left ventricular anatomy and function in essential hypertension. Cardiovasc Med 1977; 2: 477–491.

14. SAVAGE DD, DRAYER JM, HENRY WL, et al: Echocardiographic assessment of cardiac anatomy and function in hypertensive subjects. Circulation 1979; 59: 623–632.

15. SAFAR ME, LEHNER JP, VINCENT MI, PLAINFOSSE MT, SIMON AC: Echocardio-

graphic dimensions in borderline and sustained hypertension. Am J Cardiol 1979; 44: 930–935.

16. MURRAY PA, VATNER SF: Reduction of maximal coronary vasodilator capacity in conscious dogs with severe right ventricular hypertrophy. Circ Res 1981; 48: 27–33.

17. BACHE RJ, ARENTZEN CE, SIMON AB, VROBEL TR: Abnormalities in myocardial perfusion during tachycardia in dogs with left ventricular hypertrophy: Metabolic evidence for ischemia. Circulation 1984; 69: 409–417.

18. SAVAGE DD, KANNEL WB, GARRISON RJ, et al: Longterm retrospective blood pressure correlates of various forms of left ventricular hypertrophy. Preliminary findings: The Framingham study (abstr). J Am Coll Cardiol 1983; 1: 622.

19. REICHEK N, DEVEREUX RB: Left ventricular hypertrophy: Relationship of anatomic, echocardiographic and electrocardiographic findings. Circulation 1981; 63: 391–407.

6

Hyperdynamic Beta-Adrenergic Circulatory State

EDWARD D. FROHLICH, M.D.

An Historical Perspective

Over the years, the medical literature has been replete with clinical descriptions of the broad spectrum of a syndrome that has intrinsic to it and variously: clinical complaints of cardiac awareness, cutaneous flushing, greater or lesser degrees of anxiety, and clinical findings of an altered physiologic state that is induced by increased adrenergic activity. Perhaps the first evidence of such an abnormality may be found in Avicenna's work of the latter part of the 10th century and earlier part of the 11th in which he described the clinical characteristics of the patient with a rapid and pounding pulse, a fearsome expression, and dilated pupils.[1] In more recent years, descriptions of this problem were prompted by the clinical findings in young men evaluated by physicians for the military service. Thus, in 1864, Hartshorne[2] described a cardiac abnormality in a sizable number of Union Army soldiers, referring to the condition as "cardiac muscular exhaustion." Seven years later, Da Costa[3] referred to this "functional" disorder as the "irritable heart syndrome." Sir Thomas Lewis reported on the soldier's heart during World War I.[4,5] Several groups of workers wrote of neurocirculatory asthenia at the same time, which was characterized by a variety of symptoms, few signs, a familial predisposition, but mostly cardiovascular complaints and anxiety.[6,7] Others described similar clinical observations: Starr and Jonas[8] described essential hyperkinesis; Holmgren et al,[9] vasoregulatory asthenia; and others the athletic heart syndrome, as physicians became involved with otherwise healthy young athletes with innocent murmurs or elevated blood pressure.[10–12] As these findings became of clinical concern to physicians evaluating athletes and other individuals who seemed otherwise normal and well, patients were referred for cardiac evaluation because of clinical complaints, a systolic murmur, or borderline or mild hypertension.

This concern was heightened at the time of another war; during the Korean conflict, Gorlin and associates[13,14] described hyperkinetic heart syndrome that was manifested by a hyperdynamic circulation, usually with a faster heart rate, but with an increased left ventricular ejection rate. This was followed by a series of other reports describing similar patients, each with a different descriptive appellation suggesting the same problem.[15–17] However, in one early report Page[18] described 9 patients with arterial hypertension having a syndrome resembling "archaic emotional patterns, possibly having their genesis in the thalamus and hypothalamus."

Hyperdynamic Beta-Adrenergic Circulatory State

More recently, we became interested in a similar subset of normotensive and hypertensive patients having similar clinical findings, but they predominantly had hypertension—labile, borderline, or fixed.[19–24] We reasoned that if we could provoke the symptoms and clinical and physiologic findings in these patients, even when they were asymptomatic, with intravenous infusion of the beta-adrenergic receptor agonist isoproterenol, we could possibly ameliorate or even prevent these symptoms and findings with specific therapy with beta-adrenergic receptor blocking drugs. We did, in fact, provoke these findings by demonstrating increased beta-adrenergic site responsiveness and therefore "dubbed" this syndrome as a beta-adrenergic hyperdynamic circulatory state.[19,20]

A Common Thread: All of the syndromes already described seem to have a common thread that relates them all. The patients, in fact, probably represent varying degrees of a broad clinical spectrum. It seems reasonable, however, to assume that the individual differences of the various syndromes probably reflect the referral characteristics of the physicians whose patients become part of their practice, the emphasis of the problem in which that clinical investigator has focused upon disease, and the variety of manifestations elicited by systemic adrenergic stimulation. Nevertheless, each syndrome is expressed by specific clinical, physical, and pathophysiologic manifestations of increased participation of the adrenergic nervous system in cardiovascular function. Clinically, the patients may describe an increased heart rate, palpitations, other symptoms of cardiac awareness, flushing, sweating, tight muscles, and anxiety. Physically, the clinician may detect cardiac murmurs or systolic clicks, abnormal cardiac rhythm and rate, altered electrocardiographic findings, and perhaps elevation of systolic and diastolic pressures.

The diagnosis varies, depending again on the patient "mix" of the physician's practice, but more frequently it may suggest valvular heart disease, mitral valve prolapse, myocardiopathy, and borderline systolic or established essential hypertension. At other times, it may also suggest pheochromocytoma, thyrotoxicosis, porphyria, and even so-called "autonomic epilepsy."

Pathophysiology: Hemodynamically, these patients demonstrate a faster heart rate and a greater resting cardiac output and myocardial contractility.[13,14,19,20] On physiologic or pharmacologic stimulation, we have observed an accentuated hemodynamic response of the foregoing hemodynamic indices and arterial pressure during upright tilting or stimulation with beta-adrenergic receptor agonists.[19,20] It was of great interest to find that during infusion of very small doses of the beta-adrenergic receptor agonist

TABLE I   Resting Hemodynamic Characteristics of Patients with the Hyperdynamic Beta-Adrenergic Circulatory State Compared with Normotensive and Essential Hypertensive Subjects*

	Hyperdynamic Beta-Adrenergic Circulatory State	Normal Subjects	Essential Hypertension
Mean arterial pressure (mmHg)	109 (7)	93 (1)	122 (5)
Heart rate (bpm)	85 (4)	68 (2)	71 (2)
Cardiac index (liters/min/m$^{(2)}$)	3.6 (0.7)	3.0 (0.1)	2.9 (0.1)
Stroke index (ml/b/m$^{(2)}$)	42 (1)	45 (2)	41 (2)
Mean rate left ventricular ejection (ml/s/m$^{(2)}$)	158 (8)	151 (4)	142 (7)
Total peripheral resistance (U)	19 (6)	17 (1)	24 (2)

*Each value represents the mean (± 1 SEM).

isoproterenol (0.1 to 0.3 μg/kg/min), doses that might increase heart rate normally up to 12 beats/minute at the highest dose, the heart rate increased by significantly greater amounts (at submaximal infusion rates), and an emotional outburst was also provoked in these patients. It was of further interest to note that if a parasympatholytic agent such as atropine was administered (intravenously) in doses that increased heart rate by the same degree as the isoproterenol infusion, an emotional response was not observed. It seemed at the time that the emotional response could be secondary to the cardiac stimulation although a primary effect centrally, in the brain, was also deemed highly possible. The primary effect of central beta-adrenergic stimulation was considered more likely, since atropine failed to evoke similar emotional findings. Most noteworthy from the physiologic point of view were the resting hemodynamic indices which were elevated to significantly greater levels than other normotensive and hypertensive individuals not having the complaints or symptoms of hyperdynamic circulation, but also receiving the isoproterenol infusion, as control subjects (Table I). We observed these findings not only in patients with hyperdynamic beta-adrenergic circulatory state but also in similarly symptomatic patients with idiopathic mitral valve prolapse syndrome.[24] Associated with these clinical and physiologic findings, we and others observed higher circulating levels of catecholamines,[24–26] and others have reported increased excretion of cyclic adenosine monophosphate in the urine of these patients.[27]

Concept: In general, most physicians have reasoned that these patients have complaints consistent with what is generally held to be an emotional disturbance that is the underlying pathologic abnormality accounting for the altered behavior, the secondary increased catecholamine levels, the hyperdynamic cardiovascular findings, and the other clinical manifestations. An alternative hypothesis might be the existence of an underlying condition of altered autonomic function in which there is a net increase in adrenergic function. The augmented adrenergic cardiovascular input produces not only hyperdynamic circulation and cardiovascular symptoms, but also the emotional response. Support for this concept might be offered by the observations that induction of a hyperdynamic circulation with inhibition of para-sympathetic activity does not produce the emotional response one finds with isoproterenol or in those conditions in which catecholamines may be elevated. In addition, psychiatrists have found that these anxiety symptoms may also be provoked by lactate infusion.[28] Also supporting the physiologic findings are the observations in patients with hypertension of reduced parasympathetic and augmented adrenergic components of the autonomic nervous system.[29,30] In some of these patients, increased adrenergic outflow or nerve activity has been measured;[31] in others, increased circulating levels of catecholamines.[32,33]

Therapeutic Implications: The importance of these observations suggested that beta-adrenergic receptor inhibitory therapy might be efficacious in this spectrum of patients with a hyperdynamic beta-adrenergic circulatory state.[19,20,23,25,26,34] Indeed, beta-blocking drugs have been quite useful in these patients, not only in preventing the symptoms, but also in normalizing the physiologic alterations.[19,20,23,34–42] It was of great interest to find that even in patients without this syndrome beta-blocking therapy may induce a state of up-regulation of beta-adrenergic receptor sites.[43] When beta-blocking therapy is suddenly withdrawn from these individuals all of the findings, clinical complaints as well as physiologic observations, become manifest, either as findings suggestive of the return of the hyperdynamic circulatory state, hyperthyroidism, or, in individuals with preexisting coronary disease, angina pectoris.[44,45]

Summary

Over the years, a syndrome comprising a spectrum of patient clinical findings and physiologic alterations suggestive of increased participation of adrenergic input to cardiovascular and other organ functions has evolved. The clinical observations have been "dubbed" with a variety of clinically descriptive diagnoses. The fundamental alteration, however, seems to be associated with increased responsiveness of beta-adrenergic receptor sites and possibly increased circulating catecholamine levels and to be amenable to beta-adrenergic receptor blocking therapy. It is hoped that fundamental pathogenetic mechanisms may be elucidated in this centuries-old clinical enigma that may suggest prevention and better treatment.

References

1. AVICENNA: Avicennae Arabum medicorum principis. Ex Gerardia Cremonensis versione and Andreae Alpasi Belunensis castisatione. Per Fabium Paulinum Utinensem. Venetiis, Apud Juntas, 1608 (in three volumes).

2. HARTSHORNE H: On heart disease in the Army. Am J Med Sci 1864; 48: 89–92.

3. DA COSTA JM: On irritable heart: a clinical study of a form of functional cardiac disorder and its consequences. Am J Med Sci 1871; 61: 17–52.

4. LEWIS T: Medical Research Committee. Report upon soldiers returned as cases of "disordered action of the heart" (D.H.A.) or "valvular disease of the heart" (V.D.H.). London: His Majesty's Stationery Office, 1917.

5. LEWIS T: The soldier's heart and the effort syndrome. London: Shaw and Sons; New York: Paul B. Hoeber, 1918.

6. LEWIS T: Report of neurocirculatory asthenia and its management. Milit Surg 1918; 42: 409–426.

7. COHEN ME, WHITE PD: Neurocirculatory asthenia: 1972 concept. Milit Med 1972; 137: 142–144.

8. STARR I, JONAS L: Supernormal circulation in resting subjects (hyperkinemia) with study of relation of kinemic abnormalities to basic metabolic rate. Arch Intern Med 1943; 71: 1–22.

9. HOLMGREN A, JONSSON B, LEVANDER M, LINDERHOLM H, SJÖSTRAND T, STRÖM G: Low physical working capacity in suspected heart cases due to inadequate adjustment of peripheral blood flow (vasoregulatory asthenia). Acta Med Scand 1957; 158: 413–436.

10. REINDELL H, ROSKAMM H, STEIN H: The heart and blood circulation in athletes. Med Welt 1960; 31: 1557–1563.

11. BULYCHEV VV, KHMELEOSKII VA, RUTMAN IV: Roentgenological and instrumental examination of the heart in athletes. Klin Med 1965; 43: 108–114.

12. GOTT PH, ROSELLE HA, CRAMPTON RS: The athletic heart syndrome: Five-year cardiac evaluation of a champion athlete. Arch Intern Med 1968; 122: 340–344.

13. GORLIN R: The hyperkinetic heart syndrome. JAMA 1962; 182: 823–829.

14. GORLIN R, BRACHFELD N, TURNER JD, MESSER VJ, SALAZAR E: The idiopathic high cardiac output state. J Clin Invest 1959; 38: 2144–2153.

15. GABOR G: Cardiovascular hyperkinetic syndrome. Acta Med Acad Sci Hung 1961; 17: 781–792.

16. GOTTSEGEN G, OKOS G, ROMODO T: Essential circulatory hyperkinesis. Am J Cardiol 1962; 10: 785–791.

17. MATOS L, TÖRÖK E: Essential circulatory hyperkinesis: epicritical studies. Acta Med Acad Sci Hung 1969; 26: 207–212.

18. PAGE IH: A syndrome simulating diencephalic stimulation occurring in patients with essential hypertension. Am J Med Sci 1935; 190: 9–14.

19. FROHLICH ED, DUSTAN HP, PAGE IH: Hyperdynamic beta-adrenergic circulatory state. Arch Intern Med 1966; 117: 614–619.

20. FROHLICH ED, TARAZI RC, DUSTAN HP: Hyperdynamic beta-adrenergic circulatory state: increased beta receptor responsiveness. Arch Intern Med 1969; 123: 1–7.

21. FROHLICH ED, KOZUL VJ, TARAZI RC, DUSTAN HP: Physiological comparison of labile and essential hypertension. Circ Res 1970; 27: 55–69.

22. FROHLICH ED, DUSTAN HP, TARAZI RC: Hyperdynamic beta-adrenergic circulatory state. An overview. Arch Intern Med 1970; 126: 1068–1069.

23. FROHLICH ED: Beta-adrenergic blockade in the circulatory regulation of hyperki-

netic states. Am J Cardiol 1971; 27: 195–199.

24. DE CARVALHO JGR, MESSERLI FH, FROHLICH ED: Mitral valve prolapse and borderline hypertension. Hypertension 1979; 1: 518–522.

25. BOUDOULAS H, REYNOLDS JC, MAZZAFERRI E, WOOLEY CF: Metabolic studies in mitral valve prolapse syndrome: a neuroendocrine-cardiovascular process. Circulation 1980; 61: 1200–1205.

26. PASTERNAC A, TUBERN JF, PUDDU PE, KRAL RB, DE CHAMPLAIN J: Increased plasma catecholamine levels in patients with symptomatic mitral valve prolapse. Am J Med 1982; 73: 783–790.

27. HAMET P, KUCHEL O, GENEST J: Effect of upright posture and isoproterenol infusion on cyclic adenosine monophosphate excretion in control subjects and patients with labile hypertension. J Clin Endocrinol Metab 1973; 36: 218–226.

28. PITTS FNJ, McCLURE JN JR: Lactate metabolism in anxiety neurosis. N Engl J Med 1967; 277: 1329–1336.

29. JULIUS S, RANDALL OS, ESLER MD, KASHIMA T, ELLIS C, BENNETT J: Altered cardiac responsiveness and regulation in the normal cardiac output type of borderline hypertension. Circ Res 1975; 36: 199–207.

30. FROHLICH ED, PFEFFER MA: Adrenergic mechanisms in human and SHR hypertension. Clin Sci Mol Med 1975; 48: 225s–238s.

31. WALLIN BG, DELIUS W, HAGBARTH KE: Comparison of sympathetic activity in normo- and hypertensive subjects. Circ Res 1921; 33: 9–21.

32. DE QUATTRO F, MIURA Y: Neurogenic factors in human hypertension: mechanism or myth? Am J Med 1973; 55: 362–378.

33. KUCHEL O, BUU NT, HAMET P, LAROCHELLE P, BOURGUE M, GENEST J: Dopamine surges in hyperadrenergic essential hypertension. Hypertension 1982; 4: 845–852.

34. FROHLICH ED, TARAZI RC, DUSTAN HP: Beta-adrenergic blocking therapy in hypertension: selection of patients. Int J Pharmacol Ther Toxicol 1970; 4: 151–156.

35. NORDENFELT O: The orthostatic ECG changes and the adrenergic and beta-receptor blocking agent, propranolol (Inderal). Acta Med Scand 1965; 178: 393–401.

36. BOLLINGER A, GANDER M, PYLKKANEN PO, et al: Treatment of the hyperkinetic heart syndrome with propranolol. Cardiologia 1966; 42: 68–82.

37. GRANVILLE-GROOSMAN KL, TURNER P: The effect of propranolol in anxiety. Lancet 1966; 1: 788–790.

38. LOHMÖLLER G, LYDTIN H: Das hyperkinetische Herzsyndrom. Fortschr Med 1971; 89: 864–867.

39. TÖRÖK E, BAJKAY G, GULYÁS A, ISTVÁNFFY M, MATOS L: Long-term propranolol therapy in essential circulatory hyperkinesis. Int J Clin Pharmacol Ther Toxicol 1972; 6: 364–374.

40. WOLF E, BRAUN K, STERN S: Effects of beta-receptor blocking agents propranolol and practolol on ST-T changes in neurocirculatory asthenia. Br Heart J 1974; 36: 872–879.

41. GUAZZI M, POLESE A, MAGRINI F, FIORENTINI C, OLIVARI MT: Long-term treatment of the hyperkinetic heart syndrome with propranolol. Am J Med Sci 1975; 270: 465–474.

42. NEFTEL KA, ADLER RH, KÄPPELL L, et al: Stage fright in musicians: a model

illustrating the effect of beta blockers. Psychosom Med 1982; 44: 461–469.

43. STILES GL, CARON MG, LEFKOWITZ RJ: β-adrenergic receptors: biochemical properties of physiological regulation. Physiol Rev 1984; 64: 665–743.

44. SHAND DG, WOOD AJJ: Editorial: Propranolol withdrawal syndrome—why? Circulation 1978; 58: 202–203.

45. SHENKMAN L, PODRID P, LOWENSTEIN J: Hyperthyroidism after propranolol withdrawal. JAMA 1977; 238: 237–239.

PART II
EPIDEMIOLOGY OF
LEFT VENTRICULAR
HYPERTROPHY

7

Prevalence and Natural History of Electrocardiographic Left Ventricular Hypertrophy*

WILLIAM B. KANNEL, M.D., M.P.H.
ANDREW L. DANNENBERG, M.D., M.P.H.

The electrocardiographic pattern of left ventricular hypertrophy (ECG-LVH) is a well-recognized clinical finding in hypertension, coronary heart disease, and other forms of cardiovascular disease. Although its diagnostic importance is generally known, its prognostic implications are not as widely appreciated.

Most estimates of the incidence and prognosis associated with ECG-LVH are based on selected clinical samples and small amounts of data. However, longitudinal data from the Framingham Heart Study provide estimates of prevalence and incidence of ECG-LVH in a general population sample. These data also allow assessment of the relationship of ECG-LVH to blood pressure levels in the cohort and of its prognostic significance with regard to specific types of cardiovascular morbidity and mortality.

Occurrence

Based on more than 20 years of follow-up of the 5,209 persons in the Framingham cohort, the prevalence of ECG-LVH increases steeply with age from less than 2% among subjects age 49 to 54 years to about 10% among subjects 75 to 82 years old.[1–4] The ECG-LVH and cardiac enlargement on radiographs do not correspond closely. The latter is present in only 35% to 50% of those with ECG-LVH.[1] The prevalence of cardiac enlargement on radiographs is about twice that of ECG-LVH, and in only about 16% of those with the former condition does ECG-LVH subsequently develop over a decade of follow-up. These results suggest that radiographs and ECG measure somewhat different phenomena or that ECG-LVH is a less sensitive measure of cardiac enlargement.

The incidence rate of ECG-LVH is higher than the prevalence data would suggest, because of the high associated mortality and the fact that the finding

*This chapter is adapted and updated from Kannel WB, Prevalence and Natural History of Electrocardiographic Left Ventricular Hypertrophy. Am J Med 1983; 75 (suppl 3A): 4–11.

does not necessarily persist. Incidence is higher in men than women and increases with age in both sexes. Based on a 26-year follow-up of the Framingham cohort, the 10-year incidence rate per 100 persons for men less than age 40 years was 1.2, for ages 40 to 49 years it was 3.1, and for age 50 or greater it was 10.7. For women, the corresponding rates were 0.3, 1.1, and 6.4.

From the 1950s to the 1970s, the age-specific prevalence of ECG-LVH among members of the Framingham Study cohort declined.[3] This decrease has been observed in both sexes and at all ages. It coincides with a decline in the prevalence of hypertension in the cohort, as might be expected given the close link between ECG-LVH and blood pressure level.

ECG Criteria for Left Ventricular Hypertrophy

In this chapter, ECG-LVH is defined by the combined voltage and repolarization criteria,[2] except where specified otherwise. The ECG-LVH based on voltage criteria alone carries only half the risk of ECG-LVH that also includes repolarization ST and T-wave changes. Nonspecific ST and T-wave abnormalities alone are not associated with any greater risk than that associated with voltage ECG-LVH alone.[3]

Voltage-only ECG-LVH appears to reflect chiefly the severity and duration of the associated hypertension. Hence, when adjustment is made for the coexistent hypertension, the excess cardiovascular risk associated with this type of ECG-LVH is virtually obliterated.[2,3] On the other hand, the excess risk associated with ECG-LVH with a repolarization abnormality persists, showing a substantial net effect after blood pressure is taken into account.[3]

Not all studies have indicated an independent contribution of ECG-LVH to cardiovascular disease, very likely because of the predominant use of voltage criteria.[5] The precise pathologic and anatomic meaning of ECG-LVH is unclear. Some 33 sets of criteria proposed for this condition have been checked against individual heart chamber dissections at autopsy and have been found wanting.[6] Studies of ECG-LVH voltage in relation to left ventricular (LV) muscle mass determined in the living by ventriculography and echo have produced varied results.[7-9] Nevertheless, as judged by necropsy, radiographs, echo, and ventriculogram, ECG-LVH does reflect anatomic hypertrophy of the left ventricle to a moderate degree.

Theoretical mathematical models of cardiac electrical activity indicate that increased cardiac cell size is characterized by increased QRS amplitude, increased ventricular activation time, and flattened or inverted T–waves.[10] Some have concluded that increased voltage primarily reflects hypertrophy, whereas the appearance of ST and T-wave repolarization abnormalities is related to coronary insufficiency.

Increased R-wave amplitude and coronary atherosclerosis are both related to hypertension and should occur together. Repolarization ST and T-wave abnormalities have been shown to be related to ventricular hypertrophy, hemodynamic overload, and myocardial ischemia and injury. There is not a high correlation between ECG-LVH and autopsy or other measures of cardiac hypertrophy in the living; this may be a reflection of the fact that ECG aberrations are a product of both ischemic myocardial damage and hypertrophy.

Autopsy data from the Framingham Study indicate a correlation between the degree of ECG-LVH and the weight of the heart as well as the thickness of the left ventricle.

Determinants

Although ECG-LVH does occur in the course of rheumatic and coronary heart disease, hypertension is the major determinant of this condition in the general population. The relationship of ECG-LVH to systolic blood pressure is stronger than to diastolic blood pressure; such a relationship seems reasonable when LVH is viewed as the physiologic response of the myocardial muscle to the stress of elevated blood pressure.[11] At systolic pressures exceeding 180 mmHg, some manifestation of ECG-LVH appeared within 12 years in half of the Framingham subjects. Abnormalities in repolarization were more common among persons with higher blood pressures. As seen in Figure 1, the risk of developing ECG-LVH is strongly related to hypertensive status at baseline. The trends for increased risk of developing ECG-LVH at higher blood pressures are highly significant ($p < 0.001$) in both men and women.

Cardiovascular Disease

In general, the appearance of ECG-LVH heralds the onset of serious cardiovascular disease. Specifically, the risks of coronary heart disease, myocardial infarction (MI), stroke, congestive heart failure, and intermittent claudication are increased in persons who develop ECG-LVH (Table I). For most of these forms of cardiovascular disease, there is a substantial residual effect of ECG-LVH on this risk after adjusting for the hypertension that is commonly present with ECG-LVH.

ECG-LVH appears to identify candidates for cardiovascular disease who have progressed to a stage of compromised coronary circulation and myocardial damage. Persons with ECG-LVH are at an increased risk for most major manifestations of coronary heart disease, including angina, MI, or coronary fatality (Fig. 2). Thirty percent of those with ECG-LVH can expect to have a major cardiovascular event within 5 years. The incidence of angina, MI, and sudden death is approximately as high in asymptomatic patients with ECG-LVH as in patients who have recovered from myocardial infarctions.

Myocardial Infarction

In the course of 26 years of follow-up, Framingham subjects with ECG-LVH experienced 2.6 to 5 times as many MIs as those without the abnormal-

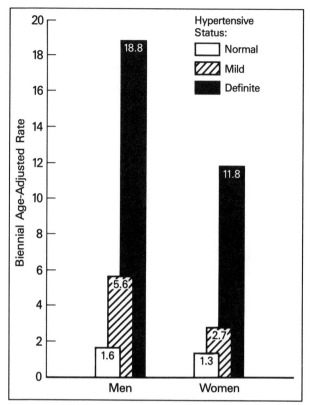

Figure 1. *Development of ECG-LVH by hypertensive status of 30-year follow-up of the Framingham Study of subjects 35 to 84 years of age. Trends significant at p < 0.001.*

Radiographic evidence of LVH carried a lesser degree of risk. This excess risk persists in multivariate analysis taking other risk factors, including hypertension, into account. Only for sudden death in women is this not true.

Whether coronary heart disease in the absence of hypertension can produce anatomic cardiac hypertrophy or ECG-LVH is in dispute.[12] Evaluation of the pathologic correlates of ECG-LVH is confounded by the frequent coexistence of hypertension and coronary artery disease.

Prognosis after the onset of overt coronary heart disease is also greatly affected by the occurrence of signs of LVH. When either cardiac enlargement on radiographs or ECG-LVH is noted, the risk of death is further increased. Following an MI, the onset of ECG-LVH in a patient increases the risk of death to four times that of a patient without that finding. Enlargement on radiographs doubles the risk. Following angina pectoris, cardiac enlargement on radiographs and ECG-LVH each increase the risk fourfold. The adverse prognostic influence of ECG-LVH after MI has also been demonstrated in the Coronary Drug Project.[13]

TABLE I   **Risk of Clinical Atherosclerotic Events by ECG-LVH Status***

Event	ECG-LVH Absent	ECG-LVH Present	Risk Ratio
Intermittent claudication			
Men	6.9	17.2	2.5[†]
Women	3.4	16.8	4.9[‡]
Brain infarction			
Men	4.0	14.6	3.7[‡]
Women	2.8	22.0	7.8[‡]
Coronary heart disease			
Men	27.3	86.4	3.2[§]
Women	13.8	61.3	4.4[§]
Congestive heart failure			
Men	6.4	76.2	11.9[§]
Women	4.4	39.9	9.1[§]
Total cardiovascular disease			
Men	34.1	144.9	4.2[§]
Women	19.4	107.7	5.6[§]

*Framingham Study of subjects 35 to 84 years old with a 26-year follow-up. Age-adjusted biennial rate per 1,000.
[†]$p < 0.05$.
[‡]$p < 0.01$.
[§]$p < 0.001$.

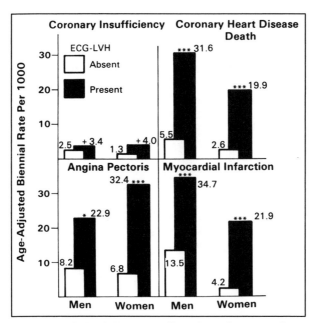

Figure 2. *Risk of clinical manifestations of coronary heart disease by ECG-LVH status in subjects 35 to 84 years old in a 26-year follow-up of the Framingham Study. *Difference significant at $p < 0.05$; ***difference significant at $p < 0.001$.*

Stroke

Hypertension is the chief risk factor for stroke; hence, it can be expected that ECG-LVH is a powerful stroke predictor. To some extent, this is a reflection of the severity and duration of associated hypertension. However, the effect of ECG-LVH is substantial even after adjustment for a coexistent increase in blood pressure. The excess risk associated with ECG-LVH (fourfold to eightfold) (Table I) is more than double that for radiographic evidence of LVH (twofold to threefold). In addition to its reflection of hypertensive hypertrophy of the heart, ECG-LVH may contribute independently to increased stroke risk due to associated myocardial damage.

Cardiac Failure

In keeping with the theory that ECG-LVH indicates the onset of myocardial damage, risk of cardiac failure is increased ninefold to twelve-fold in persons who exhibit this evidence of hypertrophy, and the risk exceeds the fivefold excess of cardiac failure noted in hypertensive persons (Table I). Also, after adjustment for the impact of associated blood pressure level, there is a significant effect of ECG-LVH. Likewise, there is a net effect of hypertension on taking this condition into account. Hence, the combination of these two significant independent contributors powerfully predisposes the patient to cardiac failure, conferring a fifteenfold excess risk. The appearance of ECG-LVH doubles the risk of cardiac failure in hypertensive persons.

It is difficult to determine when compensatory hypertrophy ceases to be beneficial. The process of hypertrophy in essential hypertension is slow, continuous, and progressive, and there is a parallel decline in ventricular function after the early physiologic and later anatomic adaptive changes take place.[14]

The maximal weight of the normal athletic heart is about 500 g, which may represent the critical heart weight beyond which there is an increasing frequency of chronic heart failure.[14] In the concentric hypertrophic phase, the heart can continue to function as an effective pressure pump. When coronary insufficiency develops, the ischemic myocardium tends to hypertrophy eccentrically, with a progressive tendency to chronic dilation and cardiac failure. The epidemiologic data suggest that voltage criteria of ECG-LVH may apply more to the concentric hypertrophic phase and that repolarization changes may ensue when the ischemic or dilatory eccentric enlargement occurs.

Peripheral Arterial Disease

Peripheral arterial disease often occurs as a cardiovascular correlate of ECG-LVH. The impact in women is greater (4.9-fold) than in men (2.5-fold), comparing those with and without ECG abnormality. For women (but not men) there is a significant residual effect, taking blood pressure levels into account. The impact of ECG-LVH in women exceeds that for hypertension. In men as well as women, hypertension contributes to the risk of occlusive peripheral arterial disease, taking ECG-LVH into account.

It is difficult to postulate a direct influence of ECG-LVH on the incidence of intermittent claudication, the chief clinical manifestation of occlusive peripheral arterial disease. It is possible that the finding reflects general vascular vulnerability to hypertension. It is also possible that subclinical impairment of cardiac output with exercise is involved.

Mortality

Despite the lack of symptoms, ECG-LVH is a lethal risk attribute. It preceded 30% of all deaths and 45% of the cardiovascular deaths in the Framingham Study. Based on 26 years of follow-up, the risk ratios for Framingham cohort subjects with definite ECG-LVH with repolarization abnormalities for overall mortality were 5.1 for men and 5.4 for women. These risk ratios for cardiovascular mortality were 8.2 and 11.5, respectively; for coronary heart disease mortality, they were 5.7 and 7.7, respectively; and for stroke mortality, they were 5.5 and 4.0, respectively. Each of these risk ratios is statistically significant ($p < 0.001$).

Within 5 years of its appearance, 35% of men and 20% of women with ECG-LVH were dead, a relative risk comparable to that of persons with overt clinically manifested coronary heart disease. The excess mortality associated with the ECG abnormality is not attributable to often-related hypertension, since ECG-LVH carried three times the risk of hypertension alone. Risk of sudden coronary death in particular was increased almost sixfold in men, but the proportion of sudden deaths from coronary heart disease was no different from that of persons without ECG-LVH.

These mortality risks were only half as great in those whose ECG-LVH was based solely on voltage criteria. Radiographic evidence of cardiac enlargement carried only a third of the risk of cardiovascular death of ECG-LVH.

Electrocardiographic Left Ventricular Hypertrophy in the Elderly

There is no evidence of a waning impact of ECG-LVH with advancing age, either in relative or absolute risk. The occurrence of ECG-LVH in the elderly (older than age 65 years) is particularly ominous. Elderly persons in whom this abnormality developed in the Framingham cohort had a 5-year mortality rate of about 50% for men and 35% for women. A major cardiovascular event occurred within 5 years in about 45% of the subjects who exhibited the ECG finding. This is especially important, since 10% of the population (aged 70 years) are affected by LVH. Cardiovascular morbidity and mortality is increased four- to sevenfold in elderly persons with definite ECG-LVH.

Preventive Implications

ECG-LVH is associated with an increased risk of a major cardiovascular event even in the absence of any of the conventional cardiovascular risk factors. In the presence of ECG-LVH, the risk of a cardiovascular event varies widely, depending on the level of coexistent risk factors. This suggests that the risk associated with ECG-LVH may be reduced by correction of coexisting risk factors.

In a number of studies ECG-LVH has been found to be associated with an increased risk of coronary heart disease and death.[2,3,5,15] Failure of some to indicate an independent contribution to risk of cardiovascular disease very likely stems from the use of only voltage criteria.[5] Coronary candidates with a poor coronary risk profile in whom ECG-LVH with repolarization abnormalities develops require management equivalent to that prescribed for persons with established coronary heart disease. This is justified because ECG-LVH appears to be a hallmark of a compromised coronary circulation and carries a risk of mortality and coronary heart disease events similar to that of overt coronary heart disease.

In any event, the appearance of ECG-LVH must be regarded as a grave prognostic sign in the course of hypertension or coronary heart disease. It carries a high risk of stroke, cardiac failure, coronary events, and premature death. Persons with hypertension and ECG-LVH should be treated promptly and vigorously.[16] Such treatment of coexisting hypertension has been shown to partially reverse LVH in some cases.[17,18] Although it has not been demonstrated that this is associated with an improved prognosis over that found for control of hypertension alone, this is possible. A comprehensive approach, including, in addition to antihypertensive treatment, weight control, elimination of cigarette smoking, improvement of serum lipids values, and supervised exercise would seem indicated. Preventive experimental measures that may be considered include beta blockers, platelet aggregation inhibitors, and calcium channel blockers. Trials to demonstrate the efficacy of all of the foregoing in subjects with this lethal manifestation of cardiovascular disease would seem long overdue.

References

1. KANNEL WB, GORDON T, OFFIT D: Left ventricular hypertrophy by ECG. Prevalence, incidence and mortality in the Framingham Study. Ann Intern Med 1969; 71: 89–105.
2. KANNEL WB, GORDON T, CASTELLI WP, MARGOLIS JR: ECG-left ventricular hypertrophy and risk of CHD. The Framingham Study. Ann Intern Med 1970; 72: 813–822.
3. KANNEL WB, SORLIE P: Left ventricular hypertrophy in hypertension: prognostic and pathogenetic implications. The Framingham Study. In: Strauer BNE, ed. The heart in hypertension. Berlin: Springer-Verlag, 1981; 223–242.

4. GORDON T, SHURTLEFF D: Means at each examination and inter-examination variation of specified characteristics: Framingham Study, Exam 1 to Exam 10. In: Kannel WB, Gordon T, eds. The Framingham Study: an epidemiological investigation of cardiovascular disease. Section 29. DHEW Publication (NIH) No. 74-478. Washington, DC, Government Printing Office, 1973.

5. BLACKBURN H, TAYLOR HL, KEYS A: The ECG in prediction of 5 year CHD incidence among men aged 45–59. Circulation 1970; 41, 42 (suppl 1): 154–161.

6. ROMHILT DW, BOVE KE, NORRIS RJ, et al: A critical appraisal of the ECG criteria for the diagnosis of left ventricular hypertrophy. Circulation 1969; 40: 185–195.

7. BENNETT DH, EVANS DW: Correlation of left ventricular mass determined by echocardiography with vectorcardiographic and electrocardiographic voltage measurements. Br Heart J 1974; 36: 981–987.

8. BAXLEY WA, DODGE HT, SANDLER H: A quantitative angiographic study of left ventricular hypertrophy and the electrocardiogram. Circulation 1968; 37: 509–517.

9. HOLT JH JR, BARNARD ACL, KRAMER JO: Multiple dipole ECG. A comparison of electrically and angiographically determined left ventricular mass. Circulation 1978; 57: 1129–1133.

10. THIRY PS, ROSENBERG RM, ABBOT JA: A mechanism for the electrocardiogram response to left ventricular hypertrophy and acute ischemia. Circ Res 1975; 36: 92–104.

11. TARAZI RC, GIFFORD RS: Left ventricular hypertrophy and hypertension (editorial). JAMA 1983; 250: 1319.

12. FRIEDBERG CK: Diseases of the heart. 2nd ed. Philadelphia: W.B., Saunders, 1956.

13. The Coronary Drug Project Research Group: Left ventricular hypertrophy and prognosis. Experience postinfarction in the Coronary Drug Project. Circulation 1974; 49: 862–869.

14. LINZBACK AJ: Structural adaptation of the heart in hypertension and the physical consequences. In: Strauer BE ed. The heart in hypertension. Berlin: Springer-Verlag, 1981; 243–249.

15. BLACKBURN H, PARLIN RW: Antecedents of disease. Insurance mortality experience. Ann NY Acad Sci 1966; 134: 965–1017.

16. Hypertension, risk, and left ventricular hypertrophy (editorial). Lancet 1984; 1: 941–942.

17. FOUAD FM, NAKASHIMA Y, TARAZI R, SALCEDO EE: Reversal of left ventricular hypertrophy in hypertensive patients treated with methyldopa. Lack of association with blood pressure control. Am J Cardiol 1982; 49: 795–801.

18. CHERCHI A, SAU F, SEGURO C: Regression of left ventricular hypertrophy after treatment of hypertension by chlorthalidone for one year and other diuretics for two years. J Hypertension 1983; 1(suppl 2): 278–280.

8

Prevalence and Evolution of Echocardiographic Left Ventricular Hypertrophy

DANIEL D. SAVAGE, M.D., Ph.D.

Clinical and epidemiologic data have documented that electrocardiographic left ventricular hypertrophy (ECG-LVH) is a lethal marker. It is apparently a late finding in the natural history of hypertension and various cardiac disorders. Echo is much more sensitive than ECG for detecting LVH and permits detection of LVH much earlier in the course of hypertension and other disorders. Moreover, echo apparently accomplishes this increased sensitivity without a loss of specificity. Echo, unlike ECG, also permits assessment of various forms of LVH, including eccentric, concentric, and disproportionate septal LVH. This sensitivity and specificity suggests the possibility that echo might be useful in identifying subjects with LVH in need of preventive measures before irreversible muscle damage. This possibility had led us and others to explore the prevalence, characteristics, and evolution of LVH in various populations. The prognostic significance of various markers for echo-LVH should be forthcoming from a number of ongoing studies. This will help put these initial data into proper perspective.

Echo Reference Criteria for LVH in Adults

There is a lack of consensus concerning criteria for echo-LVH. Until more is known about the diagnostic and prognostic significance of echo-LVH, it is advisable to use such criteria only for reference purposes as opposed to using them for labeling subjects as "abnormal or normal." For now, the use of continuous variables, such as left ventricular mass index, should be emphasized rather than the categorical variable, LVH.

Echo reference data for LV mass and criteria for LVH have been derived recently in Framingham.[1-3] Inadequacies of published criteria include: (1) their being based on relatively small numbers of subjects, thus being less generalizable; (2) their lack of adequate adjustment for the effects of sex, body size (men and women), and age (women), thus giving faulty estimates of LVH prevalence in various sex-age groups; and (3) their not being based on general population samples, again making them less generalizable.

Our criteria were based on 864 apparently healthy subjects from a large free-living population-based sample of about 5,000 subjects with adequate M-mode echoes.[3] The 864 subjects included individuals with no overt evidence of cardiopulmonary disease or major systemic illness by history, physical examination, echo, ECG, and (for most subjects) recent chest radiographic evaluations. Subjects were excluded if their blood pressures exceeded 139/89 mmHg, if they were taking antihypertensive medications, or if they were obese or underweight (weight for height greater than 20% above or below that recommended for medium frame in the Metropolitan Life Insurance Company Table).[4] These most recent criteria for normal weight[3] are more stringent than those we[2] and others (R.B. Devereux, M.D., personal communication) have previously used because they eliminate mildly obese and underweight individuals.

Interventricular septal (IVST) and LV posterior wall thickness (LVPWT) in diastole and LV internal diastolic dimension (LVIDD) were measured using American Society of Echocardiography (ASE) recommendations.[5] For calculation of LV mass, LVIDD, LVPWT and IVST, measurement conventions ("Penn") and formula described by Devereux and Reichek were used:[6]

$$LV \text{ mass (g)} = 1.04[(LVIDD + LVPWT + IVST)^3 - (LVIDD)^3] - 13.6$$

For disproportionate septal LVH, National Institutes of Health measurement criteria were used.[7,8] Chamber dimensions are given in centimeters. The mean LV mass index (Penn LV mass divided by body surface area) for the apparently healthy Framingham men was 92.5 ± 19 g/m^2 (S.D.); for women 72 ± 14 g/m^2. Thus, the upper limit for LV mass index (mean plus two standard deviations) is 131 g/m^2 for men and 100 g/m^2 for women.[3] When comparing young women (e.g., age 20 to 30 years) with older women (e.g., age 70 to 80 years), age adjustments may be necessary. Although these cut points are useful as reference values, the actual value of the LV mass index (as noted above) is a much more informative description of the status of LVH than simply indicating the presence or absence of LVH. One may also need to take leisure-time activity level into account as a possible confounder in certain groups such as young men (R. Washburn, et al, personal communication).

Upper 95% confidence limits for LVIDD index (ASE)
(LVIDDI = LVIDD/body surface area)
= 3.2cm/m^2 for women and 3.1cm/m^2 for men.

The relation of LV wall thickness to LV internal radius (relative wall thickness (RWT = 2LVPWT/LVIDD)) was calculated.

Four types of echo-LVH were defined as follows:[3]

Disproportionate septal LVH is defined as echo-LVH with IVST/LVPWT of 1.3 or greater.

Concentric LVH is defined as echo-LVH with RWT 45% or greater without disproportionate septal LVH.

Eccentric dilated LVH is defined as echo-LVH with RWT less than 45% and LVIDDI more than upper confidence limits in the absence of disproportionate septal LVH.

Eccentric nondilated LVH is defined as echo-LVH in the absence of criteria for other types of LVH (i.e., with RWT less than 45% and LVIDDI less than upper confidence limits in the absence of disproportionate septal LVH).

Prevalence of Echo Left Ventricular Hypertrophy in Adults

As already suggested, discussion of the prevalence of echo-LVH in adults is best deemphasized until more information is available regarding the significance of the various echo markers for such hypertrophy. In addition, the prevalence is critically dependent on the specific criteria used for hypertrophy as well as the population under consideration. Despite these precautions, it is useful to review some recent data that give order-of-magnitude prevalence estimates for echo-LVH found in a large population-based sample.[1–3,9]

Routine application of M-mode echo (guided by two-dimensional echo) during the 16th biennial examination of the original Framingham cohort and the second examination of their offspring (and spouses of the offspring) permitted such population-based prevalence estimates. Using the criteria described, 676 (13.6%) of 4,975 Framingham subjects had echo-LVH. The prevalence of echo-LVH ranged from less than 6% in those under age 50 years to up to 31% (men) and 67% (women) in those 80 years and older (Figs 1 and 2). Less than 0.3% of the offspring group and less than 5% of the cohort subjects

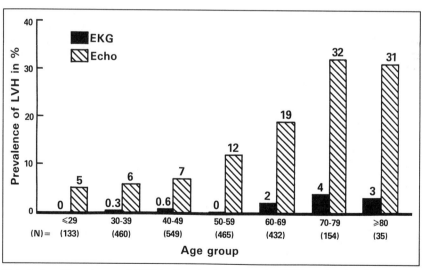

Figure 1. *Prevalence of LVH in Framingham men by ECG and echo. Prevalence should be viewed only as order of magnitude, since the population samples are not ideal probability samples. (Adapted from Savage et al.[3])*

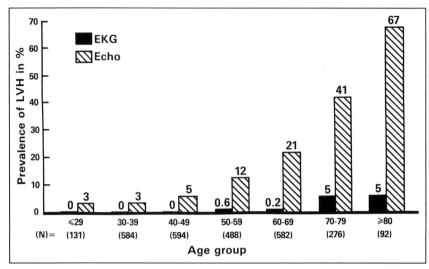

Figure 2. *Prevalence of LVH in Framingham women by ECG and echo. Prevalence should be viewed only as order of magnitude, since the population samples are not ideal probability samples. (Adapted from Savage et al.[3])*

had ECG-LVH.[1–3] Using Framingham reference criteria, echo-LVH was found in 273 (7.6%) of the 3,610 offspring study subjects (mean age, 44 years) and in 403 (29.5%) of the 1,365 original cohort subjects (mean age, 71 years).[3] The prevalence estimates for echo-LVH in offspring study subjects and the older cohort subjects were 9% and 16%, respectively, when previously published non-sex-specific reference values[8] were used. The prevalence of echo-LVH was less in cohort men than women when Framingham sex-specific reference values were used for comparison.[3]

Not only was the prevalence of echo-LVH greater in the elderly than in the young, but the degree of echo-LVH was substantially greater in the elderly with echo-LVH. For example, men less than age 30 years with echo-LVH had an average LV mass index of 144 g/m^2, whereas men older than 80 years with echo-LVH had an average LV mass index of 193 g/m^2. This again points to the value of treating LV mass as a continuous variable.[3]

Eccentric LVH was the most common form of echo-LVH in the relatively young offspring study subjects. Concentric echo-LVH constituted a somewhat larger proportion of the echo-LVH in the elderly cohort (particularly in women) than in the younger subjects (Table I). Disproportionate septal LVH was found in 0.1% to 0.3% of the offspring study subjects and in 1% to 2% of the elderly cohort.[9] Elderly women had the highest prevalence of disproportionate septal LVH. Systolic anterior mitral leaflet motion was found in roughly 30% of elderly subjects who had disproportionate septal LVH. None of the subjects less than age 60 years had both disproportionate septal LVH and systolic anterior mitral leaflet motion.

TABLE I **Prevalence of Various Forms of Echo-LVH in Framingham Subjects***

	No.	%	E		C		DS	
			No.	%*	No.	%	No.	%
Original cohort								
Men	121/510	24	62	51	54	45	5	4
Women	282/855	33	130	47	136	48	16	6
Offspring-spouse								
Men	148/1718	9	86	58	59	40	3	2
Women	125/1892	7	88	70	34	27	3	3

E = eccentric dilated and nondilated LVH; C = concentric LVH; DS = disproportionate septal LVH.
*New Framingham reference data used (adapted from Savage et al[3]).

Available data from the studies mentioned, and others with similar results, make it possible to outline some of the sequential cardiac structural and functional changes in hypertension.[10]

Evolution of Echo Left Ventricular Hypertrophy in Black Hypertensive and White Hypertensive Subjects

The studies cited and numerous others have suggested the following overall pattern for the evolution of echo findings in hypertensive subjects. The most commonly described initial echo finding in hypertensive subjects is a concentric increase in ventricular septal and free-wall thickness. Thus, LV mass is moderately augmented. Echo may detect this in a large percentage of hypertensive subjects before it is otherwise apparent. Abnormalities in diastolic function may precede the more obvious echo findings, such as increased LV mass. At this stage, LVIDD, wall stress, left atrial dimension, mitral valve E-F slope, and indexes of LV systolic function remain within normal limits. At an early stage, the increased mass of myocardium in combination with the stimulating effect of humoral factors, such as catecholamines, may actually allow ventricular performance to exceed that found in normotensive persons.

Subsequent to the diagnosis of hypertension, the effect of treatment may be reflected by changes in LV mass, which in general increases with inadequate control of blood pressure and decreases if blood pressure is substantially reduced.[11,12] Differential effects of various antihypertensive regimens on LV mass are under intense investigation. Despite apparently equivalent lowering of blood pressure, some agents may cause less regression in LV mass than others (or may actually lead to increased LV mass).[11,12] Relative wall thickness may also increase enough to exceed the normal range if hypertension is not adequately controlled,[13] indicating progression of concentric LVH. The effect of nonpharmacological antihypertension therapy on LV mass should be investigated further.

With persistence or progression of hypertension, LVH becomes severe enough to be recorded on the ECG, and the echo may reveal functional decompensation well before clinical symptoms of congestive heart failure develop. Substantially augmented LV wall thickness may occur with a small LV chamber.[14] Symptoms suggesting congestive failure may occur secondary to diastolic LV dysfunction.[14] On the other hand, LV wall stress may be increased with augmented LV internal dimensions and reduced ventricular systolic function evident on the echo. Left atrial enlargement and depressed mitral valve E-F slope may be evident. The chest radiograph may show cardiac enlargement. Finally, with progressive systolic dysfunction, the echo may show further LV dilation without an accompanying increase in LV wall thickness. Accordingly, relative wall thickness may decline in relation to blood pressure, further increasing wall stress. The prognostic importance of symptoms and signs of congestive heart failure is indicated by the finding some years ago in Framingham of a 50% mortality in 5 years in hypertensive subjects with congestive heart failure.[15]

Although this outline of the course of hypertensive cardiac changes has been oriented around the effects of mounting hypertension, numerous other factors besides the level of blood pressure may alter the course of these cardiac structural and functional changes in hypertensive patients. Included among these are:

Hemodynamic factors (heart rate, alterations of cardiac output, physical activity, and obesity related factors, among others)
Neurohumoral and endocrine factors (the renin-angiotensin system, catecholamines, prostaglandins, thyroid and growth hormone, among others)
Concomitant processes (aging or other cardiac disorders)
Genetic factors
Altered cardiac composition (such as increased collagen)[16]
Alcohol intake

Echo study of cardiac structural adaptations in hypertension has answered some questions but has raised others. It is possible that in the young, the echo findings reflect types and level of physical activity as much as does blood pressure.[2] More information is needed regarding determinants and significance of various types of LVH. Safar et al[17] postulated that disproportionate septal LVH is a common feature of borderline hypertension. Niederle et al[18] reported similar findings. On the other hand, Criley et al[19] hypothesized that disproportionate septal LVH is a common feature of malignant hypertension since they found it in 14 (47%) of 30 subjects with such hypertension. All three groups speculated that the disproportionate septal LVH might be the result of neurohumoral adrenergic stimulation. Some have considered this form of LVH to be a potentially important risk marker for sudden death, particularly in young athletes.[20–26]

In our study of 234 persons with mild to moderate hypertension, 9 patients (4%) had disproportionate septal LVH.[26] In addition, half of the hypertensive first-degree relatives of the latter group also had disproportionate septal

LVH. In these persons, disproportionate septal LVH showed similarities to genetically transmitted hypertrophic cardiomyopathy.[27] Thus, the cause or causes and significance of disproportionate septal LVH in hypertensive persons remain unclear.

Systolic anterior motion of the anterior mitral leaflet may appear under basal conditions in a variable number of hypertensive persons with disproportionate septal LVH[9,28] and in an occasional patient with concentric LVH and dynamic ventricular function.[29] This may be provoked (with ventricular outflow gradients) in other patients by sympathomimetic agents.[29] This echo finding may influence choice of therapy in hypertensive subjects since diuretic use could potentially provoke or aggravate left ventricular outflow obstruction.[9] Sympatholytic agents would thus be preferred in such subjects. Again, more information is needed regarding the prognostic significance of these echo findings.

References

1. SAVAGE DD, ABBOTT RD, ANDERSON SJ, PADGETT SJ: Determinants of left ventricular mass based on a large population-based sample of apparently healthy subjects. The Framingham Study (abstr.). Circulation 1983; 68: III-36.

2. SAVAGE DD, ABBOTT RD, PADGETT SJ, GARRISON RJ: Epidemiologic aspects of left ventricular hypertrophy in normotensive and hypertensive subjects in Cardiac Ventricular Hypertrophy. In: ter keurs HEDJ, Schipperheyn JJ, eds. The Hague: Martinus-Nijhoff Publishing, 1983: 3–15.

3. SAVAGE DD, GARRISON RJ, KANNEL WB, et al: The spectrum of left ventricular hypertrophy in a general population sample—the Framingham Study. Circulation (in press).

4. ROBINSON CH: Normal and therapeutic nutrition. 14th ed. New York: Macmillan, 1972; 703.

5. SAHN DJ, DeMARIA A, KISSLO J, WEYMAN: Recommendations regarding quantitation in M-mode echocardiography: results of a survey of echocardiographic measurements. Circulation 1978; 58: 1072.

6. DEVEREUX RB, REICHEK N: Echocardiographic determination of left ventricular mass. Anatomic validation of the method. Circulation 1977; 55: 613–618.

7. HENRY WL, CLARK CE, EPSTEIN SE: Asymmetric septal hypertrophy: echocardiographic identification of the pathognomonic anatomy of IHSS. Circulation 1973; 47: 225–233.

8. GARDIN JM, HENRY WL, SAVAGE DD, WARE JH, BURN C, BORER JS: Echocardiographic measurements in normal subjects: evaluation of an adult population without clinically apparent heart disease. J Clin Ultrasound 1979; 7: 439–447.

9. SAVAGE DD, CASTELLI WP, ABBOTT RD, et al: Hypertrophic cardiomyopathy and its markers in the general population: the great masquerader revisited: the Framingham Study. J Cardiovasc Ultrasonogr 1983; 2: 41–47.

10. SAVAGE DD, DEVEREUX RB: Echocardiography and hypertension. Primary Cardiol 1981; 7: 137–152.

11. DEVEREUX RB, SAVAGE DD, SACHS I, LARAGH JH: Effect of blood pressure control on left ventricular hypertrophy and function in hypertension (abstr). Circulation 1980; 62 (part 2): III-36.

12. TARAZI RC: Regression of left ventricular hypertrophy by medical treatment: present status and possible implications. Am J Med 1983; 75: 80–86.

13. KARLINER JS, WILLIAMS D, GORWIT J, CRAWFORD MH, O'ROURKE RA: Left ventricular performance in patients with left ventricular hypertrophy caused by systemic arterial hypertension. Br Heart J 1977; 39: 1239–1245.

14. TOPOL EJ, TRAILL TA, FORTUIN NJ: Hypertensive hypertrophic cardiomyopathy of the elderly. N Engl J Med 1985; 312: 1277–1283.

15. KANNEL WB, CASTELLI WP, MCNAMARA PM, MCKEE PA, FEINLEIB M: Role of blood pressure in the development of congestive heart failure. N Engl J Med 1972; 287: 781–787.

16. FROHLICH ED, TARAZI RC: Is arterial pressure the sole factor responsible for hypertensive cardiac hypertrophy? Am J Cardiol 1979; 44: 959–963.

17. SAFAR ME, LEHNER JP, VINCENT MI, PLAINFOSSE MT, SIMON AC: Echocardiographic dimensions in borderline and sustained hypertension. Am J Cardiol 1979; 44: 930–935.

18. NIEDERLE P, WIDIMSKY J, JANDOVA R, RESSL J, GROSPIC A: Echocardiographic assessment of the left ventricle in juvenile hypertension. Int J Cardiol 1982; 2: 91–101.

19. CRILEY JM, BLAUFUSS AH, ABBASI AS: Nonobstructive IHSS. Circulation 1975; 52: 963.

20. SAVAGE DD, SEIDES SF, MARON BJ, MYERS DJ, EPSTEIN SE: Prevalence of arrhythmias during 24-hour electrocardiographic monitoring and exercise testing in patients with obstructive and nonobstructive hypertrophic cardiomyopathy (ASH). Circulation 1979; 59: 866–875.

21. MARON BJ, SAVAGE DD, WOLFSON JK, EPSTEIN SE: Prognostic significance of 24-hour ambulatory electrocardiographic monitoring in patients with hypertrophic cardiomyopathy: a prospective study. Am J Cardiol 1981; 48: 252–257.

22. MCKENNA WJ, ENGLAND D, DOI YL, DEANFIELD JE, OAKLEY C, GOODWIN JF: Arrhythmia in hypertrophic cardiomyopathy. I. Influence on prognosis. Br Heart J 1981; 46: 168–172.

23. MARON BJ, LIPSON LC, ROBERTS WC, SAVAGE DD, EPSTEIN SE: "Malignant" hypertrophic cardiomyopathy: identification of a subgroup of families with unusually frequent premature deaths. Am J Cardiol 1979; 41: 1133–1140.

24. MCKENNA W, DEANFIELD J, FARUQUI A, ENGLAND D, OAKLEY C, GOODWIN J: Prognosis in hypertrophic cardiomyopathy: role of age and clinical, electrocardiographic and hemodynamic features. Am J Cardiol 1981; 47: 532–538.

25. MCMANUS BM, WALLER BF, GRABOYS TB, et al: Exercise and sudden death—Part II. Curr Probl Cardiol 1982; 6: 1–57.

26. MARON BJ, ROBERTS WC, MCALLISTER HA, ROSING DR, EPSTEIN SE: Sudden death in young athletes. Circulation 1980; 62: 218–229.

27. SAVAGE DD, DEVEREUX RB, SACHS I, LARAGH JH: Disproportionate ventricular septal thickness in hypertensive patients. J Cardiovasc Ultrasonogr 1982; 1: 79–85.

28. SAVAGE DD, DRAYER JIM, HENRY WL, et al: Echocardiographic assessment of

cardiac anatomy and function in hypertensive subjects. Circulation 1979; 59: 623–632.

29. Maron BJ, Gottdiener JS, Roberts WC, Henry WL, Savage DD, Epstein SE: Left ventricular outflow obstruction due to systolic anterior motion of the anterior mitral leaflet in patients with concentric left ventricular hypertrophy. Circulation 1978; 57: 527–533.

PART III
MORPHOLOGY AND
BIOCHEMICAL CHANGES

9

Morphology of the Heart in Left Ventricular Hypertrophy

VICTOR J. FERRANS, M.D., Ph.D.,
E. RENÉ RODRÍGUEZ, M.D.

Cardiac hypertrophy is defined as an increase in the mass of the heart, and it is present when the weight of the heart exceeds the accepted limits of normal for age, sex, and body weight (average, 295 g for adult men and 250 g for adult women). The most accurate estimation of cardiac weight is based on its relationship to body weight (0.43% in men and 0.40% in women). Hypertrophied human hearts can weigh up to four times as much as normal hearts. Patients with coronary arterial narrowing but with no other evidence of cardiovascular disease can have cardiac weights of up to 500 g. Cardiac weights in systemic hypertension rarely exceed 1,000 g. Hearts weighing more than 1,000 g are uncommon and are found mostly in patients with aortic regurgitation or with hypertrophic cardiomyopathy.

Types of Hypertrophy

Depending on the specific cause, the increase in cardiac mass that occurs in cardiac hypertrophy is associated with characteristic alterations in the volume of the cardiac cavities and in the thickness of the chambers (normal for left ventricular (LV) free wall and ventricular septum, 10 to 12 mm; for right ventricular wall, 3 mm). On the basis of these changes, cardiac hypertrophy can be classified anatomically as being either concentric (hearts with small cavities and thick walls) or eccentric (hearts with large cavities and walls that are relatively thin, although they actually may be thicker than normal). Concentric hypertrophy is usually associated with conditions that cause pressure overloading (aortic stenosis or systemic hypertension), and eccentric hypertrophy, with conditions that cause volume overloading, such as aortic or mitral regurgitation and congestive or ventricular-dilated cardiomyopathy. Eccentric hypertrophy also develops as the result of congestive heart failure and dilation in the late, decompensated stages of pressure overloading.[1]

"Asymmetric hypertrophy" is the term that designates the bizarre type of hypertrophy that develops in hypertrophic cardiomyopathy and in a few rare disorders. This hypertrophy characteristically causes a degree of ventricular septal thickening that is greater than that observed in the free wall of the left ventricle (measured by echo at the level of the free margin of the posterior mitral leaflet) by a factor of 1.3 or greater (normal, 1.0).

Cardiac hypertrophy also can be classified according to whether it occurs as a consequence of increased physiologic activity (physiologic hypertrophy) or of disease states (pathologic hypertrophy). In either of these circumstances, hypertrophy represents a phenomenon of adaptive growth, which occurs in response to mechanical or chemical alterations in cardiac function. A distinction between concentric and eccentric types of hypertrophy can be made in hearts undergoing either pathologic or physiologic hypertrophy. Athletes participating in strenuous isotonic exercise tend to have increased LV mass with changes similar to those present in patients with chronic pressure overloading.[2]

Stages of Hypertrophy

A very useful way of classifying hypertrophy relates to the fact that cardiac morphology and function undergo a series of progressive changes during the time course of hypertrophy. Three distinct stages of hypertrophy can be recognized in this series of changes: transient breakdown or damage of the muscle cells and rapid increases in energy production and protein synthesis; stable hyperfunction of compensated hypertrophy; and finally, gradual exhaustion of the heart in association with failure to synthesize proteins and renew myofibrils and mitochondria.[3,4]

Gross Anatomic Changes in Cardiac Hypertrophy

The two most important gross anatomic features of cardiac hypertrophy are thickening of the ventricular walls (which can exceed 2 cm in thickness) and cavity dilation. The degree of wall thickening or thinning observed in left ventricular hypertrophy (LVH) is dependent on two main factors: the extent to which myocytes increase in size, and the pattern of arrangement that they have in the LV wall.[5] The latter factor is of particular importance. It should be emphasized that chronic dilation of the left ventricle is not accomplished by overstretching of the sarcomeres of the myocytes but by a rearrangement of the orientation of the layers of myocytes. Normally, these layers are oriented somewhat obliquely to the epicardium-endocardium axis, and they become more and more obliquely oriented as dilation progresses, thus allowing the wall to become thinner and more stretched.

Dilation of the LV cavity is accompanied by lengthening of the chamber in the apex-to-base direction. This dilation involves the apical portion of the left ventricle to a greater extent than the region in front of the anterior leaflet of the mitral valve; the portion behind the posterior leaflet of the mitral valve is least affected. Thus, the left ventricle becomes less conical and more hemispheric in shape as it dilates, and the papillary muscles appear to originate more cephalad on the wall than is the case in concentric hypertrophy; the trabeculae carneae tend to flatten out. The change in position of the papillary muscles and the change in the angle that they form with the plane of the mitral valve orifice eventually lead to inadequate closure of the mitral valve and to mitral valvular regurgitation. This can occur in LVH of any cause, but is very often found in congestive cardiomyopathy.

Cellular Basis of Cardiac Hypertrophy

The mass of the heart increases in hypertrophy as the result of an increase in the sizes of the myocytes and an increase in the number of cellular (connective tissue cells and vascular elements) and extracellular (collagen, elastic fibers, proteoglycans) components of connective tissue.[1] In the early stages of hypertrophy, the growth of myocytes exceeds or equals that of connective tissue components. In the late stages of hypertrophy, myocardial interstitial fibrosis may become prominent as a consequence of progressive deposition of connective tissue, particularly of collagen, and of atrophy and degeneration of the myocytes.

During the normal embryonic growth of the heart, most of the increase in cardiac mass is due to an increase in the number of myocytes, which reproduce by mitosis (Fig. 1). Mitoses in myocytes cease to occur soon after birth, after which the growth of the heart is mediated by increases in the sizes of the individual myocytes.[6,7] Synthesis of DNA continues to occur in myocytes after birth, and results either in binucleation, multinucleation, or polyploidy.[8] The latter can be greatly exaggerated in cardiac hypertrophy.

The quantitative studies of Linzbach[9] and Astorri et al[10] have suggested that hypertrophy of myocytes (without an increase in number) can account for an increase in cardiac mass of up to 500 g, and that further increments in mass are mediated by an additional increase in the number of myocytes. The mechanism by which this occurs is not clear; it has been suggested that amitotic division may occur in myocytes.[9] On the other hand, experimental evidence suggests that the ability of cardiac myocytes to undergo cell division is not irretrievably lost after birth.[11,12]

The increase in myocyte size that mediates cardiac hypertrophy is due to an increase in the sizes of some cellular components (nuclei, Golgi complexes) and to an increase in the number of others (myofibrils, mitochondria). From the quantitative standpoint, the mitochondria and the myofibrils account for the largest portions of the volume of the myocytes.[1,4]

The formation of sarcomeres and myofibrils is a complex event that involves the synthesis of appropriate amounts of a variety of proteins. These proteins then must become aggregated into filaments which in turn become organized into specific three-dimensional arrays and become aligned with respect to other contractile elements already present in the cell. A continuous process of synthesis and breakdown of proteins goes on in the fully developed sarcomeres of normal cardiac muscle, as shown by studies demonstrating that the half-life of actin and myosin is less than 2 weeks.

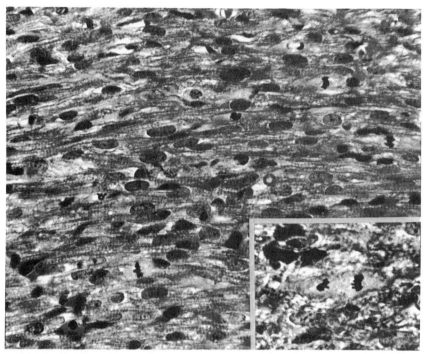

Figure 1. *Section of left ventricle of newborn rat showing several myocytes undergoing mitotic division. Section of tissue embedded in glycol methacrylate and stained with alkaline toluidine blue is 1 μ thick. The inset shows higher magnification view of a myocyte undergoing mitosis. As shown here, the contractile material in such myocytes is disrupted; it becomes organized again after mitosis is completed. (× 800.)*

Accumulations of material similar to that present in mature Z bands are thought to play an organizer role in the formation of sarcomeres. These accumulations appear to serve as sites for attachment and subsequent orientation of myofilaments, both in normal growth and in the process of hypertrophy.[1,4,13]

Histologic Changes in Cardiac Hypertrophy

On histologic study, the most readily recognizable indications of cardiac hypertrophy are increases in the transverse diameters of the muscle cells and in the size and basophilia of their nuclei (Fig. 2). Normal ventricular muscle cells range up to 15 μ in diameter. In hypertrophy, the diameters of many of the myocytes exceed 20 μ, although cells with diameters exceeding 50 μ may be found. Ultrastructural studies have confirmed that such large cells are single cells and not groups of cells with boundaries that are not recognizable by light microscopy.

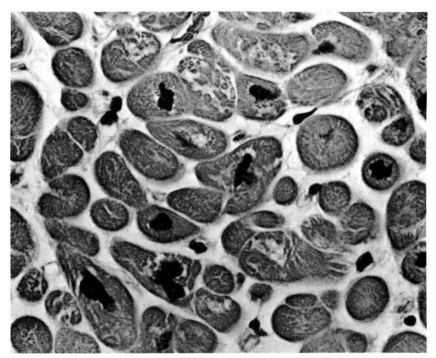

Figure 2. *Histologic section of myocardial biopsy specimen from a patient with dilated cardiomyopathy, showing enlarged myocytes with large, irregularly shaped, hyperchromatic nuclei. (H & E stain; X 600.)*

In histologic preparations, the cytoplasm of hypertrophied myocytes may or may not show abnormal features. The orderly arrangement of myocytes is maintained in hypertrophy due to either pressure or volume overloading; however, this arrangement is abnormal (myocardial fiber disarray) in focal areas, usually well in excess of 5% of the tissue, in the ventricles of patients with hypertrophic cardiomyopathy.[14,15] The nuclei of hypertrophied myocytes usually appear enlarged, more darkly stained than normal (more basophilic in preparations stained with hematoxylin and eosin), and vary in shape from oval or rectangular with blunted ends to highly irregular and convoluted. The increase in the density of the nuclear staining is considered to be related to polyploidy of nuclear DNA. As hypertrophy becomes more severe, the shapes of hypertrophied myocytes tend to become more irregular and less cylindrical than those of normal myocytes. These irregularities of shapes may represent sites of localized addition of new sarcomeres during the process of cellular growth.

In addition to the changes of cellular enlargement just cited, hearts with long-standing hypertrophy often also show some degree of atrophy and degeneration of the myocytes as well as interstitial fibrosis and some degree of thickening of mural endocardium. Atrophic muscle cells often are isolated from adjacent cells by fibrous connective tissue and may be altered to the point that they are difficult to recognize as muscle cells. This is particularly true of the myocytes in the giant, dilated left atria of patients with severe mitral valvular disease of long duration.[16] Degenerative changes in the cytoplasm of the myocytes include loss of myofibrils and vacuolization. These changes may be difficult to appreciate in tissues that have undergone postmortem autolysis and are best evaluated by electron microscopic study of tissue obtained by myocardial biopsy.[4]

Ultrastructural Changes in Cardiac Hypertrophy

In the first stage of hypertrophy (Fig. 3) the myocytes show evidence of increased synthesis of proteins, in the form of nuclear and nucleolar alterations (particularly the formation of coiled, ribbonlike nucleoli). Furthermore, the numbers of cisterns of endoplasmic reticulum and free ribosomes increase, the Golgi complexes enlarge, and the width and extent of the folding of the intercellular junctions is increased. The myocytes also exhibit accumulations of Z band material (suggestive of the formation of new sarcomeres), and small mitochondria with features frequently suggestive of budding. The hexagonal array of the myofilaments, the dimensions of the sarcomeres, and the diameters of the thick and thin myofilaments are similar in normal and in hypertrophied myocytes. Therefore, hypertrophy is not mediated by increases in the sizes of the contractile elements.[1,4]

After hypertrophy has developed for a certain time, the rate of cellular enlargement appears to decrease and the changes described tend to be less prominent. Therefore, in the second or stable stage of hypertrophy, the myocytes usually are larger than normal and contain greater numbers of myofibrils and mitochondria but show few or no qualitative abnormalities in their organelles. They may differ from normal myocytes in the percentage of the total cell volume occupied by myofibrils and mitochondria. Detailed studies of these changes have indicated that the different organelles of hypertrophying myocytes do not increase in size or number synchronously or to the same ultimate extent and their relative growth may differ according to the nature of the stimulus to hypertrophy.[1,4]

In the late stage of hypertrophy (Fig. 4) degenerative changes occur that involve the myofibrils, the sarcoplasmic reticulum, mitochondria, T-tubules, intercellular junctions, and most other organelles. The most important degenerative changes are those that affect the myofibrils and result in loss or lysis of the myofilaments. The intercellular junctions tend to undergo some degree of dissociation, especially in areas of fibrosis. This dissociation often is accompanied by the formation of numerous spherical microparticles in areas of interstitium in the immediate vicinity of the cells. The tubules and cisterns of sarcoplasmic reticulum frequently undergo proliferation and tend to fill those areas of the myocytes from which the myofibrils have been lost. The T-tubules often lose their cylindrical shape and become shallow,

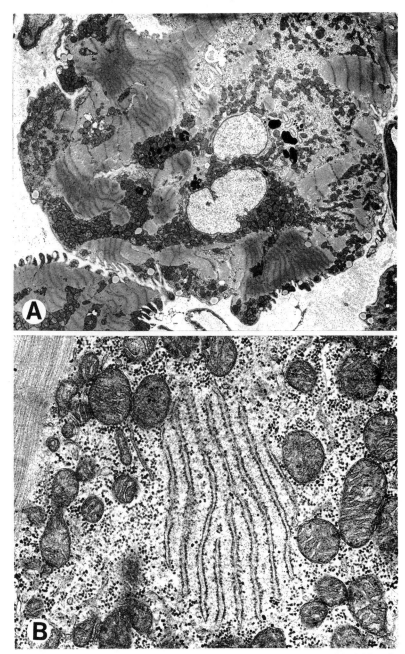

Figure 3. **A.** *Low magnification electron micrograph of hypertrophied, binucleated myocyte without degenerative changes. (Uranyl acetate and lead citrate stain; × 4,500.)* **B.** *Detail of cell similar to that shown in* **A.** *Note the cisterns of endoplasmic reticulum, the abundance of small, dark particles of glycogen, and the marked variation in the size of the mitochondria. (Uranyl acetate and lead citrate stain; × 24,000.)*

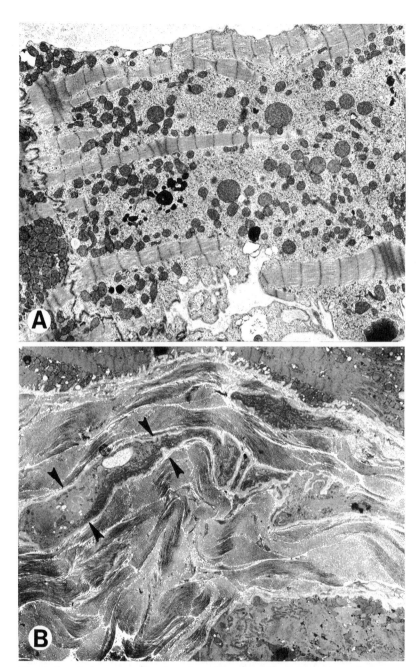

Figure 4. **A.** *Low magnification view of hypertrophied, degenerated myocyte that has lost many myofibrils from its central portion, now filled with mitochondria of irregular sizes and numerous particles of glycogen. (Uranyl acetate and lead citrate stain; × 6,000.)* **B.** *Area of severe interstitial fibrosis, with dense bundles of collagen fibrils separating the myocytes. Note the small, atrophic myocyte (arrowheads) that appears isolated in the area of fibrosis. (Uranyl acetate and lead citrate stain; × 5,000.)*

widened invaginations without a clear relationship to the T-bands of the myofibrils.

The degenerative changes cited occur in left as well as in right ventricular hypertrophy and tend to be related to the duration and severity of the hypertrophy rather than to its specific etiologic basis.[4,17,18] Thus, they constitute a clear reason for early and effective treatment of the underlying conditions (congenital heart disease, systemic hypertension) that lead to hypertrophy in the hope of avoiding the irreversible myocardial degeneration and failure that characterize the late stage of hypertrophy.

References

1. FERRANS VJ: Morphological aspects of cardiac hypertrophy. In: Zak, R. ed. Growth of the heart in health and disease. New York: Raven Press, 1984; 185–237.

2. MORGANROTH J, MARON BJ, HENRY WL, EPSTEIN SE: Comparative left ventricular dimensions in trained athletes. Ann Intern Med 1975; 82: 521–524.

3. MEERSON FZ, ZALETAYEVA TA, LAGUTCHEV SS, PSHENNIKOVA MG: Structure and mass of mitochondria in the process of compensatory hyperfunction and hypertrophy of the heart. Exp Cell Res 1964; 36: 568–578.

4. FERRANS VJ, BUTANY JW: Ultrastructural pathology of the heart. In: Trump BF, Jones RT, eds. Diagnostic electron microscopy, vol 4. New York: John Wiley & Sons, 1983; 319–473.

5. SPOTNITZ HM, SPOTNITZ WD, COTTRELL TS, SPIRO D, SONNENBLICK EH: Cellular basis for volume related wall thickness changes in the rat left ventricle. J Mol Cell Cardiol 1974; 6: 317–331.

6. BUGAISKY L, ZAK R: Cellular growth of cardiac muscle after birth. Tex Rep Biol Med 1979; 39: 123–135.

7. ZAK R: Development and proliferative capacity of cardiac muscle cells. Circ Res 1974; 35: 17–27.

8. ADLER CP: DSN in Kinderherzen. Biochemische und zytophotometrische Untersuchungen. Beitr Pathol 1976; 158: 173–202.

9. LINZBACH AJ: Heart failure from the point of view of quantitative anatomy. Am J Cardiol 1960; 5: 370–382.

10. ASTORRI E, BOLOGNESI E, COLLA B, CHIZZOLA A, VISIOLI O: Left ventricular hypertrophy: a cytometric study on 42 human hearts. J Mol Cell Cardiol 1977; 9: 763–775.

11. OBERPRILLER JO, FERRANS VJ, CARROLL RJ: Changes in DNA content, number of nuclei and cellular dimensions of young rat atrial myocytes in response to left coronary artery legation. J Mol Cell Cardiol 1983; 15: 31–42.

12. RUMYANTSEV PP: Interrelations of the proliferation and differentiation processes during cardiac myogenesis and regeneration. Int Rev Cytol 1977; 51: 187–273.

13. MARKWALD RR: Distribution and relationship of precursor Z material to organizing myofibrillar bundles in embryonic rat and hamster ventricular myocytes. J Mol Cell Cardiol 1973; 5: 341–350.

14. MARON BJ, ROBERTS WC: Quantitative analysis of cardiac muscle cell disorganization in the ventricular septum of patients with hypertrophic cardiomyopathy. Circulation 1979; 59: 689–706.

15. MARON BJ, ANAN TJ, ROBERTS WC: Quantitative analysis of distribution of cardiac muscle cell disorganization in the left ventricular wall of patients with hypertrophic cardiomyopathy. Circulation 1981; 63: 882–894.

16. THIEDEMANN K-U, FERRANS VJ: Left atrial ultrastructure in mitral valvular disease. Am J Pathol 1977; 89: 575–604.

17. JONES M, FERRANS VJ: Myocardial ultrastructure in children and adults with congenital heart disease. In: Roberts WC, ed. Congenital heart disease in adults. Philadelphia: F.A. Davis, 1979; 501–530.

18. MARON BJ, FERRANS VJ, ROBERTS WC: Ultrastructural features of degenerated cardiac muscle cells in patients with cardiac hypertrophy. Am J Pathol 1975; 79: 387–434.

PART IV
PATHOPHYSIOLOGY OF
LEFT VENTRICULAR
HYPERTROPHY

10

Physiologic Considerations in Left Ventricular Hypertrophy

EDWARD D. FROHLICH, M.D.

Prospective data provided from the Framingham Study have demonstrated that hypertension is the most common cause of congestive heart failure in the United States.[1] When one considers the natural history of hypertensive heart disease and its duration in man,[2] its apparent early onset in childhood and adolescence,[3] and the magnitude of the prevalence of hypertension,[4] these data are not too astonishing. What is perhaps more surprising is the general impression among clinicians that the problem of cardiac failure in hypertension is less frequently encountered.

In part, this clinical conclusion is somewhat justified: more patients are being treated for hypertension and, therefore, fewer patients should be experiencing the consequences of pressure overload on the left ventricle. However, the problem of left ventricular (LV) failure may be obscured by lack of recognition of the chronically and severely elevated arterial pressures; it may not infrequently develop in patients with a coexistent cardiac disease (most often ischemic heart disease); and it may be obscured and attributed to intravascular volume expansion from antihypertensive therapy in the patient with associated preexistent or concomitant cardiac enlargement.

This discussion is concerned with certain physiologic aspects of the heart in hypertension: as an adaptive organ that is forced to perform against an increasing and unrelenting pressure overload, as a target organ of other possible coexisting diseases, and as an organ that may be affected by coexisting factors that may also be associated with cardiac enlargement independent of the factor of hypertensive vascular disease. We shall also consider the physiologic roles of the heart: in initiating or responding to reflexive readjustments, in adapting to, or perhaps even participating in, total body volume homeostasis, as a possible endocrine organ, and as a target organ not only affected by the hypertensive disease process but also by the antihypertensive therapy (Table I).

Much of the pertinent information is only presently being accumulated through careful clinical and experimental study. Several of these subjects will be discussed in more extensive detail in other chapters in this book. Moreover, it is possible that much that is presently known may only be germane to the normal heart and may not at all be analogous to the circumstances under which ventricular hypertrophy exists.[2] Therefore, it may not be valid to ex-

TABLE I   Considerations of Cardiac Function in Left Ventricular Hypertrophy

Myocardial adaptability
  Homeometric autoregulation
  Increased myocardial contractility
  Ventricular hypertrophy
Other factors in cardiac enlargement
  Role of pressor substances
  Collagen deposition
  Aging
  Sexual factors
  Racial factors
  Associated diseases (such as, coronary
  artery disease, diabetes mellitus, obesity)
Other physiologic factors
  Neural reflexes of cardiac origin
  Cardiac role in volume regulation
  Endocrine function of the heart
  Reversal of ventricular hypertrophy

tend conclusions as to the function of the heart with hypertrophy to the function of the heart hypertrophied from long-standing pressure overload. Moreover, the knowledge that has been learned from heart with ventricular hypertrophy (produced by one form of pressure or volume overload) may not at all be analogous to the left ventricle hypertrophied over an extended time period from an insidiously progressive pressure overload produced by naturally occurring systemic arterial hypertension. Thus, we must remember that information concerning pressure overload hypertrophy was derived from certain experimental and clinical situations in which the hypertrophy was initiated through a myriad of mechanisms or interventions that were not always similar to the slowly progressing situation found in genetic experimental (for example, spontaneously hypertensive rat) or clinical (for example, essential hypertensive man) hypertension. Even under these situations, the pathophysiologic alterations are not homogeneous.[5]

Myocardial Adaptability

Homeometric Autoregulation: One characteristic of both normal as well as hypertrophied myocardium is its ability to increase its force of contraction in response to increased end-diastolic pressure (or volume) or to certain interventions that serve to augment its external performance.[6] Thus, under a wide variety of controlled experimental situations (as well as in clinical circumstances), the heart is able to adapt to changes in venous return, to augmented adrenergic input, and to levels of catecholamines or other circulating substances by shifting from one force-volume relationship to another as a family of parallel curves that relate to one another in proportion to the intervention introduced.[7] Ultimately, the load or the degree of stress imposed on the ventricle may be so great that the myocardium can no longer adapt and the shift of this Frank-Starling relationship to the right achieves a descending limb of the curve.[8]

Hypertrophy: The ability of the myocardium to adapt structurally to the increased tension by the process of hypertrophy permits the Frank-Starling curve to be shifted more rightward. Eventually, the myocardium can no longer sustain the force necessary to overcome the load imposed on it, and a descending limb to the curve can be demonstrated. In a recent study from our laboratory, rats with two kidneys were made hypertensive by placing a clip around only one renal artery.[9] Myocardial hypertrophy soon occurred, but when a volume load was rapidly given intravenously after only 4 weeks of hypertension, the heart was no longer able to maintain a normal cardiac output at any end-diastolic pressure. In fact, at the maximal volume load (at the end of the 1-minute infusion), end-diastolic pressure exceeded the pressures achieved by the normal hearts of sham-operated rats. When the same experiment was performed on rats with hypertension for 6 weeks, a definite descending limb of this Frank-Starling relationship was demonstrated, and this was seen at still higher end-diastolic pressures. Indeed, using a similar volume-loading intervention as a functional test of ventricular pumping ability, spontaneously hypertensive rats (older than 1 year of age) with marked concentric left ventricular hypertrophy (LVH) failed to perform as well as two groups of normotensive rats matched according to age and sex.[10,11] Thus, under rigidly controlled experimental circumstances, there is a progressive adaptability of the heart seen in hypertension, first seen as a stage of increased function; this is followed by structural adaptation, or hypertrophy, of the myocardium permitting a stable functioning ventricle that is able to cope with the increased wall tension and stress. Ultimately, a relationship consistent with a failing left ventricle is demonstrated that, unless reversed therapeutically (with drugs or by unclipping the renal artery), will be followed by frank congestive heart failure and pulmonary edema. This sequence of pathophysiologic events has been lucidly described by Meerson.[12] Moreover, although in lesser controlled circumstances, a similar course of pathophysiologic events has been described in the patient with essential hypertension.[5,13,14]

Clinical Adaptability: Under the conditions of clinical investigation, it is essential not to compromise the individual patient's well-being, and thus patient groups with as similar a degree of homogeneity of clinical and demographic criteria as possible are essential. For this reason patient grouping is necessary. In studies from our laboratory, patients with only essential hypertension were asked to remain off all therapy for at least 4 weeks while they were followed carefully in our clinic.[13,14] Patients suspected of having other coexisting diseases, such as ischemic heart (that is, coronary arterial atherosclerotic) disease or diabetes mellitus are excluded from study. The following describes our present understanding of the pathophysiologic changes, but these observations are described with some historic perspective.

As Freis[15] described in 1960, the hemodynamic hallmark of hypertension is an increased total peripheral resistance (TPR) that results from generalized arteriolar constriction. He also suggested coexisting venoconstriction in essential hypertension. Now, more than 20 years later, investigators have confirmed that in addition to the arteriolar constriction there is indeed a significant venular constriction that serves to redistribute blood from the peripheral circulations to the cardiopulmonary area.[16–18] This serves to increase venous return and add to the hyperfunction of the heart early in hypertension that is provoked by the increased contractility necessary to overcome the ventricular afterload and perhaps the net increased adrenergic activity that is also imposed on the heart.[19–21] Julius et al[20] demonstrated this in man with essential hypertension, and we have also shown in the spontaneously hypertensive rat that there is evidence of increased adrenergic activity associated with reduced parasympathetic control.[21] In addition, Tarazi et al[22] reported that not only in milder forms of hypertension but even in more severe forms of essential hypertension there is evidence of increased myocardial contractility, just as if isoproterenol were administered to normotensive patients. Thus, in these individuals the Frank-Starling relationship is shifted upward and to the left.

Adrenergic factors are important in augmenting myocardial contractility, but other naturally occurring humoral agents may also participate in increasing the inotropic and chronotropic function of the heart. These agents include other catecholamines, angiotensin II, increased ionizable calcium, and perhaps vasopressin and other substances.[23] As we learn more about the participation of other pressor mechanisms in hypertension, we shall become more aware of the complexity of the interrelationship of the many agents that participate in myocardial contractility.

A number of years ago we compared patients with essential hypertension of increasing severity with normal normotensive individuals. These studies demonstrated that as arterial pressure and clinical evidence of vascular disease increased in severity, so did the TPR.[24] Later, we classified patients according to evidence of cardiac involvement and compared each group with normotensive subjects.[13] As severity of hypertension progressed from one group to the next (that is, from the normotensive subjects to the patients with essential hypertension without cardiac involvement, to those with left atrial abnormality, and then to those with LVH), there was also a progressive increase in arterial pressure following pari passu the increased TPR. Normal resting cardiac output (CO) was maintained in patients until LVH was demonstrated. However, when left atrial abnormality was demonstrated electrocardiographically, the LV ejection rate index was impaired, even though resting CO was normal. Moreover, there were significant increases in tension time index, LV work, and pressure time per beat with each group of more severe cardiac involvement.

There will be considerable discussion in this book on the echo in hypertension; but the first study in this area of clinical investigation was reported from our group by Dunn et al.[14] In that study patients were classified using the same criteria that were used earlier (electrocardiogram and chest radiographs), but echo indices were also measured. The same parallel progression of arterial pressure with elevation of TPR and normal cardiac index (CI) was maintained until severe hypertrophy ensued. However, using a better index of myocardial contractility than LV ejection rate, significant impairment of LV function was demonstrated in patients with only left atrial abnormality. These patients had a severely reduced LV ejection fraction and fiber shortening rate that was associated with a definitely enlarged left atrium. Furthermore, even though the electrocardiogram and chest radiograph failed to show hypertrophy of the left ventricle in these patients, greater LV mass, septal wall thickness, and posterior wall thickness were demonstrable by echo. Increased left atrial mass was also present in the patients with ventricular hypertrophy; its presence before obvious ventricular hypertrophy occurred provided further credibility to the concept that the left atrial abnormality merely reflected the lesser compliance of the left ventricle as it underwent hypertrophy. Thus, the enlarged left atrium provided the first clinical evidence of LVH. More recent studies documented still earlier echo evidence of hypertrophy, even before demonstration of left atrial abnormality. Thus, impaired (diastolic) filling of the left ventricle provides an index of reduced compliance of the stiffer, early hypertrophying left ventricle.[25]

These clinical findings parallel the same sequence of physiologic changes suggested by Meerson,[12] a stage of ventricular hyperfunction that preceded a longer stage of stable hyperfunction with hypertrophy, but eventually a stage of depressed myocardial contractility followed by one of overt LV failure.

Other Factors Associated with Increased Cardiac Mass

Notwithstanding the considerable amount of evidence that has been amassed to support the hemodynamic basis for increased cardiac mass in hypertension, a variety of other factors are associated with cardiomegaly (Table I).

Pressor Substances: Over and above the pathogenetic factor of each of the myriad of pressor substances producing myocardial hypertrophy through the hypertensive hemodynamic process that involves elevating pressure and increasing ventricular afterload is the possibility that these agents may have a direct role in the initiation of new myocardial protein synthesis. Several of the known pressor agents have been shown to produce increased myocardial mass even in the absence of an actual increase in arterial pressure. For examples, addition of angiotensin II to myocardial cell tissue culture will increase cellular protein synthesis,[26] and subpressor infusions of catecholamines will also increase myocardial protein synthesis and initiate development of ventricular hypertrophy as well as produce increased collagen deposition and myocardial fibrosis.[27,28]

Age, Sex, and Race: In recent years a considerable body of information has accumulated, from large population studies as well as from prospective epidemiologic data, that demonstrates that cardiac enlargement may be directly related to aging, racial, and sexual factors independent of the level of arterial pressure and other hemodynamic alterations.[29,30] Thus, pathologic data have demonstrated that aging itself is related to increased cardiac mass and ventricular wall thickness.[31] Moreover, the male patient has a greater prevalence of LVH than the female patient who may tolerate the elevated pressure better than the male and have less prevalence of cardiac failure.[29,30] These epidemiologic studies are supported by recent controlled experimental studies that indicate that hemodynamic factors may be dissociated from sexual characteristics in response of cardiac mass to pharmacotherapy or hormonal manipulation.[32,33] Other epidemiologic studies have indicated that the black patient with hypertension may have more severe cardiac and vascular disease than the white patient.[29,30] However, a recent hemodynamic study from our laboratory involving black and white patients with hypertension matched with respect to age, sex, height of arterial pressure, body habitus, and (if possible) duration of hypertension showed no differences in systemic hemodynamics.[34] However, black patients seemed to have larger left ventricles that were related in mass to the level of arterial pressure[35] and more severe renal vascular disease.[36] These demographic characteristics point to other physiologic factors that may relate to development of cardiac enlargement and suggest new areas of investigation that should provide rewarding information.

Coexisting Diseases: These findings bring to mind the question of whether complicating diseases associated with aging may also participate in the process of cardiac enlargement. Increased collagen deposition may be related to aging, and coexistent ischemic heart disease provides yet another strong possible explanation. In addition to these factors are the findings of a high prevalence of carbohydrate intolerance (if not actual diabetes mellitus) and hyperuricemia (if not gout).[29,30] With respect to the latter, recent studies from our laboratory have related the finding of elevated serum uric acid levels not to a metabolic disease but to progressively more severe hemodynamic involvement of the kidney by hypertensive vascular disease.[37] Thus, patients with higher uric acid levels had more severely increased total peripheral and renal vascular resistances and lower renal blood flow. Since the functions relate also to the afterload imposed on the left ventricle, it seems reasonable that further investigation into these associations with ventricular hypertrophy will be rewarding.

An additional problem frequently associated with hypertension is that of exogenous obesity.[38] Indeed, overweight is a true characteristic of patients with hypertension in addition to sodium sensitivity and more rapid heart rate.[29] In other studies from our laboratory, we have shown that the obesity associated with essential hypertension is related to expanded intravascular (plasma) volume, higher CO in proportion to the degree of volume expansion, and elevated TPR.[39] Thus, the hearts of patients with obesity and essential hypertension are subjected to a dual workload: increased ventricular preload related to the volume overload and increased ventricular afterload related to the elevated arterial pressure and TPR. It is therefore reasonable to assume that the left ventricle adapts to this twofold load in a more complex structural manner. Further studies in this area are clearly necessary, but these early pathophysiologic characteristics may provide some understanding of the increased risk of cardiovascular morbidity and mortality in these patients.

Additional Physiologic Considerations

Reflex Mechanisms: As arterial pressure increases in the normotensive situation, there is a predictable response on the part of the heart to decrease its rate, reduce its minute output and its vigor of contraction, and for the peripheral arterioles to dilate and reduce TPR. One would, therefore, expect that in the hypertensive state there might be a slower heart rate and a lesser CO to compensate for the increased vascular resistance; however, this is not the case. On the contrary, heart rate is frequently faster in most experimental and clinical forms of hypertension and, at least in the earlier stages of hypertension, hyperdynamic circulation is found.[2] These findings, as well as altered baroreceptor nerve traffic, have led physiologists to conclude that in chronic hypertension a state of "reset" baroreceptors exists.[40] Less information is available as to whether this resetting is corrected with reversal of hypertension. Moreover, there is little to support any thesis that the locus of resetting is within the carotid baroreceptor, the brain stem, or elsewhere. We do know that there is an alteration in the carotid reflex mechanism but there are no specific studies to indicate that this defect also involves the high-pressure LV receptors in hypertension or to indicate that these receptors are altered in the ventricle with hypertrophy. Moreover, if these receptors are altered in hypertension and/or hypertrophy, do they alter blood flow distribution to the peripheral circulations?

These foregoing conjectures are related to the effects of hypertension on high-pressure receptors in the great vessels and left ventricle. However, other investigators have been concerned with how cardiogenic reflexes might induce hypertension.[41] How these relate to the clinical forms of hypertension is purely speculative, but there is ample evidence to indicate that hypertension (and presumably LVH) may follow myocardial infarction (MI).[42] Still another related consideration may concern the physiologic mechanisms that might explain the antihypertensive actions of certain therapeutic agents, including the beta-adrenergic receptor blocking drugs.[43]

Endocrine and Volume Regulating Mechanisms: What of the role of atrial receptors? Several years ago Braunwald et al[44] published a provocative editorial referring to the heart as an endocrine organ. In those days they considered primarily the storage capacity of the myocardium for norepinephrine and how this ability was diminished in the failing ventricle. We now know, through the work of James and his associates,[45] that serotonin also participates in cardiac pressor reflexes. This report suggested that a pressor response in MI could be initiated by the release of serotonin from platelet aggregrates, but whether there are differences in responses to serotonin in the normal myocardium and the ventricle with hypertrophy or fibrosis is not known.

Recently, physiologists have been concerned about a natriuretic factor that originates in atrial granules.[46] Investigators in our institution have partially purified this substance, isolated from the atria of rats, rabbits, dogs, monkeys, and man (but not from the ventricle), and have shown that it does produce a very profound natriuresis.[47] These findings suggest that the heart may be a volume-responding or volume-controlling organ through humoral as well as neural mechanisms. We already know that episodes of paroxysmal atrial tachycardia are followed by significant diuresis. Current thinking explains this phenomenon through a reflex initiated by the distended atrium.[48] However, an additional explanation might be a natriuretic factor that is released.

We have already referred to the role of intravascular volume and vascular capacity (peripheral venoconstriction) in hypertension, but the question has also been raised as to the role of the heart in response to volume overload, particularly as it might relate to the phenomenon of exaggerated natriuresis in hypertension. Ulrych et al[49] related this exaggerated sodium excretion in patients with hypertension to the increased CO provoked by the intravascular volume expansion. They suggested that the CO increased more in patients with hypertension, largely because of a venoconstricted periphery, and that greater sodium excretion resulted from some factor over and above an intrarenal factor. Perhaps this is produced by low-pressure volume receptors or even the recently postulated atrial natriuretic factor.

Reversal of Ventricular Hypertrophy: Later in this book we will learn about the response of the hypertrophied left ventricle associated with treatment of the hypertensive condition. Some consider this response to therapy as "good;" whether this is good or bad is more of a moral judgment. However, we do know that the ventricular hypertrophy is a phenomenon that permits the heart to work more efficiently at higher pressure loads over a long term. This process is subject to therapeutic reversal and especially to the vagaries of man while taking antihypertensive therapy. Thus, we may produce regression of ventricular hypertrophy therapeutically; but if that therapy is discontinued abruptly by the patient, this might not be good. To explain, development of LVH is a slow and "normal" response to the progressively increasing pressure and ventricular afterload. Certain antihypertensive drugs, such as methyldopa, beta-adrenergic receptor blocking drugs, converting enzyme inhibitors, and perhaps the slow-channel calcium antagonists, may regress this process, leaving a greater proportion of collagen,[9,50–54] whereas other agents, such as vasodilators, that may have more salutary hemodynamic effects on the myocardium and may even control pressure better may have little effect on the hypertrophy.[52,54] This suggests the possibility of a therapeutic dilemma: we may regress hypertrophy, but what happens when the arterial pressure abruptly increases if the patient discontinues therapy? Is that heart able to meet the demand of the suddenly increased pressure load without the opportunity to undergo a more long-term, adaptive change? Is it possible for the myocardium to develop appropriate hypertrophy once the initial hypertrophy has regressed?

It is therefore apparent from this overview discussion that although much is known about the pathophysiology of the heart in the normal and hypertrophied state, much more remains to be learned. Is this not the expected result of disciplined inquiry?

References

1. KANNEL WB, CASTELLI WP, MCNAMARA PM, MCKEE PA, FEINLEIB M: Role of blood pressure in the development of congestive heart failure. N Engl J Med 1972; 287: 781–787.
2. FROHLICH ED: The heart in hypertension. In: Genest J, Kuchel O, Hamet P, Cantin M, eds. Hypertension: physiopathology and treatment. New York: McGraw-Hill, 1983; 791–810.
3. Report of the National Heart, Lung, and Blood Institute's Task Force on Blood Pressure Control in Children. Pediatrics 1977; 59: 797–820.
4. U. S. Department of Health, Education, and Welfare National Health Survey: Hypertension and hypertensive heart diseases in adults. United States 1960–1962. National Center for Health Statistics, U. S. Public Health Service Publication No. 1000, Series 11, No. 13, Washington, DC: Superintendent of Documents, 1966.
5. TRIPPODO NC, FROHLICH ED: Controversies in cardiovascular research: similarities of genetic (spontaneous) hypertension. Man and rat. Circ Res 1981; 48: 309–319.
6. BRAUNWALD E: Pathophysiology of heart failure. In: Braunwald E, ed. Heart disease. Philadelphia: W. B. Saunders, 1980; 453–471.
7. SARNOFF SJ: Myocardial contractility as described by ventricular function curves: observations on Starling's law of the heart. Physiol Rev 1955; 35: 107–122.
8. BRAUNWALD E, ROSS J JR, SONNENBLICK EH: Mechanisms of contraction in the normal and failing heart, 2nd ed. Boston: Little, Brown, 1976.
9. KUWAJIMA I, KARDON MB, PEGRAM BL, SESOKO S, FROHLICH ED: Regression of left ventricular hypertrophy in two-kidney, one-clip Goldblatt hypertension. Hypertension 1982; 4 (part II): 113–118.
10. PFEFFER MA, PFEFFER JM, FROHLICH ED: Pumping ability of the hypertrophying left ventricle of the spontaneously hypertensive rat. Circ Res 1976; 92: 423–429.
11. PFEFFER JM, PFEFFER MA, FISHBEIN MC, FROHLICH ED: Cardiac function and morphology with aging in the spontaneously hypertensive rat. Am J Physiol 1979; 237: H461–H468.
12. MEERSON FZ: Compensatory hyperfunction of the heart and cardiac insufficiency. Circ Res 1962; 10: 250–258.
13. FROHLICH ED, TARAZI RC, DUSTAN HP: Clinical-physiological correlations in the development of hypertensive heart disease. Circulation 1971; 44: 446–455.
14. DUNN FG, CHANDRARATNA PN, DE CARVALHO JGR, BASTA LL, FROHLICH ED: Pathophysiologic assessment of hypertensive heart disease with echocardiography. Am J Cardiol 1977; 39: 789–795.
15. FREIS ED: Hemodynamics of hypertension. Physiol Rev 1960; 40: 27–53.

16. FROHLICH ED: Haemodynamics of hypertension. In: Genest J, Koiw E, Kuchel O, eds. Hypertension: physiopathology and treatment. New York: McGraw-Hill, 1977; 15–49.

17. ULRYCH M, FROHLICH ED, DUSTAN HP, PAGE IH: Cardiac output and distribution of blood volume in central and peripheral circulations in hypertensive and normotensive man. Br Heart J 1969; 31: 570–574.

18. FROHLICH ED: Hemodynamic factors in the pathogenesis and maintenance of hypertension. Fed Proc 1982; 41: 2400–2408.

19. FROHLICH ED: The adrenergic nervous system and hypertension. Mayo Clin Proc 1977; 52: 361–368.

20. JULIUS S, PASCUAL AV, LONDON R: Role of parasympathetic inhibition in the hyperkinetic type of borderline hypertension. Circulation 1971; 44: 413–418.

21. FROHLICH ED, PFEFFER MA: Adrenergic mechanisms in human and SHR hypertension. Clin Sci Mol Med 1975; 48: 225s–238s.

22. TARAZI RC, IBRAHIM MM, DUSTAN HP, FERRARIO CM: Cardiac factors in hypertension. Circ Res 1974; 34 (suppl 1): 213–221.

23. DUNN FG, FROHLICH ED: Hypertension and angina pectoris. In: Yu PN, Goodwin JF, eds. Progress in cardiology. vol. 7. Philadelphia: Lea & Febiger, 1978; 163–196.

24. FROHLICH ED, KOZUL VJ, TARAZI RA, DUSTAN HP: Physiological comparison of labile and essential hypertension. Circ Res 1970; 27: 55–69.

25. DRESLINSKI GR, FROHLICH ED, DUNN FG, MESSERLI FG, SUAREZ DH, REISIN E: Echocardiographic diastolic ventricular abnormality in hypertensive heart disease: atrial emptying index. Am J Cardiol 1981; 47: 1087–1090.

26. KHAIRALLAH PA, SEN S, TARAZI RC: Angiotensin, protein biosynthesis and cardiovascular hypertrophy (abstr). Am J Cardiol 1976; 37: 148.

27. GORDON AL, INCHIOSA MA JR, LEHR D: Isoproterenol-induced cardiomegaly: assessment of myocardial protein content, actomyosin ATPase and heart rate. J Mol Cell Cardiol 1972; 4: 543–557.

28. SZAKACS JE, MEHLMAN B: Pathologic changes induced by 1-norepinephrine: quantitative aspects. Am J Cardiol 1960; 5: 619–627.

29. KANNEL WB, GORDON T, SCHWARTZ MJ: Systolic versus diastolic blood pressure and risk of coronary heart disease: the Framingham Study. Am J Cardiol 1971; 27: 335–346.

30. POOLING PROJECT RESEARCH GROUP: Relationship of blood pressure, serum cholesterol, smoking habit, relative weight and ECG abnormalities to incidence of major coronary events: final report of the Pooling Project. J Chronic Dis 1978; 31: 201–306.

31. LAKATTA EG: Alterations in the cardiovascular system that occur in advanced age. Fed Proc 1979; 38: 163–167.

32. PFEFFER MA, PFEFFER JM, WEISS AD, FROHLICH ED: Development of SHR hypertension and cardiac hypertrophy during prolonged beta blocking therapy. Am J Physiol 1977; 39: 789–795.

33. CAMBOTTI LJ, COLE FE, GERALL AA, FROHLICH ED, MACPHEE AA: Neonatal gonadal hormones and blood pressure in the spontaneously hypertensive rat. Am J Physiol 1984; 247: E258–E264.

34. MESSERLI FH, DE CARVALHO JGR, CHRISTIE B, FROHLICH ED: Essential hypertension in blacks and whites: hemodynamic findings and fluid volume state. Am J Med 1979; 7: 27–31.

35. DUNN FG, OIGMAN W, DRESLINSKI GR, et al: Racial differences in cardiac adaptation to essential hypertension. J Am Coll Cardiol 1983; 1: 1348–1351.

36. FROHLICH ED, MESSERLI FH, DUNN FG, OIGMAN W, VENTURA H, SUNGAARD-RIISE K: Greater renal vascular involvement in the black patient with essential hypertension. Mineral Electrolyte Metab 1984; 10: 173–177.

37. MESSERLI FH, FROHLICH ED, DRESLINSKI GR, SUAREZ DH, ARISTIMUNO GG: Serum uric acid in essential hypertension: an indicator of renal vascular involvement. Ann Intern Med 1980; 93: 817–821.

38. KANNEL W, BRAUD N, SKINNER J, DAWLZER T, MCNAMARA P: Relation of adiposity to blood pressure and development of hypertension: the Framingham Study. Ann Intern Med 1967; 67: 48–59.

39. MESSERLI FH, CHRISTIE B, DE CARVALHO JGR, ARISTIMUNO GG, SUAREZ DH, DRESLINSKI GR, FROHLICH ED: Obesity and essential hypertension: hemodynamics, intravascular volumes, sodium excretion and plasma renin activity. Arch Intern Med 1981; 141: 81–85.

40. MCCUBBIN JW, GREEN JH, PAGE IH: Baroreceptor function in chronic renal hypertension. Circ Res 1956; 4: 205–210.

41. LIARD JF, TARAZI RC, FERRARIO CM, MANGER WM: Hemodynamic and humoral characteristics of hypertension induced by prolonged stellate stimulation in conscious dogs. Circ Res 1975; 36: 455–468.

42. GIBSON TC: Blood pressure levels in acute myocardial infarction. Am Heart J 1978; 96: 475–480.

43. FROHLICH ED: Beta-adrenergic receptor blockade in the treatment of essential hypertension. In: Strauer BE, ed. The heart in hypertension. Berlin: Springer-Verlag, 1981; 425–435.

44. BRAUNWALD E, HARRISON DC, CHIDSEY CA: The heart as an endocrine organ. Am J Med 1964; 36: 1–4.

45. JAMES TN, ISOBE JH, URTHALER F: Analysis of components in a hypertensive cardiogenic chemoreflex. Circulation 1975; 52: 179–192.

46. DE BOLD AJ, BORENSTEIN HB, VERESS AT, SONNENBERG H: A rapid and potent natriuretic response to intravenous injection of atrial myocardial extract in rats. Life Sci 1981; 28: 89–94.

47. TRIPPODO NC, MACPHEE AA, COLE FE, BLAKESLEY HL: Partial chemical characterization of a natriuretic substance in rat atrial heart tissue. Proc Soc Exp Biol Med 1982; 170: 502–508.

48. HENRY JP, GAUER OH, REEVES JL: Evidence of the atrial location of receptors influencing urine flow. Circ Res 1956; 4: 85–92.

49. ULRYCH M, HOFMAN J, HEJL Z: Cardiac and renal hyperresponsiveness to acute plasma volume expansion in hypertension. Am Heart J 1964; 68: 193–203.

50. SEN S, TARAZI RC, KHAIRALLAH PA, BUMPUS FM: Cardiac hypertrophy in spontaneously hypertensive rats. Circ Res 1974; 35: 775–781.

51. SEN S, TARAZI RC, BUMPUS FM: Reversal of cardiac hypertrophy in renal hypertensive rats: medical versus surgical therapy. Am J Physiol 1981; 240: H408–H412.

52. Sen S, Tarazi RC, Khairallah PA, Bumpus FM: Cardiac hypertrophy and its reversal by antihypertensive drugs in spontaneously hypertensive rats (SHR). Clin Exp Pharmacol Physiol 1976; 3: 173–177.

53. Sen S, Bumpus FM: Collagen synthesis in development and reversal of cardiac hypertrophy in spontaneously hypertensive rats. Am J Cardiol 1979; 44: 954–958.

54. Pegram BL, Ishise S, Frohlich ED: Effects of methyldopa, clonidine, and hydralazine on cardiac mass and hemodynamics in Wistar-Kyoto and spontaneously hypertensive rats. Cardiovasc Res 1982; 16: 40–46.

11

Echo Assessment of Left Ventricular Structure and Function in Hypertension: Methodology

NATHANIEL REICHEK, M.D.

Echo provides an array of methods for the study of left ventricular (LV) structure and function in hypertension. In applying these methods, a fundamental distinction must be made between hypertensive hearts with and without coronary artery disease, since inhomogeneity of myocardial structure and function due to coronary disease invalidates a number of otherwise valuable techniques. This brief review will describe those techniques applicable in the absence of coronary disease that form the basis for many recent clinical studies of the regulation of left ventricular hypertrophy (LVH) in hypertension.

Left Ventricular Volume and Pump Function

Using M-mode echo, left ventricular (LV) size and systolic pump function can be expressed as LV diameter and percent change in LV diameter (%D) from end-diastole to end-systole. The diameter correlates closely with volume by the so-called cube function in normally shaped ventricles.[1] Thus, %D has a good relationship to ejection fraction in hypertensive subjects without clinical cardiac dysfunction. However, LV dysfunction is frequently associated with changes in LV shape that alter the relationship of %D to ejection fraction, even in the absence of coronary disease. Typically, the left ventricle becomes more spherical as it dilates.[2] Furthermore, %D is less useful when right ventricular dilation or left bundle branch block alters interventricular septal motion.[3,4] In the absence of these factors, %D can be used to determine effects of antihypertensive agents on LV pump performance.

Two-dimensional echo ejection fraction is more generally applicable than M-mode %D and can be used despite LV shape abnormalities, left bundle branch block, or segmental dysfunction due to myocardial ischemia.[5-8] Many methods have been described, but the most successful have been biplane Simpson's rule and area-length models that have given good agreement with angiographic and radionuclide results. Recently, a simplified area-length approach has been described based on multiple dimensional measurements without planimetry.[9]

In interpreting pump function indices in hypertension the roles of afterload and pharmacologic milieu must be appreciated. The LV pump function is the product of the interaction of contractility, hemodynamic load, and the amount of myocardium available to support that load. Both contractility and hemodynamic load can be changed acutely by antihypertensive therapy, whereas hypertrophy changes relatively slowly, over months.[10] A reduction in afterload, with constant contractile state and myocardial mass, can produce increased ejection fraction. Conversely, increases in contractility or muscle mass with constant hemodynamic load can also enhance pump function indices. Many antihypertensive agents, such as the beta blockers, affect both contractility and hemodynamic load acutely and myocardial mass more gradually. In consequence, alterations in pump function must be interpreted with great caution and cannot be assumed to reflect either contractile state or hemodynamic load alone.

Ejection fraction is a relative measure of systolic and diastolic LV volumes. Its reliability need not be impaired by systematic, proportional errors in both volume estimates. Such errors have been shown in vitro with two-dimensional echo data.[11,12] The results indicate systematic underestimation of LV cavity volume by roughly 30%. Two-dimensional echo estimates of absolute LV volume can be corrected by an appropriate regression calibration formula. Unfortunately, the correction appears to differ for different echo instruments.[13] Thus, it may be necessary to calibrate each instrument individually to obtain valid absolute results. Applicability of this regression correction approach to clinical echo images has been demonstrated prospectively.[14]

The ejection fraction is a reliable but relatively insensitive index of LV systolic pump function. Measurement of the rate of ejection expressed as the velocity of circumferential fiber shortening (VCF) is a potentially more sensitive approach to systolic function.[15] The mean VCF can be determined from M-mode measurements and agrees closely with angiographic VCF values. In addition, because of the high sampling rate, M-mode permits determination of instantaneous VCF throughout the cardiac cycle. Hence, peak systolic VCF can be identified and appears to be useful in recognition of mild LV dysfunction.[16] Similar analysis of diastolic VCF and wall thinning in relation to mitral valve opening may be useful in assessment of depressed diastolic LV cavity function.[17]

Afterload and Mechanics

Quantitation of afterload is central to the analysis of cardiac function in hypertension. Although it is common to use either arterial pressure or calculated systemic vascular resistance as afterload indices in studies of hypertension, neither accurately reflects afterload at the myocardial level. The after-

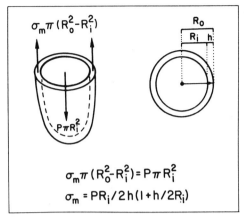

$$\sigma_m \pi (R_o^2 - R_i^2) = P \pi R_i^2$$

$$\sigma_m = PR_i / 2h(1 + h/2R_i)$$

Figure 1. *Derivation of wall stress in the meridional plane. Wall stress (σ_m) can be determined if ventricular pressure (P), wall thickness (h), ventricular chamber radius (R_i) and total ventricular radius ($R_o = R_i + h$) are known. The product of pressure and ventricular chamber area in this plane ($P\pi R_i^2$) must equal the product of stress and myocardial area ($\sigma_m\pi[R_o^2 - R_i^2]$). (Reprinted with permission from Grossman et al.[20])*

load seen by the myocardium is actually systolic wall force. Because of compensatory hypertrophy, this source is generated by different amounts of myocardium in different hypertensive hearts. Therefore, it is important to normalize load for the amount of myocardium available to support it, using the concept of wall stress, or force per unit of myocardial area. Wall stress, which varies continuously throughout the cardiac cycle, can be estimated using the law of Laplace if LV pressure and geometry are known.[18] Furthermore, wall stress is different in different planes through the three-dimensional left ventricle.[19] M-mode echo provides the dimensional data needed for wall stress determination in the meridional plane and can be extrapolated to the circumferential plane if the ratio of LV minor axis to LV length is known or a reasonable estimate assumed.[20-22] Two-dimensional echo permits direct determination of the geometric variables needed for wall stress determination in both the meridional and circumferential planes.[23] The derivation of meridional stress is shown in Figure 1.[20] Using M-mode echo, this derivation can be reexpressed as:

Meridional stress = 0.33PD/T(1 + T/D) (units = 10^3 dynes/cm^2)

where P = instantaneous LV pressure; T = instantaneous posterior wall thickness; D = instantaneous LV diameter. The corresponding two-dimensional derivation yields the results:

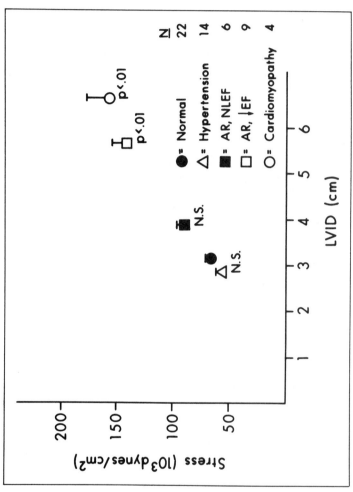

Figure 2. *Mean values for end-systolic stress and left ventricular diameter (LVID) in groups of normal subjects, hypertensive patients with normal LV function, aortic regurgitation (AR) with normal and reduced ejection fraction (EF), and congestive cardiomyopathy. This index of after-load is normal in hypertension and AR with normal ejection fraction but elevated in the two groups with impaired LV function. (Reprinted with permission from Reichek et al.[21])*

$$\text{Meridional stress} = \frac{1.33P \ Ac}{At - Ac}$$

$$\text{Circumferential stress} = \frac{1.33P \ \sqrt{Ac}}{\sqrt{At} - \sqrt{Ac}} \left(1 - \frac{4Ac^{(1.5)}/\pi L^2}{\sqrt{At} - \sqrt{Ac}}\right)$$

where At = total LV short axis area, including the myocardium; Ac = LV short-axis cavity area, and L = cavity length.

Complete assessment of LV wall stress by any approach requires simultaneous recording of dimensional data and high-fidelity pressure via an LV micromanometer catheter.[20,21] The one wall stress index that can be determined reliably by totally noninvasive means is end-systolic stress.[21-24] This is due to the fact that cuff auscultatory systolic pressure corresponds closely to LV high-fidelity end-systolic pressure. As it happens, end-systolic stress is a most important value of instantaneous stress to measure, since it represents the critical afterload value that terminates LV ejection.[25,26] Increases in ejection fraction in a given ventricle with constant contractile state and preload can only occur if end-systolic stress decreases. Thus, end-systolic stress is a good index to represent the role of afterload in determining LV pump function. Using end-systolic stress, the normalization of afterload by hypertrophy is readily demonstrated (Fig. 2).

Another potential use of end-systolic stress is the construction of a load-independent index of contractile state. In the isolated working heart, the relationship of end-systolic wall stress to LV diameter is linear over the physiologic range, as is the relationship of end-systolic pressure to end-systolic volume. The slope and intercept of this line can be shifted only by an alteration in contractile state.[25,26] Similar phenomena have been demonstrated in the intact human circulation.[24,27] Administration of a vasodilator, such as sublingual nitroglycerin, or an alpha-adrenergic agonist, such as intravenous phenylepherine, may permit noninvasive characterization of this end-systolic force-length relationship.[21-25]

Assessment of Hypertrophy

When LV pressure is chronically elevated, LV hypertrophy occurs as an adaptive mechanism and keeps the force generated by each unit of myocardium or LV wall stress within the normal range (Fig. 2), whether measured as peak, mean, or end-systolic stress.[20] In hypertension, this results from the specific adaptive pattern of concentric hypertrophy, which, in the compensated phase, increases LV wall thickness but keeps LV cavity size unchanged. Quantitation of this process of concentric hypertrophy can be approached by echo in two ways.

First, echo can be used to estimate the actual weight of LV myocardium. In relatively symmetrical ventricles, without LV aneurysm or diastolic shape abnormality due to marked dilation of the right side of the heart, this can be

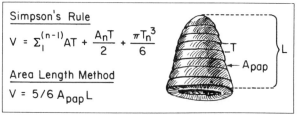

Figure 3. *Left ventricular volume or mass reconstruction by short-axis area-length and Simpson's rule methods. The ventricle is sectioned into disk-like short-axis slices. For Simpson's rule, these are simply summated with an ellipsoid treatment of the apex. The volume of each section is the product of area (A) and thickness (T). The area-length method estimates volume from an ellipsoid model as the product of midventricular area at the papillary muscle level (Apap) and length (L). (Reprinted with permission from Helak and Reichek.[11])*

accomplished successfully with M-mode echo dimensional data.[28] In such ventricles, ventricular volume is roughly proportional to the cube of the echo LV minor axis.[1] Although this relationship is not sufficiently close to permit determination of absolute LV cavity volume or ejection fraction accurately in abnormal ventricles, there is a good relationship between echo estimates of LV muscle mass from cube function analyses at end-diastole and angiographic estimate of LV mass.[29] Subsequent autopsy validation studies demonstrated that angiographically based methods for such estimates did not in fact correlate closely with actual postmortem LV weight.[28] However, a minor modification of the measurement technique used to determine mean myocardial thickness and a regression correction do permit accurate prediction of postmortem LV weight from M-mode echo data. The resultant equation is:

$$\text{LV mass} = 1.04 \, (\text{LVID} + \text{T} + \text{S})^3 - 13.6 \text{ g}; r = 0.96, \text{SD} = 29 \text{ g}$$

where LVID = LV diameter; T = posterior wall thickness; and S = septal thickness. The results obtained are as statistically reliable as those obtained with biplane ventriculography.[28,30]

Two-dimensional echo estimation of LV mass is more complex, since two-dimensional images tend to overestimate LV myocardial cross-sectional area in in vitro studies.[11] Further application of both Simpson's rule and area-length analyses has been complicated by the poor endocardial resolution obtained in the apical four-chamber and two-chamber views that provide most extensive geometric information. To date, short-axis image-based reconstructions of LV mass have proved more successful. A short-axis Simpson's rule approach (Fig. 3) would be optimal, but one cannot obtain enough short-axis sections to implement this method clinically. Fortunately, a short-axis area-length method (Fig. 3) based on a single short-axis cross-section at papillary muscle level and measurement of ventricular length from the four-chamber apical view appears to be reliable in both experimental models and in man.[11,13,14] Prospective data derived from clinical echo studies have been compared with postmortem LV weight using a regression correction derived from in vitro imaging. Despite inclusion of hearts with marked LV shape abnormalities, such as ventricular aneurysm and marked septal flattening due to right ventricular enlargement, early results indicate an excellent agreement between predicted and actual LV weight (r = 0.93, slope = 0.85, (Standard error of the estimate = 31 g).[14] The two-dimensional method may further reduce the error of LV mass estimates in normally shaped hearts compared with the M-mode technique. This is of consequence because the mean increase in LV mass encountered in untreated hypertensive patients is only 100 g, or 67% above the mean normal value in healthy control subjects.[10,31]

Quantitation of LV mass is of great value in studies of hypertensive heart disease, but the determination of relative wall thickness may be a more sensitive expression of concentric hypertrophy in response to LV pressure elevation. Relative wall thickness (RWT) is the ratio of wall thickness to chamber diameter and is usually expressed as twice echo LV posterior wall thickness divided by LV diameter on M-mode echo.[32] The analogous two-dimensional index is the ratio of myocardial area to LV chamber area in a short-axis section above the papillary muscles. In normal populations, RWT at end-diastole RWT has 95% confidence limits of 0.33 ± 0.06 (SD) from age 10 to age 70 years in normotensive subjects of both sexes.[33] A ratio of 0.45 or higher is highly predictive of an LV systolic pressure above 140 mmHg.[32,33] End-systolic RWT can be used similarly and has been used to estimate LV pressure in children with aortic stenosis with good results.[34,35] However, the end-systolic index appears to be quite sensitive to depression of contractile state and has not been helpful in adult populations with pressure overload hypertrophy.[32,36] In contrast, the end-diastolic index may be applicable even in heterogeneous populations, including subjects with mild clinical congestive heart failure.[32] However, it is important to point out that there is sufficient biologic variability to the concentric LV hypertrophic response that subjects with moderate untreated hypertension often have RWT values that fall within the upper normal range. Nonetheless, RWT is more sensitive than absolute LV mass values in detecting early concentric LV hypertrophy. If LV volume is small, it is quite possible to have obvious LV hypertrophy by the RWT index but an absolute LV mass within the upper normal range. An important limitation of M-mode echo RWT is the extreme sensitivity of the index to small variations in measured wall thickness. It is hoped that substitution of a two-dimensional area method for the M-mode technique will greatly enhance the stability of the RWT index.

Summary

M-mode and two-dimensional echo now provide noninvasive techniques that permit assessment of LV pump function (%D, two-dimensional echo ejection fraction, mean and peak VCF), quantitation of afterload (end-systolic stress), a load-independent assessment of contractile state (end-systolic stress-diameter relationship), and quantitation of pressure overload hypertrophy (LV mass and relative wall thickness). Combined application of these methods to problems in the assessment of hypertensive heart disease can clarify both disease mechanisms and therapeutic effects by identifying the role of changes in myocardial mass, alterations in contractile state, and variations in afterload in a given setting. Application of these methods in clinical research on hypertensive heart disease is in its early phases.[36-38] Their applicability to decision making in individual patients remains to be determined.

Acknowledgements

Supported in part by a Commonwealth of Pennsylvania Health Services Contract and by grants from Merck Sharpe & Dohme. I am indebted to Mary Johnson for her invaluable assistance with manuscript preparation.

References

1. FEIGENBAUM H, WOLFE SB, POPP RL, HAINE CL, DODGE HT: Correlation of ultrasound with angiocardiography in measuring left ventricular diastolic volume. Am J Cardiol 1969; 23: 111.

2. LEWIS RP, SANDLER H: Relationship between changes in left ventricular dimensions and the ejection fraction in man. Circulation 1971; 44: 548–557.

3. DIAMOND MA, DILLON JC, HAINE CL, CHANG S, FEIGENBAUM H: Echocardiographic features of atrial septal defect. Circulation 1971; 43: 129–135.

4. DILLON JC, CHANG S, FEIGENBAUM H: Echocardiographic manifestations of left bundle branch block. Circulation 1974; 49: 876–880.

5. SCHILLER NB, ACQUATELLA H, PORTS TA, et al: Left ventricular volume from aired biplane two-dimensional echocardiography. Circulation 1979; 60: 547–555.

6. FOLLAND ED, PARISI AF, MOYNIHAN BS, JONES DR, FELDMAN CL, TOW DE: Assessment of left ventricular ejection fraction and volumes by real-time, two-dimensional echocardiography. Circulation 1979; 60: 760–766.

7. CARR KW, ENGLER RL, FORSYTHE JR, JOHNSON AD, GOSINK B: Measurement of left ventricular ejection fraction by mechanical cross-sectional echocardiography. Circulation 1979; 59: 1196–1206.

8. ERBEL R, SCHWEIZER E, MEYER J, GRANNER H, KREBS W, EFFERT S: Left ventricular volume and ejection fraction determination by cross-sectional echocardiography in patients with coronary artery disease: a prospective study. Clin Cardiol 1980; 3: 377–383.

9. QUINONES MA, WAGGONER AD, REDUTO LA, et al: A new, simplified and accurate method for determining ejection fraction with two-dimensional echocardiography. Circulation 1981; 64: 744–753.

10. REICHEK N, FRANKLIN BB, CHANDLER T, MUHAMMAD A, PLAPPERT T, ST. JOHN SUTTON M: Reversal of left ventricular hypertrophy by antihypertensive therapy. Eur Heart J 1982; 3 (suppl A): 165–169.

11. HELAK JW, REICHEK N: Quantitation of human left ventricular mass and volume by two-dimensional echocardiography: in vitro anatomic validation. Circulation 1981; 63: 1398–1407.

12. BARRETT MJ, JACOBS L, GOMBERG J, HORTON L, WOLF NM, MEISTER SF: Simultaneous contrast imaging of the left ventricle by two-dimensional echocardiography and standard ventriculography. Clin Cardiol 1982; 5: 208–213.

13. HELAK JW, PLAPPERT T, MUHAMMAD A, REICHEK N: Two-dimensional echocardiographic imaging of the left ventricle: comparison of mechanical and phased-array systems *in vitro*. Am J Cardiol 1981; 48: 720–727.

14. REICHEK N, HELAK J, PLAPPERT T, ST. JOHN SUTTON M: Anatomic validation of left ventricular mass estimates from clinical two-dimensional echocardiography: initial results. Circulation 1983; 67: 348–352.

15. COOPER R, KARLINER JS, O'ROURKE RA, PETERSON KL, LEOPOLD GR: Ultrasound determinations of mean fiber-shortening rate in man. Am J Cardiol 1972; 29: 257.

16. WILSON JR, REICHEK N: Echocardiographic indices of left ventricular function: a comparison. Chest 1979; 76: 441–447.

17. UPTON MT, GIBSON DG, BROWN DJ: Echocardiographic assessment of abnormal left ventricular relaxation in man. Br Heart J 1976; 38: 1001.

18. SANDLER H, DODGE HT: Left ventricular tension and stress in man. Circulation 1963; 13: 91–104.

19. GOULD KL, LIPSCOMB K, HAMILTON GW, KENNEDY JW: Relations of left ventricular shape, function and wall stress in man. Am J Cardiol 1974; 34: 627–634.

20. GROSSMAN W, JONES D, McLAURIN LP: Wall stress and patterns of hypertrophy in the human left ventricle. J Clin Invest 1975; 56: 56–64.

21. REICHEK N, WILSON J, ST. JOHN SUTTON M, PLAPPERT T, GOLDBERG S, HIRSHFELD J: Noninvasive determination of left ventricular end-systolic stress: validation of the method and initial applications. Circulation 1982; 65: 99–109.

22. QUINONES MA, MOKETOFF DM, NOURI S, WINTERS WL JR, MILLER RR: Noninvasive quantification of left ventricular wall stress. Am J Cardiol 1980; 45: 782–790.

23. ST. JOHN SUTTON MG, PLAPPERT TA, HIRSHFELD JW, REICHEK N: Assessment of left ventricular mechanics in patients with asymptomatic aortic regurgitation: a two-dimensional echocardiographic study. Circulation 1984; 69: 259–268.

24. MARSH JD, GREEN LH, WYNNE J, COHN PF, GROSSMAN W: Left ventricular end-systolic pressure dimension and stress-length relations in normal human subjects. Am J Cardiol 1979; 44: 1311–1317.

25. WEBER KT, JANICKI JS, HEFNER LL: Left ventricular force-length relations of isovolumic and ejecting contractions. Am J Physiology 1976; 231: 337–343.

26. WEBER KT, JANICKI JS: Instantaneous force-velocity length relations: experimental findings and clinical correlates. Am J Cardiol 1977; 40: 740–747.

27. GROSSMAN W, BRAUNWALD E, MANN T, McLAURIN LP, GREEN LH: Contractile state of the left ventricle in man as evaluated from end-systolic pressure-volume relations. Circulation 1977; 56: 845–852.

28. DEVEREUX RB, REICHEK N: Echocardiographic determination of left ventricular mass in man: anatomic validation of the method. Circulation 1977; 55: 613–618.
29. TROY BL, POMBO J, RACKLEY CE: Measurement of left ventricular wall thickness and mass by echocardiography. Circulation 1972; 45: 602–611.
30. KENNEDY JW, REICHENBACH DD, BAXLEY WA, DODGE HT: Left ventricular mass. Am J Cardiol 1967; 19: 221–223.
31. REICHEK N, ST. JOHN SUTTON M, PLAPPERT T, WILSON J, HIRSHFELD J: Echocardiographic recognition of afterload excess: relationship to ejection fraction (abstr). Am J Cardiol 1982; 49: 918.
32. REICHEK N, DEVEREUX RB: Reliable estimation of peak left ventricular systolic pressure by M-mode echographic-determined end-diastolic relative wall thickness: identification of severe valvular aortic stenosis in adult patients. Am Heart J 1982; 103: 202–209.
33. ST. JOHN SUTTON M, REICHEK N, LOVETT J, KASTOR JA, GUILIANI E: Effects of age, body size and blood pressure on the normal human left ventricle. Circulation 1980; 62: III-305.
34. GEWITZ MH, WERNER JC, KLEINMAN CS, HELLENBRAND WE, TALNER NS, TAUNT KA: Role of echocardiography in aortic stenosis: pre- and post-operative studies. Am J Cardiol 1979; 43: 67–73.
35. GALNZ S, HELLENBRAND WE, BERMAN MA, TALNER NS: Echocardiographic assessment of the severity of aortic stenosis in children and adolescents. Am J Cardiol 1976; 38: 620–625.
36. SCHWARTZ A, VIGNOLA PA, WALKER JH, KING ME, GOLDBLATT A: Echocardiographic estimation of aortic-valve gradient in aortic stenosis. Ann Intern Med 1978; 89: 329–335.
37. REICHEK N, FRANKLIN BB, CHANDLER T, MUHAMMAD A, PLAPPERT T, ST. JOHN SUTTON M: Reversal of left ventricular hypertrophy by antihypertensive therapy. Eur Heart J 1982; 3 (suppl A): 165–169.
38. SCHLANT RC, FELNER JM, BLUMENSTEIN BA, et al: Echocardiographic documentation of regression of left ventricular hypertrophy in patients treated for essential hypertension. Eur Heart J 1982; 3 (suppl A): 171–175.

12

Determinants of Left Ventricular Hypertrophy and Function in Hypertensive Patients
An Echocardiographic Study

FREDDY ABI-SAMRA, M.D.
FETNAT M. FOUAD, M.D.
ROBERT C. TARAZI, M.D.

Recent studies have emphasized the multifactorial role played by the heart in hypertension[1] as well as the serious prognostic significance associated with the development of left ventricular hypertrophy (LVH).[2] It is not surprising, therefore, that the relationship of cardiac hypertrophy and function to systemic hypertension has come under closer scrutiny.[3] Most of the early studies of the heart in hypertensive patients were based on some estimate of hypertrophy by electrocardiography (ECG) and of function by measurements of cardiac output (CO); they, therefore, suffered from the limitations inherent in those methods.[3,4] Because of the difficulty of justifying invasive studies in asymptomatic patients, there was a tendency to extend many of the conclusions developed from other types of cardiac hypertrophy to hypertension. These extensions, however, may not necessarily be appropriate because of the demonstrated heterogeneity among different types of cardiac hypertrophy[5] and of the many differences between hypertension and other types of pressure overload[3].

The widespread use of echo has allowed a noninvasive and more precise investigation of LV mass and has thus helped to identify different forms of LVH among hypertensive patients. Moreover, it has allowed a noninvasive calculation of LV wall stress based on the concepts developed by Grossman et al[6] and extended by the observations of Quinones et al[7] and of Wilson et al[8] who described a simple method for quantification of LV meridional wall stress. Most reports utilizing these methods dealt with patients having valvular heart disease, and many of those describing hypertensive patients have included treated patients.[9,10] In the present study, we have examined different aspects of the LV structural and functional changes in 74 hypertensive patients with no clinical evidence of coronary arterial disease. A clear distinction was made between treated and untreated subjects, and the results in both groups were compared with each other as well as with those in normotensive healthy subjects. A wide spectrum of ventricular structure abnormalities was revealed. A close relationship was found between end-systolic stress and LV performance in both hypertensive and normotensive patients.

Methods

Patient Population; Hypertensive subjects: The data on all echo examinations made in hypertensive patients between 1979 and 1981 at the Research Division, Cleveland Clinic Foundation, were reviewed. All patients with tracings determined to be of excellent quality by separate double-blind examination were included provided they had no evidence of coronary arterial disease, congestive heart failure, chronic renal failure, or other hemodynamically significant diseases.

The total number of patients who fit these criteria was 74; half of these patients (37) were either untreated or had discontinued all antihypertensive treatment for at least 2 weeks prior to examination. The remaining 37 were still receiving various antihypertensive drugs at the time of study. The two groups were analyzed separately to determine the influence, if any, of therapy on the relation between LVH and LV function. There was no significant difference between the two groups in regard to sex distribution (22 men, 15 women in the untreated group versus 17 men, 20 women in the treated group) or age (range, 17 to 69 years in both groups, with a median of 50 in the first and 55 in the second). In each group there happened to be 30 patients with essential hypertension and with either renal arterial disease or primary aldosteronism. The known duration of hypertension ranged from 1 month to 39 years and did not differ significantly between the treated and untreated subjects. At the time of study, mean arterial pressure (MAP) ranged from a low of 90 mmHg to a high of 162 mmHg; this wide range of blood pressure reflected the effects of treatment in some of these patients and the borderline labile type of hypertension in others.

Normotensive subjects. All echo records from all healthy normotensive subjects studied during the same period of time were examined by the same investigators using exactly the same criteria; 19 records obtained from 10 men and 9 women, aged 23 to 61 years (median, 30), were found suitable for subsequent analysis. These same normal subjects were restudied 2 weeks later to evaluate the reproducibility of the echo measurements.

Methodology: All subjects were studied after at least ½ hour of supine rest in the postabsorptive state. The echo methods used have been described in detail previously.[11] All records were obtained under two-dimensional control with a Toshiba SSH-IDA phased array ultrasonic sector scanner. The two-dimensional technique was used for accurate localization of the plane of measurement and for detection of areas of dyskinesia. This approach allowed repeated comparable examinations as well as a clear definition of septal echoes and delineation of papillary muscles.[11] The LV dimensions were measured from at least 10 cardiac cycles at precisely the same level in all (tip of the mitral valve leaflets),[12] using the standard leading edge method.[13] The beginning of the QRS complex was used to time end-diastole; end-systole was marked at the point of maximal excursion of the posterior LV wall. In our experience, cycle-to-cycle variability did not exceed 5% to 6% for measurements of interventricular septum, or LV posterior wall thickness or of the end-systolic diameter; it was less than 4% for measurements of the end-diastolic diameter.

Arterial blood pressure levels were determined in all subjects by auscultation before and at the end of the echo examination, using a cuff appropriate to the arm size and a mercury manometer; systolic and diastolic pressures were defined by Korotkoff phase 1 and 5, respectively.[14] Two to four measurements were obtained each time, at 1- to 2-minute intervals, and averaged to yield the single reading used in subsequent calculations of ventricular wall stress. Observations in our laboratory have confirmed previous reports by others[7,8,15] that auscultatory cuff systolic blood pressure correlated very closely with intraventricular pressure ($r = 0.96$, $p < 0.001$).

Derived echo data included:

1. Left ventricular volume and mass: End-diastolic LV cavity volume was calculated by classic formulas assuming an idealized ellipsoidal model[16] and utilizing the Teichholtz correction[17] for both the outer and inner LV volumes. The results were normalized for body surface area and expressed as ml/m^2 for LV volume and g/m^2 for LV mass.

2. Left ventricular wall stress: The LV meridional wall stress was calculated as an index of afterload.[6] End-systolic and peak systolic meridional wall stress (end-systolic stress and peak systolic stress, respectively) were calculated by the noninvasive method of Wilson and Reicheck.[8] In addition, a third index of LV wall stress was calculated from measurements obtained at the end of isovolumetric contraction when intraventricular pressure reaches the aortic diastolic level; at that point, LV internal diameter is still at or near its maximum (end-diastolic diameter) and the LV wall has not yet substantially increased in thickness (h_d). In contrast to peak-systolic stress, which combines peak systolic pressure with diastolic LV measurements, this index has the theoretic advantage of combining pressure and dimension data obtained at the same temporal point in the cardiac cycle. This end-isovolumetric systolic stress (EISS) was calculated on the same basis as the other two indices of stress:

$$EISS = \frac{0.334 \text{ end-diastolic diameter} \times \text{diastolic blood pressure}}{h_d(1 + h_d/\text{end-diastolic diameter})}$$

3. As an index of preload, we used the LV end-diastolic volume normalized for body surface area. Left ventricular performance was evaluated by the standard echo index of fractional shortening. The ratio of systolic blood pressure to end-systolic volume was calculated as an index of LV contractility, since this ratio has been shown by many to be relatively independent of changes of preload and afterload.[18,19]

Statistical Analysis: Data were analyzed with the help of PROPHET, a national computer service resource supported by the National Institutes of Health. In addition to the standard statistical methods for statistical analysis of differences between groups and of linear regression equations, multiple regression analysis techniques were applied to evaluate the relative contributions of different factors (load and contractility) to overall LV performance in both hypertensive and normotensive subjects. The values are reported mean ± 1 SD of the mean.

Results

A wide spectrum of values for LV dimensions was found in both treated and untreated hypertensive patients (Table I). More than 40% of our hypertensive subjects had normal LV dimensions by M-mode echo; disproportionate septal thickening was observed in 8 of 37 treated patients; of the 37 untreated patients, 8 had disproportionate septal thickening with a normal end-diastolic diameter and 2 had disproportionate septal thickening with LV dilation. Thus, a total of 18 of 74 patients had disproportionate septal thickening, a prevalence of 24%, almost as high as that of symmetric LVH, which was seen in 20 of 74, or 27%. None of the patients with disproportionate septal thickening had systolic anterior motion of the mitral valve. Left ventricular dilation with or without increased wall thickness was a common finding (12 of 74 patients, or 16%); it was seen in 4 of 37 untreated and 8 of 37 treated patients. Statistical analysis showed no significant difference ($p > 0.05$) in the prevalence of any of these categories between the treated and untreated patients. None of the 19 healthy normotensive volunteer subjects showed any of the aforementioned indices of LV abnormalities.

TABLE I   Left Ventricular Abnormalities in 74 Hypertensive Patients

Patient Groups	Normal LV Dimension	LV Hypertrophy Concentric	ASH*	LV Dilation With Thickened LV Walls	LV Wall Thickness Within Normal Range
Untreated (n = 37)	19	6	8	4	0
Treated (n = 37)	12	9	8	3	5
Total	31	15	16	7†	5

NOTE: The echo diagnoses were defined as follows: left ventricular (LV) hypertrophy (concentric left ventricular hypertrophy without dilation) included patients with a diastolic septal wall thickness 1.2 cm or greater and posterior wall thickness 1.2 cm or greater but an end-diastolic diameter less than 5.5 cm. ASH meant a septal wall in diastole 1.2 cm or greater *and* a ratio of diastolic septal to posterior wall thickness 1.3 or greater. Left ventricular diameter meant an end-diastole diameter greater than 5.5 cm; of these 12 patients, 7 had thickened ventricular walls, either symmetric or dyssymmetric, and 5 had no measurable increase in thickness of the wall.
*ASH = asymmetric septal hypertrophy. None had abnormal motion of mitral valve.
†Only 2 of the former group (2 of 7) had left ventricular diameter with asymmetric septal hypertrophy and both were untreated.

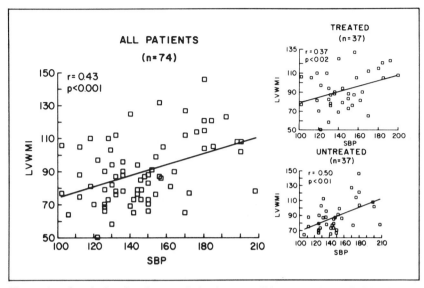

Figure 1. *Graph showing the correlation between LV mass and systolic blood pressure in all 74 hypertensive patients; the smaller insets show similar results obtained in separate analysis of treated and untreated patients.*

Calculated ventricular mass was normal (less than 90 g/m²) in all but 1 of the 31 hypertensive patients recorded as having a "normal left ventricle" by unidimensional criteria; it measured 92 g/m² in that patient, whereas it ranged from 64 to 88 g/m² in all the others. In patients with concentric LVH, with or without dilation, LV mass was increased in all but 1. In contrast with this uniformity among patients with global hypertrophy, only 7 of the 16 patients with disproportionate septal thickening had an increased LV mass.

Hemodynamic Correlates of Left Ventricular Hypertrophy: Left ventricular mass showed a weak but significant positive correlation with systolic blood pressure in hypertensive patients (r = 0.43, n = 74, p < 0.001) (Fig. 1). Both treated and untreated patients showed the same correlation between these two indices; the r value was slightly greater in the untreated group (r = 0.50, p < 0.01) than in the treated group (r = 0.37, p < 0.02). In both groups, a weak negative correlation was observed between peak systolic stress and LV mass index (r = −0.30, p < 0.05).

All indices of LV wall stress were significantly higher in hypertensive patients, both treated and untreated, than in normal subjects (Table II). However, the wide variance (SD/X̄) found among hypertensive patients (from 29% to 42%) pointed to the wide range of individual LV responses to high blood pressure in different subjects. More important, therefore, than group averages was the correlation between blood pressure or indices of stress and overall cardiac performance as estimated from LV percent shortening. No significant correlation was found between that index of performance and ei-

TABLE II   Indices of Left Ventricular Meridional Wall Stress in Normotensive Subjects and Hypertensive Patients

	Normotensive Subjects Untreated (n = 19)	Hypertensive Patients Treated (n = 37)	Hypertensive Patients Untreated (n = 37)
Index			
End-systolic stress (10^3 dynes/cm^2)	49 ± 10	62 ± 22[†]	59 ± 25[*]
Peak systolic stress (10^3 dynes/cm^2)	157 ± 26	181 ± 48[*]	185 ± 52[*]
End-isovolumetric systolic stress (10^3 dynes/cm^2)	100 ± 17	119 ± 33[*]	117 ± 34[*]

NOTE: Values = average ± 1 SD. Differences between hypertensive and normotensive groups were significant.
[*]$p < 0.02$.
[†]$p < 0.005$.

ther systolic blood pressure, peak systolic stress or end isovolumetric systolic stress ($r < 0.20$ in all groups for all these indices; Table III). In marked contrast, end-systolic stress was significantly correlated with fractional shortening in all subjects, both normotensive and hypertensive (Fig. 2).

Left ventricular "contractility" was estimated from the systolic blood pressure to end-systolic volume ratio.[18,19] This index was strongly and positively correlated with percent shortening in both treated and untreated hypertensive patients as well as in the group of normotensive subjects ($r = 0.65, 0.75, 0.75$, respectively, $p < 0.001$ for all) (Fig. 3). In contrast only a weak correlation was found between preload and ventricular performance; the correlation coefficient between diastolic left ventricular volume and fractional shortening was only -0.36 in hypertensive subjects ($p < 0.05$) and did not even attain statistical significance in the small normotensive group ($r = -0.30, p = 0.10$).

TABLE III   Left Ventricular Performance (Percent Shortening) in Relation to Different Indices of Left Ventricular Wall Stress

Group	Correlation Coefficient (r) of Percent Shortening with End-Systolic Stress	End-Isovolumetric Systolic Stress	Peak Systolic Stress
Normotensive	−0.65	−0.13	−0.02
(n = 19)	(<0.005)	(NS)	(NS)
Hypertensive			
Untreated (n = 37)	−0.66	−0.03	−0.03
	(<0.001)	(NS)	(NS)
Treated (n = 37)	−0.75	−0.19	−0.13
	(<0.001)	(NS)	(NS)

NS = not statistically significant.

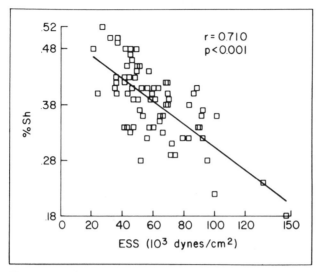

Figure 2. *A highly significant inverse correlation (r = −0.710, p <0.001) was found among all 74 subjects between end-systolic left ventricular wall stress (ESS) and left ventricular percent shortening; this also held in separate analysis of each individual group (normotensive as well as untreated and treated hypertensive) (Table III), with no significant difference in sign or slope of the regression equation.*

Multivariate Analysis of Determinants of Left Ventricular Performance:

A multiple regression analysis was performed in order to evaluate the relative role of preload, afterload, and ventricular contractility as determinants of overall left ventricular performance (dependent variable). LV end-diastolic volume (normalized for body surface area), was taken as an index of preload, end-systolic blood pressure to end-systolic volume ratio as an index of contractility. LV fractional shortening was used as an estimate of LV performance. The correlation coefficient obtained in each group was highly significant ($p < 0.001$ at least) with indices of determination ranging from 64% to 89% (Table IV). However, the components entering this multiple correlation formed a different pattern in the various groups. Whereas the index of contractility (systolic blood pressure to end-systolic volume) was the major component in normotensive subjects, it was afterload (end-systolic stress) that appeared as the major component among hypertensive subjects with either normal echo or symmetric LVH, afterload was particularly important in patients with LVH and dilatation, in whom it accounted for 75% of variations in fractional shortening. In contrast, hypertensive patients with asymmetric septal hypertrophy showed a pattern similar to that of normotensive subjects (Table IV).

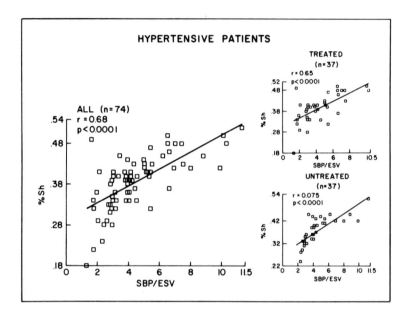

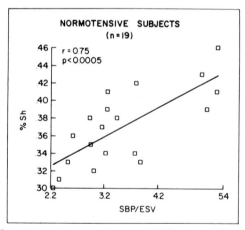

Figure 3. *Correlation between indices of LV contractility (systolic blood pressure/end-systolic volume) and of LV function (percent shortening) in hypertensive patients, and normotensive subjects.*

TABLE IV   Multivariate Analysis of Factors Influencing Left Ventricular
Contraction (Percent Shortening)

Group	Multiple Correlation* r	Multiple Correlation* r²	Major Component (r²)† (%)		Other Significant Component	Added Contribution (%)
Normotensive (n = 19)	0.879	0.77	SBP/ESV	55	LVCI	+19
Hypertensive						
Normal LV (n = 31)	0.082	0.64	ESS	49	SBP/ESV	+14
LVH (n = 15)	0.909	0.81	ESS	49	SBP/ESV	+13
					LVCI	+19
LVD (n = 12)	0.943	0.89	ESS	74	SBP/ESV	+9
Hypertensive with						
ASH (n = 16)	0.876	0.77	SBP/ESV	64	LVCI	+6

LVH = left ventricular hypertrophy; LVD = left ventricular dilation; LV = left ventricle; ASH = asymmetric septal hypertrophy; SBP = systolic blood pressure; ESV = end-systolic volume; ESS = end-systolic stress; LVCI = left ventricular cavity index.
* The multiple correlation coefficient was highly significant (p <0.001) in all groups, as was the major component of the regression equation.
† Index of determination, estimating the contribution of the major component to the overall multiple correlation.

Comments

Left Ventricular Patterns in Hypertension: This study of 74 hypertensive patients with no clinical evidence of coronary arterial disease or heart failure revealed a wide spectrum of structural changes among both treated and untreated subjects (Table I). Fifteen patients showed only concentric LVH, 16 had asymmetric septal thickening (asymmetric septal hypertrophy without systolic anterior movement of the mitral valve and without LV end-diastolic diameter greater than 5.5 cm), and 12 had a dilated left ventricle with various types of hypertrophy. The salient feature of these results was the high prevalence of asymmetric septal hypertrophy, in agreement with some[20,21] but not all[10,22,23] studies. It is important, however, to note that earlier assumptions regarding the rarity of asymmetric septal hypertrophy among hypertensive patients are being revised. Review of more than 1,368 hypertensive subjects in the Framingham study[24] revealed an incidence of 10% of disproportionate septal hypertrophy among 190 patients with echo evidence of LVH.

Various explanations have been suggested for the occurrence of asymmetric septal hypertrophy in hypertensive patients. In borderline hypertensive young subjects it has been suggested that this might be related in some way to increased sympathetic tone.[20,21] The septum, at least in its base, seems indeed to be particularly rich in sympathetic nerve supply. A more mechanical explanation is based on the flatter aspect of the septum in comparison with the posterior LV wall; this would lead to higher local tension with subsequent hypertrophy.[25] Finally, it is possible that the rapid variations in septal wall thickness that have been described following cessation of antihypertensive therapy might lead to a higher incidence of asymmetric septal hypertrophy in patients who stopped antihypertensive treatment recently. Our data do not allow us to decide between these different hypotheses; a prospective study from many centers might be required in order to delineate precisely the prevalence and factors responsible for asymmetric septal hypertrophy in different types of hypertension. There was no evidence of subaortic stenosis in any of our patients.

It has often been stated that an otherwise normal heart responds to a long-term increase in blood pressure, first by concentric hypertrophy and only later by additional dilation. The frequency of increased LV wall thickness without LV dilation in hypertension is in accord with this concept. However, the occasional occurrence of LV dilation without measurable increase in wall thickness suggests that, in some patients at least, dilation might occur early in the evolution of hypertension. Unfortunately, serial echo tracings were not available in our population. However, this suggestion may find some support in the recent data reported from the Framingham study, particularly in the offspring of hypertensive patients.[24] Among the latter (n = 2,965), 274 had echo LVH, mostly due to eccentric hypertrophy (71%), contrary to what was expected. Observations in renovascular hypertensive rats[26] and spontaneously hypertensive rats[27] have led to similar suggestions of early dilation of the LV cavity.

Reasons for variability in incidence and pattern of LVH in hypertension are difficult to delineate. We found no apparent clinical predictors by which we could recognize which type of hypertrophy was likely to develop in which type of patient. Systolic blood pressure levels were only weakly correlated with LV mass. This finding, similar to that in many previous reports,[28–30] suggests that other factors besides blood pressure level can modulate the development of LVH in hypertensive subjects.[31] Average blood pressure level from 24-hour recordings, however, might prove to be a better predictor of LVH than single readings.[32] Electrocardiographic evidence of LVH reportedly correlated better with home than with office blood pressure recordings.[33]

Correlations between LV mass and LV wall stress are subject to conflicting influences because the development and type of hypertrophy can alter LV wall stress in various ways. In that respect, the only statistically significant correlate of LV mass in this series was peak systolic stress (r = −0.30, p < 0.01). The same negative relationship was reported in children with aortic stenosis.[34] This inverse correlation might mean that the development of hypertrophy tended to normalize peak systolic wall stress.[34] The weak correlation coefficient found among our patients suggests, however, that normalization did not occur commonly, a fact clearly demonstrated by the wide scatter of the data points around the calculated line of regression.

Left Ventricular Function and Its Correlates in Hypertension: The most striking feature of this study was the significant negative correlation between end-systolic stress and percent shortening in both hypertensive and normotensive subjects (Table III, Fig. 3). These findings confirm those in previous reports that documented that relationship, by echo as well as angiographic studies.[35] End-systolic stress was found to be a much better predictor of LV performance than either systolic blood pressure or peak systolic stress.

Since LV function can also be influenced by variations in contractility, preload conditions, or both, it was more informative to evaluate the relative importance of these various factors by multiple regression analysis involving all these factors. This approach allowed us to account, to a very large degree, for the variations in percent shortening among both normotensive and hypertensive patients ($r = 0.8$ to 0.9, $p < 0.001$; Table IV). However, there was a basic difference in the relative importance of these factors in normotensive versus hypertensive subjects. Among the normotensive subjects, myocardial contractility appeared as a major factor modulating overall cardiac function; however, among hypertensive patients, LV performance was mostly afterload-dependent. This dependence on afterload was most pronounced in those patients who had associated LVH and dilation, a pattern in keeping with the effects of a progressive reduction in cardiac performance.[36] Serial echo tracings and long-term follow-up are needed for more definite conclusions.

The important influence of variations in afterload on cardiac performance in hypertension must not, however, obscure that of variations in myocardial contractility or inotropic responsiveness.[3,26] The variables influencing ventricular function at rest might not be the same as those influencing its response to a sudden stress. Thus, the cardiac response to the load imposed by static exercise was markedly dependent on adrenergic mechanisms.[37] More studies are certainly needed to correlate the different types of structural changes uncovered by echo with changes in ventricular function not only at rest but also in response to different types of stress. Furthermore, it is not really impossible to predict the pattern of evolution of a chronic disease from an examination at a single point in time; serial prospective echo studies are needed to determine the sequence of cardiac alterations in hypertension.

Summary

This study of 74 hypertensive patients has revealed a wide spectrum of changes in both LV structure and function among hypertensive subjects. Overall cardiac performance was closely related to end-systolic LV wall stress in normotensive as well as hypertensive subjects. The finding of a greater dependency on afterload among hypertensive patients than among normotensive subjects again indicates the importance of adequate blood pressure control to prevent further deterioration of cardiac function. Whether reversal of cardiac hypertrophy should also constitute a goal of that treatment still remains to be determined.[11]

Acknowledgment

Supported in part by grant NHLBI-6835 from the National Heart, Lung and Blood Institute and by the American Heart Association, Northeast Ohio Affiliate. Dr. Abi-Samra was a research fellow supported by training grant HL-7242 from the National Institutes of Health.

References

1. TARAZI RC: The role of the heart in hypertension. Clin Sci 1982; 63: 347s–358s.
2. KANNEL WB, GORDON T, OFFUTT D: Left ventricular hypertrophy by electrocardiogram: prevalence, incidence, and mortality in the Framingham Study. Ann Intern Med 1969; 71: 89–105.
3. TARAZI RC, LEVY M: Cardiac responses to increased afterload. State-of-the-art review. Hypertension 1982; 4 (suppl II): II-8–II-18.
4. TARAZI RC, FERRARIO CM, DUSTAN HP: The heart in hypertension. In: GENEST J, KOIW E, JUCHEL O, eds. Hypertension physiopathology and treatment. 1st ed. New York: McGraw-Hill, 1977; 738–754.
5. SKELTON CL, SONNENBLICK EH: Heterogeneity of contractile function in cardiac hypertrophy. Circ Res 1974; 34, 35 (suppl II): 83–96.
6. GROSSMAN W, JONES D, McLAURIN LP: Wall stress and patterns of hypertrophy in the human left ventricle. J Clin Invest 1975; 56: 56–64.
7. QUINONES MA, MOKOTOFF DM, NOURI S, et al: Noninvasive quantification of left ventricular wall stress: validation of method and application to assessment of chronic pressure overload. Am J Cardiol 1980; 45: 782–790.
8. WILSON JR, REICHEK N, HIRSHFELD J: Noninvasive assessment of load reduction in patients with asymptomatic aortic regurgitation. Am J Med 1980; 68: 664–674.
9. KARLINER JS, WILLIAMS D, GORWIT W, et al: Left ventricular hypertrophy caused by systemic hypertension. Br Heart J 1977; 39: 1239–1245.
10. SAVAGE DD, DRAYER JIM, HENRY WL, et al: Echocardiographic assessment of cardiac anatomy and function in hypertensive subjects. Circulation 1979; 59: 623–632.
11. FOUAD FM, NAKASHIMA Y, TARAZI RC, SALCEDO EE: Reversal of left ventricular hypertrophy in hypertensive patients treated with methyldopa. Lack of association with blood pressure control. Am J Cardiol 1982; 49: 795–801.
12. FEIGENBAUM H: Echocardiography, 2nd ed. Philadelphia: Lea & Febiger, 1976.
13. HENRY WL, DE MARIA A, GRAMIAK R, et al: Report of the American Society of Echocardiography Committee on Nomenclature and Standards in Two-Dimensional Echocardiography. Circulation 1980; 62: 212–217.
14. KIRKENDALL WM, BURTON AC, EPSTEIN FH, FREIS ED: Recommendations for human blood pressure determination by sphygmomanometers. Circulation 1967; 36: 980–988.

15. EL-TOBGI SM, FOUAD FM, KRAMER JR, et al: Left ventricular function in coronary artery disease comparison of E_{max}, systolic P/V ratio and ejection fraction (abstr). J Am Coll Cardiol 1983; 1: 665.

16. TROY BL, POMBO J, RACKLEY CE: Measurement of left ventricular wall thickness and mass by echocardiography. Circulation 1972; 45: 602–611.

17. TEICHHOLZ LE, KREULEN T, HERMAN AV, GORLIN R: Problems in echocardiographic volume determinations: echocardiographic-angiographic correlations in the presence or absence of asynergy. Am J Cardiol 1976; 37: 7–11.

18. SUGA H, SAGAWA K, SHOUKAS AA: Load independence of the instantaneous pressure-volume ratio of the canine left ventricle and effects of epinephrine and heart rate on the ratio. Circ Res 1973; 32: 314–322.

19. NIVATPURMIN T, KATZ S, SCHEURER J: Peak left ventricular systolic pressure/end-systolic volume ratio: a sensitive detector of left ventricular disease. AM J Cardiol 1979; 43: 969–974.

20. SAFAR ME, LEHNER JP, VINCENT MI, et al: Echocardiographic dimensions in borderline and sustained hypertension. Am J Cardiol 1979; 44: 930–935.

21. COREA L, BENTIVOGLIO M, VERDECCHIA P, et al: Left ventricular wall thickness and plasma catecholamines in borderline and stable essential hypertension. Eur Heart J 1982; 3: 163–170.

22. ABBASSI AS, MAXALPIN RN, EBER LM, PEARCE ML: Left ventricular hypertrophy diagnosed by echocardiography. N Engl J Med 1973; 289: 118–121.

23. DUNN FG, CHANDRARATNA PN, DE CARVALHO JGR, et al: Pathophysiologic assessment of hypertensive heart disease with echocardiography. Am J Cardiol 1977; 39: 789–795.

24. SAVAGE DD, GARRISON RJ, KANNEL WB, et al: Prevalence, characteristics and correlates of echocardiographic left ventricular hypertrophy in a population-based sample—preliminary findings: the Framingham Study (abstr). Circulation 1982; 66 (suppl II): II-63.

25. BURTON AC: Transmural pressures, pressure gradients and resistance to flow in the vascular bed. In: Physiology and biophysics of the circulation. Chicago: Year Book Medical Publishers, 1965; 84.

26. SARAGOCA M, TARAZI RC: Impaired cardiac contractile response to isoproterenol in the spontaneously hypertensive rats. Hypertension 1981; 3: 380–385.

27. HALLBACK-NORDLANDER M, NORESSON E, THOREN P: Hemodynamic consequences of left ventricular hypertrophy in spontaneously hypertensive rats. Am J Cardiol 1979; 44: 986–993.

28. HARTFORD M, WIKSTRAND J, WALLENTIN I, et al: Non-invasive signs of cardiac involvement in essential hypertension. Eur Heart J 1982; 3: 75–87.

29. FROHLICH ED, TARAZI RC: Is arterial pressure the sole factor responsible for hypertensive cardiac hypertrophy. Am J Cardiol 1979; 44: 959–963.

30. DEVEREUX R, SAVAGE DD, SACHS I, LARAGH JH: Effect of blood pressure control on left ventricular hypertrophy and function in hypertension (abstr). Circulation 1980; 62 (suppl II): III-36.

31. TARAZI RC, SEN S, SARAGOCA M, KHAIRALLAH PA: The multifactorial role of catecholamines in hypertensive cardiac hypertrophy. Eur Heart J 1982; 3: 103–110.

32. DEVEREUX RB, PICKERING TG, HARSHFIELD GA, et al: Does home blood pressure

improve prediction of cardiac changes in patients with hypertension? Circulation 1982; 66 (suppl II): II-63.

33. IBRAHIM MM, TARAZI RC, DUSTAN HP, GIFFORD RW JR: Electrocardiogram in evaluation of resistance to antihypertensive therapy. Arch Intern Med 1977; 137: 1125–1129.

34. BLACKWOOD RA, BLOOM KR, WILLIAMS CM: Aortic stenosis in children. Experience with echocardiographic prediction of severity. Circulation 1978; 57: 263–268.

35. STRAUER BE: Ventricular function and coronary hemodynamics in hypertensive heart disease. Am J Cardiol 1979; 44: 999–1006.

36. COHN J: Vasodilator therapy for heart failure: the influence of impedance on left ventricular performance. Circulation 1973; 48: 5–8.

37. ALICANDRI C, FOUAD FM, TARAZI RC, BRAVO EL, GREENSTREET RL: Sympathetic contribution to the cardiac response to stress in hypertension. Hypertension 1983; 5: 147–154.

13

Systolic Function of the Hypertrophied Left Ventricle: Hypertension and Aortic Stenosis

JEFFREY S. BORER, M.D.
JEFFREY FISHER, M.D.
RICHARD B. DEVEREUX, M.D.
MICHAEL JASON, M.D.
MICHAEL V. GREEN, M.S.
STEPHEN L. BACHARACH, Ph.D.
THOMAS PICKERING, M.D.
JOHN H. LARAGH, M.D.

Chronically increased impedance to left ventricular (LV) outflow usually results in hypertrophy with increased LV mass. Abnormal wall stress due to increased ventricular pressure load is mitigated by this hypertrophic response.[1,2] These two processes, pressure loading with increased wall stress and myocardial hypertrophy, have opposing effects on LV mechanical performance. Hence, the systolic function of the chronically pressure-loaded left ventricle cannot be inferred from the existence of abnormal afterload per se. To begin to define systolic performance in the chronically pressure-loaded hypertrophied ventricle, we tabulated our preliminary data from assessments of LV function at rest and during exercise in patients with systemic hypertension and aortic stenosis.

Hypertension

Patients with systemic hypertension generally are classified according to the severity of arterial pressure elevation.[3] Although prognostic determinations and therapeutic decisions can be made from such a classification, determination of risk based on blood pressure measurement alone may be an imperfect predictor of clinical outcome for the individual patient. It is possible that by assessing the functional effects of hypertension on the heart, a more accurate determination of risk and more appropriate therapeutic decisions can be made.

To evaluate this hypothesis, we studied the relationship between arterial pressure and cardiac function in patients with essential hypertension.[4] All

60 patients thus far studied have manifested arterial diastolic pressure of 90 mmHg or greater; none had clinical or laboratory evidence of either renovascular disease or primary hyperaldosteronism. No patient had symptoms of pulmonary vascular congestion, typical angina pectoris, or evidence of valvular heart disease. Average systolic and diastolic pressures were 150 and 103 mmHg, respectively. Phamacologic therapy was withheld for at least 1 week before the study. Arterial pressure was determined by cuff sphygmomanometry in the seated position, using phases 1 and 5 of the Korotkoff sounds. Arterial pressure was recorded as the average of all readings obtained off antihypertensive therapy. M-mode echos were performed using standard techniques.[5,6] End-systolic meridional wall stress, an index of LV afterload, was calculated by the method of Wilson et al[7] using echo dimensions and cuff blood pressure. Equilibrium radionuclide cineangiography for assessment of LV function was performed with patients in the supine position at rest and during exercise after intravenous administration of 10 to 20 mCi of technetium-99m.[8,9] Exercise was begun at a load of 25 W and was increased by 25 W increments at 2-minute intervals until the development of exercise-limiting dyspnea, fatigue, or chest discomfort.

Systolic Arterial Pressure Versus Left Ventricular Function at Rest: All but 1 patient manifested a normal or supernormal LV ejection fraction at rest as determined by radionuclide cineangiography. A positive correlation existed between systolic arterial pressure and ejection fraction, confirming the finding of Blaufox et al.[10] This relationship was strongest in patients less than 50 years of age,[4] suggesting the possibility that hypertrophy in younger patients may be manifested as improved mechanical performance in the resting state, when ventricular afterload is relatively low.

Although a statistically significant linear relationship between arterial pressure and ejection fraction was demonstrated, the correlation coefficient was only 0.33 ($p < 0.01$), indicating that, in any person, LV performance at rest could not be predicted from arterial pressure alone.[4]

Systolic Arterial Pressure Versus Left Ventricular Ejection Fraction During Exercise: Prior investigations in patients with coronary and valvular heart disease have indicated that myocardial dysfunction is often inapparent with the patient at rest, but may be manifested only during the interposition of stress.[9,11,12] Therefore, we studied the relationship between resting systolic pressure and the ejection fraction, both during exercise and during the change in LV ejection fraction from rest to exercise (LV functional reserve). In normal subjects the ejection fraction invariably increases by at least 5% during exercise to an absolute level of 54% or greater. In our 60 patients with hypertension, a subnormal LV ejection fraction during exercise was seen in 6, one of whom underwent catheterization and was found to be free of coronary stenosis.[4] An additional 13 patients had subnormal LV functional reserve.

Left ventricular functional reserve manifested a significant but modest inverse linear relationship to resting blood pressure ($r = -0.35$, $p < 0.01$) (Fig. 1).[4] Hence, prediction of LV functional reserve in the individual patient cannot be made from arterial pressure measurement alone. No differences in

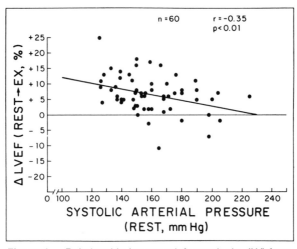

Figure 1. *Relationship between left ventricular (LV) functional reserve (change in LV ejection fraction from rest to exercise) and resting systolic arterial pressure. There is a modest inverse linear relationship between functional reserve and arterial pressure. However, for individual patients arterial pressure cannot be used for prediction of LV functional reserve.*

exercise response were attributable to age or known duration of hypertension.

Left Ventricular Wall Stress Versus Function at Rest and During Exercise: Since arterial pressure is only one component of LV afterload, it might be more reasonable to expect that ventricular performance would be predicted by a measure of total afterload rather than solely by blood pressure. Therefore, we employed echo in 43 of these patients to determine LV wall stress, a direct measure of afterload, which represents a synthesis of information, including blood pressure, LV volume and mass. A strong relationship was found between resting systolic function and afterload stress in these hypertensive patients, and systolic function could be predicted moderately well from assessment of wall stress (Fig. 2).[4] Two patients manifested subnormal systolic function for the level of afterload apparent at the time of testing. This suggests that in some asymptomatic hypertensive patients intrinsically depressed myocardial contractile function may be present. In these patients it appears that depressed systolic function is not merely a reflection of loading stresses; in these 2 patients, arterial pressures were well within the range noted in our other patients.

Moreover, these 2 patients also manifested subnormal ejection fraction responses during exercise, consistent with the presumption of the presence of depressed myocardial function. Absence of a normal ejection fraction response during exercise was additionally noted in 12 patients who manifested a normal fractional shortening response to afterload at rest.[4] It is possible

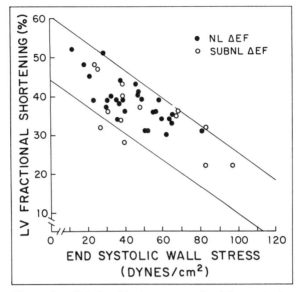

Figure 2. *Relationship between echo left ventricular (LV) fractional shortening at rest, a measure of systolic performance, and LV end-systolic wall stress. Open circles indicate patients whose LV ejection fraction response was subnormal during exercise. The 2 solid lines represent confidence limits 2 SD from the mean for the fractional shortening-end-systolic wall stress response approximating those found in our normal subjects.*

that these patients have had intrinsic myocardial damage, but that it is sufficiently mild so that it has not yet caused subnormal responses to loading stresses present at rest.

To evaluate this hypothesis, it would be necessary to measure wall stress during exercise and to evaluate directly the relationship between LV performance and afterload. Technical limitations make such determinations difficult at present. However, we found that the blood pressure component of afterload, measured as the change in systolic pressure from rest to exercise, bore no relationship to the change in ejection fraction from rest to exercise. Similarly, no relationship existed between absolute ejection fraction during exercise and systolic pressure during exercise, or between the exercise-induced change in ejection fraction during exercise and the systolic pressure during exercise.

Left Ventricular Mass and End-Diastolic Volume Versus Left Ventricular Systolic Function

The contention that abnormal LV functional reserve is attributable to the presence of intrinsically abnormal myocardium is also supported by the finding of only a modest inverse correlation between ejection fraction and LV mass and end-diastolic volume.[13]

Preliminary Conclusions: Our data suggest the possibility that we can usefully classify patients with hypertension into three groups on the basis of noninvasive assessment of LV systolic function. The first group has evidence of load-independent LV dysfunction at rest, as well as by subnormal LV functional reserve during exercise. These patients might be expected to have the poorest long-term prognosis and to require particularly aggressive pharmacologic attempts at afterload reduction, perhaps sufficient to lower arterial pressure well below levels now considered to be therapeutically acceptable. The second group does not manifest abnormalities at rest, but has subnormal LV functional reserve. The third group comprises those patients with normal LV function at rest and during exercise. These patients might be expected to have the best long-term outlook. It is of particular note that these groups cannot be separated on the basis of arterial pressure measurement alone, the current standard for stratification of risk in the hypertensive patient. These preliminary results suggest that, for purposes of designing optimal therapeutic regimens, proper categorization of hypertensive patients may need to include objective assessment of LV systolic function, rather than measurement of arterial pressure alone.

Aortic Stenosis

The studies in patients with hypertension emphasize the potential clinical importance of assessment of LV function in patients with myocardial hypertrophy, but have not as yet delineated the functional response of the hypertrophied left ventricle to therapeutic removal of the underlying afterload stress. Preliminary results of studies performed at the National Heart, Lung and Blood Institute in patients with aortic stenosis provide information regarding the functional response to therapy.[14]

Preoperative Studies: In these studies, radionuclide cineangiography was employed during exercise in 26 symptomatic patients with isolated, hemodynamically severe aortic stenosis (peak-to-peak transvalvular systolic gradient 50 mmHg or greater), to obtain an accurate assessment of LV function at rest and during exercise, and to assess the effects of aortic valve replacement on exercise-induced dysfunction. Exercise was continued until the development of moderate angina, dyspnea, severe fatigue, or a decrease in systolic blood pressure greater than 10 mmHg. All patients older than age 35 years had undergone coronary arteriography, and no patient included in this series had greater than 30% narrowing of any coronary artery.

In the patients with aortic stenosis, average ejection fraction at rest was 67%, a significantly supernormal value (average normal, 57%, $p < 0.05$); during exercise, the average ejection fraction decreased to 56%, moderately subnormal (average normal, 71%, $p < 0.05$).[14] In these patients with aortic stenosis, the LV ejection fraction ranged widely at rest and, as with our hypertensive patients, often was considerably higher than normal, particularly in younger patients. During exercise, the response was variable, with

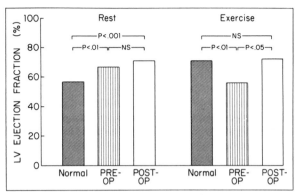

Figure 3. *Average left ventricular (LV) ejection fractions at rest and during exercise in normal subjects and in 12 patients with aortic stenosis before and after aortic valve replacement. NS = not significant.*

some patients maintaining a high normal ejection fraction during intense exercise. Most commonly, however, in contrast to the results in the patients with hypertension, the ejection fraction decreased during exercise, often to a marked degree.[14] Thus, resting ejection fraction could not be used to predict the abnormal functional reserve demonstrated during exercise.

To elucidate factors that might predict LV response to exercise, we compared the LV ejection fraction during exercise with several hemodynamic parameters. The LV ejection fraction during exercise did not show significant correlation with resting transvalvular gradient, peak LV systolic pressure, cardiac output, or LV end-diastolic pressure. However, exercise ejection fraction correlated with aortic valve area index (r = 0.60). This apparent relationship between LV functional reserve and valve area suggests that the mechanical obstruction to outflow plays an important role in determining ejection fraction during exercise in aortic stenosis. Therefore, intrinsic myocardial damage might be relatively less important as a cause of exercise-induced dysfunction in patients with aortic stenosis than is actual impedance to outflow.

Postoperative Studies: To assess this hypothesis, patients with aortic stenosis were restudied 6 months after operation. Preliminary results in the first 12 patients demonstrated that the ejection fraction was improved at rest and usually reached levels within the normal range during exercise[14] (Fig. 3). Parenthetically, these findings contrast with postoperative results in patients with aortic regurgitation, associated with hypertrophy due to volume loading, in whom LV function is often subnormal during exercise following valve replacement.[12]

Preliminary Conclusions: Thus, preliminary results indicate that even though high normal ejection fraction often is present at rest in patients with severe aortic stenosis, the stress of exercise often causes a marked decrease in this measure of ventricular performance. This finding cannot be predicted from resting hemodynamic parameters measured routinely at catheterization and may prove of prognostic importance. However, the response of ejection fraction during exercise correlates with the degree of outflow tract obstruction indicated by the calculated aortic valve area. This suggests that the reduced LV functional reserve could, in large part, be a reversible result of excessive impedance to LV outflow rather than of intrinsic myocardial damage. This possibility is supported by results of study after operation, which indicate a return to normal LV ejection fraction during exercise, even in patients with markedly depressed functional reserve before operation. Moreover, early studies indicate that such functional changes after operation are associated with at least partial resolution of LV hypertrophy.[15] Quantitative dissimilarities in the response of LV ejection fraction during exercise are apparent when results of studies in patients with aortic stenosis are compared with those in patients with systemic arterial hypertension, in that patients with aortic stenosis more uniformly manifest depressed LV ejection fraction with exercise. However, the restitution of normal function during exercise after valve replacement in patients with aortic stenosis suggests, consistent with the early data of Blaufox et al,[10] that with aggressive antihypertensive therapy, normal LV functional reserve could be restored to patients with systemic hypertension who have developed hypertrophy and LV systolic dysfunction with stress. Further studies will be necessary to verify these findings and to delineate clinical benefits.

Acknowledgment

Dr. Borer was an Established Investigator of The American Heart Association during the performance of these studies, and was supported, in part, by the American Heart Association, Dallas, Texas.

References

1. GROSSMAN W, JONES D, McLAURIN LP: Wall stress and patterns of hypertrophy in the human left ventricle. J Clin Invest 1975; 56: 56–64.
2. GUNTHER S, GROSSMAN W: Determinants of ventricular function in pressure-overload hypertrophy in man. Circulation 1979; 59: 679–688.
3. Veterans Administration Cooperative Study Group on Hypertensive Agents: Effects of treatment on morbidity in hypertension. III. Influence of age, diastolic ressure, and prior cardiovascular disease, further analysis of analysis of side-effects. Circulation 1972; 45: 991–1004.
4. JASON M, BORER JS, DEVEREUX RB, JACOBSTEIN J, PICKERING T, LARAGH JH: Load-independent left ventricular dysfunction in hypertension: noninvasive detection (abstr). Am J Cardiol 1982; 49: 996.
5. SAHN DJ, DeMARIA A, KISSLO J, WEYMAN A: Recommendation regarding quantitation in M-mode echocardiography: results in a survey of echocardiographic measurements. Circulation 1978; 58: 1072–1083.

6. Devereux RB, Reichek N: Echocardiographic determination of left ventricular mass in man: anatomic validation of the method. Circulation 1977; 55: 613–618.

7. Wilson JR, Reichek N, Hirshfeld J: Noninvasive assessment of load reduction in patients with asymptomatic aortic regurgitation. Am J Med 1980; 68: 664–674.

8. Bacharach SL, Green MV, Borer JS, Douglas MA, Ostrow HG, Johnston GS: A real-time system for multi-image gated cardiac studies. J Nucl Med 1977; 18: 79–84.

9. Borer JS, Bacharach SL, Green MV, Kent KM, Epstein SE, Johnston GS: Real-time radionuclide cineangiography in the non-invasive evaluation of global and regional left ventricular function at rest and during exercise in patients with coronary artery disease. N Engl J Med 1977; 296: 839–844.

10. Blaufox MD, Wexler, JP, Sherman RA, et al: Left ventricular ejection fraction and its response to therapy in essential hypertension. Nephron 1981; 28: 112–117.

11. Borer JS, Kent KM, Bacharach SL, et al: Sensitivity, specificity and predictive accuracy of radionuclide cineangiography during exercise in patients with coronary artery disease: comparison with exercise electrocardiography. Circulation 1979; 60: 572–580.

12. Borer JS, Bacharach SL, Green MV, et al: Exercise-induced left ventricular dysfunction in symptomatic and asymptomatic patients with aortic regurgitation: assessment by radionuclide cineangiography. Am J Cardiol 1978; 42: 351–357.

13. Jason M, Herrold E, Borer JS, et al: Depressed left ventricular functional reserve in essential hypertension: pathophysiologic implications (abstr). J Am Coll Cardiol 1984; 3: 591.

14. Borer JS, Bacharach SL, Green MV, et al: Left ventricular function in aortic stenosis, response to exercise and effects of operation. Am J Cardiol 1978; 41: 382.

15. Henry WL, Bonow RO, Borer JS, et al: Evaluation of aortic valve replacement in patients with valvular aortic stenosis. Circulation 1980; 61: 814–825.

14

Diastolic Function of the Hypertrophied Left Ventricle

JOHN WIKSTRAND, M.D., Ph.D.

For some decades, cardiologic research laboratories have focused their interest on studying isovolumetric contraction and the ejection phase, and until recently little attention was paid to diastolic heart function, an area of special interest in connection with left ventricular hypertrophy (LVH).

The purpose of this chapter is to describe the functional consequences of LVH in early primary hypertension in man, with special reference to diastolic function of the left heart. The results of different studies of this topic depend greatly on which stage of hypertension is explored, that is, by the prevailing extent of hypertensive complications, such as coronary heart disease, LV failure, kidney disorders, and other complicating diseases, such as generalized arteriosclerosis or diabetes. This chapter will concentrate mainly on the early phases before these complications are clinically detectable through signs or symptoms.

Research Studies

Table I[1–10] summarizes the results of work on LV diastolic and systolic function in early primary hypertension in man. In many of these studies the findings have not been related to LV wall thickness. In Figures 1 and 2, therefore, results are also presented from a study performed in Göteborg, Sweden, where findings regarding LV diastolic and systolic function were related to LV wall thickness.[11–14] In that study a noninvasive investigation was undertaken in 49-year-old men (n = 120, with no echo studies, for anatomic reasons, in 11 men) who had blood pressure screening in an epidemiologically defined subsample. None of the men had had antihypertensive treatment. They were divided into four groups by blood pressure: normotensive (n = 21); borderline blood pressure elevation (n = 30); mild blood pressure elevation (n = 45); and moderate blood pressure elevation (n = 24). There was a successive increase in blood pressure, LV wall thickness, and total peripheral resistance (TPR) from the normotensive subjects to the group with moderate blood pressure elevation (Fig. 2). The last group could be divided into two subgroups, one with and one without a significant increase in LV wall thickness (Fig. 2).[13]

TABLE I — **Review of Studies Dealing with Left Ventricular (LV) Diastolic and Systolic Function in Early Primary Hypertension**

Reference	Diastole				Systole
		Distensibility			
	Relaxation	Passive Filling	Atrial Contraction	Isovolumetric Contraction	Ejection Phase
Dunn et al[1]					
Finding	0	↓ (Left atrium)		0	↔
Variable	–	Left atrium		–	SV, EF, FS
Method	–	E		–	E
Guazzi et al[2]					
Finding	0	0	0	0	↑
Variable	–	–	–	–	SV, mean V_{CF}
Method	–	–	–	–	Dye/E
Savage et al[3]					
Finding	0	↓	0	0	↔
Variable	–	E-F slope	–	–	FS, EF
Method	–	E	–	–	E
Fouad et al[4]					
Finding	0	↓	0	0	↔ or ↑
Variable	–	Fill rate	–	–	ejec rate
Method	–	G	–	–	G
Dreslinski et al[5,6]					
Finding	0	↓	0	0	↑
Variable	–	AEI	–	–	Mean V_{CF}
Method	–	E	–	–	E
Devereux et al[7]					
Finding	0	↓		0	↔
Variable	–	LV wall thick/CO		–	FS/ESWS
Method	–	E		–	E
Johnsson et al[8]					
Finding	0	0	0	0	↑
Variable	–	–	–	–	FS, mean V_{CF}/PSWS
Method	–	–	–	–	E
Wikstrand et al, Hartford et al, and Hartford[9–14]					
Finding	↓	↓	↓	↑	↔ or ↑
Variable	A_2O	AEI	a/H and IV	P rise vel	SV, FS/ESWS, mean V_{CF}
Method	Ph/A	E	A and Ph	Ph/A/C	E/C/Ph

Fill = filling; ejec = ejection; thick = thickness. Methods: A = apex cardiography; C = carotid pulse tracing; E = echo; G = gated blood pool; Ph = phonocardiography. Variables: AEI = atrial emptying index; CO = cardiac output; EF = ejection fraction; ESWS = end-systolic wall stress; FS = fractional shortening; IV = fourth heart sound; PSWS = peak systolic wall stress; P rise vel = pressure rise velocity; SV = stroke volume; 0 = not studied; ↔ = normal; ↓ = prolonged or decreased; ↑ = supernormal.

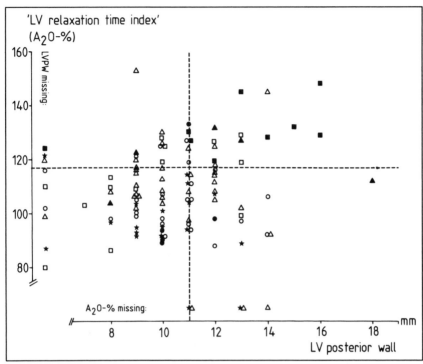

Figure 1. *Left ventricular relaxation time index (A_2O-%) in relation to left ventricular posterior wall thickness and signs of lowered left ventricular distensibility (a/H ratio more than 15%) in four groups (for explanation see text). Note the presence of a prolonged left ventricular relaxation time index (117% or greater) in several subjects with normal left ventricular wall thickness (arbitrarily defined as 11 mm or greater) and normal left ventricular distensibility (a/H ratio 15% or less). * = normotensive group; ○ = borderline group; △ = mild hypertensive group; □ = moderate hypertensive group. (Reprinted with permission from Hartford et al.[13])*

Blood Pressure and Left Ventricular Wall Thickness

No simple linear relationship exists in persons with primary hypertension between the recorded blood pressure level and the degree of LVH, whether measured as wall thickness, wall to lumen ratio, or LV mass. This may partly be explained by genetic factors and the fact that the hypertrophic process is modified by hormonal and metabolic factors with trophic influence.[15,16] The time factor is also important, but is generally unknown, both in respect to the blood pressure levels during the previous few months or years and to the diurnal variations.[17] A further factor of importance is probably the hemodynamic profile of the hypertension, wall thickness (but not necessarily LV mass, see later) being more pronounced in high-resistance hypertension

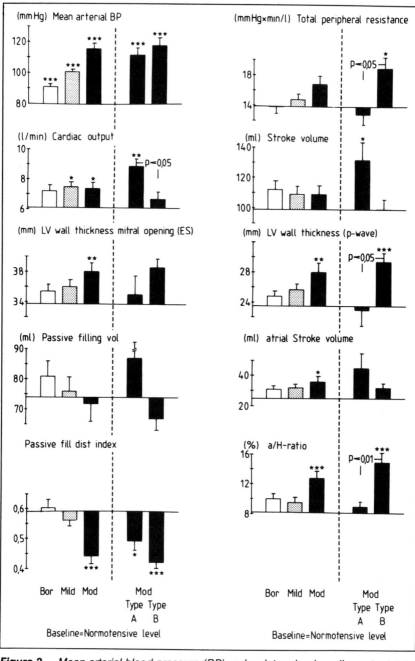

Figure 2. Mean arterial blood pressure (BP), echo-determined cardiac output, total peripheral resistance, and stroke volume in 4 groups, one of which is composed of 2 subgroups with moderate blood pressure elevation, one with high-output hypertension and the other with high-resistance hypertension. Left ventricular wall thickness at mitral valve opening (left panel) and at the p-wave in the electrocardiogram before atrial contraction (right panel) is also illustrated, together with calculated values for the respective contribution of passive filling and atrial contraction to the recorded stroke volume, and 2 indices of LV distensibility, one during passive filling (synonymous with atrial emptying index, see Table I) and the other during atrial contraction (a/H ratio). The bars indicate 1 SEM. ES = end-systolic. * = $p < 0.05$, ** = $p < 0.01$, *** = $p < 0.001$. For explanation, see text. (Reprinted with permission from Hartford and Wikstrand.[12])

than in high-output hypertension at similar blood pressure levels (Fig. 2).[14,18]

It is quite clear, therefore, that there are great individual variations in wall thickness in early primary hypertension, even in groups with comparable blood pressures. Aware that there are many variations on the theme, an attempt will be made to describe the effects of increased wall thickness on LV diastolic function.

Left Ventricular Wall Thickness and Left Ventricular Relaxation

It is clear from Table I that a prolongation of LV relaxation may be recorded despite a normal or supernormal LV systolic function in early primary hypertension.[4,10,12–14,18] Mechanical relaxation of the heart is a complex process and the exact reason for a prolonged LV relaxation time in people with early primary hypertension is not yet completely understood.[19] Data presented in Figure 1 about LV relaxation time index indicate that an increase in LV wall thickness above normal limits might be of importance for a prolonged LV relaxation in some hypertensive subjects, but not in all. Collagen and elastin endowment changing geometry of the left ventricle, regional variations in wall thickness, interstitial fibrosis, and loss of myocardial contractile elements or of normal intracellular connections are other factors suggested as being responsible for a delay in LV relaxation.[19] Any of these factors may be present in people with early primary hypertension.

The question also arises whether an impairment in the active energy-dependent intracellular shifts of calcium ions that are necessary for relaxation to occur could be of importance for a prolongation.[20,21] As discussed by Nayler and Williams,[20] there are several possible ways for an impairment in active relaxation to be effected, for instance, an inadequate supply of adenosine triphosphate (ATP), a defective calcium-accumulating activity of the sarcoplasmic reticulum, or an increased calcium influx from the extracellular space. Relaxation could well be disturbed by any of these mechanisms in the absence of an increase in LV wall thickness, as it was in many of the hypertensive subjects in the Göteborg study (Fig. 1).

A prolonged LV relaxation time reduces the time for passive LV filling, which could cause problems when heart rate is increased, for example, during physical exertion, especially if filling is also impaired because of decreased LV distensibility (see later). The situation becomes even worse if the active atrial contraction becomes weakened. The functional consequences of prolonged relaxation in early primary hypertension have hardly been studied, but it has been suggested that a prolongation of LV relaxation may be one explanation for impaired filling during the passive filling phase.[4,10,13] This in turn may have a negative impact on cardiac output (CO).

Left Ventricular Wall Thickness and Left Ventricular Filling

Increased LV wall thickness leads to reduced distensibility and an altered filling pattern of the left ventricle, as illustrated in Figure 2 (see also Table I).

Signs of reduced ventricular distensibility have been registered during the passive filling phase in the form of a reduced rate of closure of the mitral valve during diastole,[3] a reduced LV filling rate, measured by isotope techniques,[4] and a decreasing passive filling volume, measured indirectly by echo[5,12,22] (Fig. 2). Signs of reduced LV distensibility during atrial contraction have been reported in the form of an increased atrial sound and an increased a-wave on the apex cardiogram.[9,13,23] Signs of reduced LV distensibility have also been recorded in the form of an enlarged left atrium on the echo[1] and a decreasing CO with an increase in LV wall thickness[7,12] (Fig. 2).

Because of the low filling pressure of the left ventricle in relation to its wall thickness, even small changes in wall thickness will have appreciable functional consequences for the LV filling pattern. When the LV wall thickness increases, a relatively smaller part of the ventricular filling is achieved during the passive filling phases and a relatively larger part during late diastole by a more powerful atrial contraction (Fig. 2).

If the increase in wall thickness becomes more pronounced, however, the left atrium is unable to maintain the end-diastolic volume at the same level as before, which probably explains why the stroke volume (SV) decreases from the previously increased levels[2,12] (Fig. 2). This may be misinterpreted as partial heart failure, but actually only reflects a reduced diastolic volume and reduced utilization of the Frank-Starling mechanism due to reduced LV distensibility. At this stage, a reduced distensibility of the venous capacitance vessels, probably due to both functional and structural factors,[24,25] may prevent a more serious decrease in LV filling and hence in SV and CO.

End-Diastolic Volume as a Main Determinant of Cardiac Output

It is generally appreciated that CO is dependent on heart rate and LV end-systolic volume. Few observers have noted that changes in LV SV and CO are also very dependent on LV end-diastolic volume. The LV end-diastolic volume, in turn, is very dependent on LV wall thickness. Because of the low filling pressure of the left ventricle in relation to its wall thickness, even minor increases in LV wall thickness decrease LV filling and hence lead to a reduction in SV and CO, as already discussed.

For obvious reasons, these mechanisms are not easy to study prospectively in man. Repeated studies during antihypertensive treatment, however, offer a suitable model. Despite being semiquantitative, echo is an ideal tool because changes in SV may be related to changes in the two determinants of SV—end-diastolic and end-systolic LV volume.

The afterload reduction at the start of antihypertensive treatment will lead to an almost immediate decrease in end-systolic LV volume, tending to increase SV. Nevertheless, a general finding in echo studies is a simultaneous reduction in LV end-diastolic volume tending to decrease SV.[26] The reason for this initial decrease in LV end-diastolic diameter and hence LV filling recorded after starting antihypertensive treatment in most echo studies published is not yet clear, but an effect on the venous capacitance function that

decreases venous return to the heart seems likely. The net effect is a reduction in SV, and if heart rate is also reduced by the treatment, a significant
decrease in CO will be recorded[26–29] (Fig. 3).

The only way to get a significant increase in CO again from this decreased
level is to improve LV filling. This will take time, however, since it implies an
improvement in LV diastolic function with reversal of hypertrophy. Two
echo investigations have been published with repeated investigations during
antihypertensive treatment. In one study, echo was performed every 6
months over a period of 2 years[26,27] and in investigations by Schlant
et al,[28,29] it was 1 and 5 years after treatment started (Fig. 3). In these studies
an initial decrease in CO was recorded after treatment started, which was
caused by reduced heart rate and reduced SV. The tendency of SV to decrease initially was due to a reduction in LV end-diastolic diameter and hence
in end-diastolic filling volume, and not to an increase in LV end-systolic volume, which on the contrary decreased.

As shown in Figure 3, the hemodynamic condition after 1 year's treatment
differed in several important respects from that after treatment for 2 to 5
years, at which time CO was again recorded at the level before treatment
started.

As is clear from Figure 3, about 80% of the increase in CO that occurs
between 1 and 2 years'[26,27] and 1 and 5 years' treatment[28,29] is explained by
an increase in LV end-diastolic volume. This increase in end-
diastolic volume is probably explained by improved compliance of the left
ventricle secondary to the decrease in LV wall thickness. It has then been
assumed that the filling pressure has remained essentially unchanged after 1
year's treatment.

The clinically important increase in LV end-diastolic volume occurs despite
the fact that the change in LV wall thickness during the same period at first
sight seems slight. The findings, therefore, illustrate how very sensitive LV
end-diastolic volume and CO are to small changes in LV wall thickness, and
to other structural changes, (elastin and collagen endowment) that increase
LV wall stiffness in hypertension.

Left Ventricular Mass and Hemodynamics

It is clear from Figure 3 that important changes in LV wall thickness and in
CO may be recorded after the first year of antihypertensive treatment, even
when there is no change in LV mass. This is because LV mass is defined both
by LV wall thickness and LV end-diastolic diameter. Therefore, LV mass may
stay unchanged if LV end-diastolic diameter increases when LV wall thickness decreases. This type of change is to be expected because the distensibility of the left ventricle and hence LV end-diastolic diameter may increase
when LV wall thickness decreases. When studying the important functional
consequences of LV hypertrophy, it is not enough to relate these to LV mass.
The LV wall thickness and LV end-diastolic volume to LV wall thickness ratio
must be studied in order to understand the complexities.

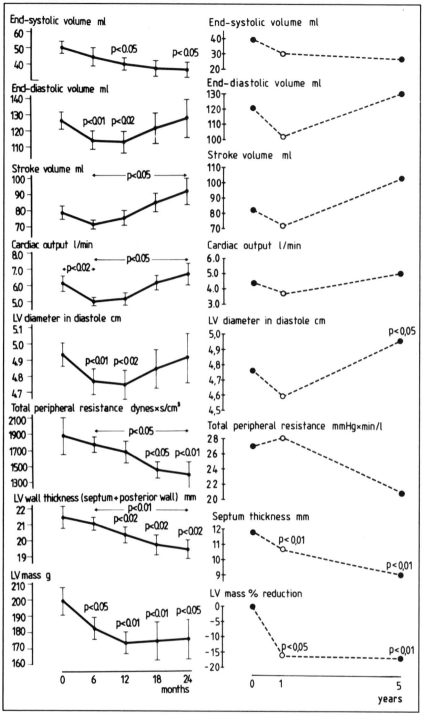

Figure 3. Echo-determined SV in relation to LV end-diastolic and end-systolic volume during antihypertensive treatment. Also illustrated are CO and total peripheral resistance and echo-determined LV mass in relation to its two determinants: LV wall thickness and LV end-diastolic diameter. Left panel: Results from Wikstrand et al.[26,27] Right panel: Results from Schlant et al.[28,29] The LV volumes given are approximations calculated from the mean values for the LV diameters by the D^3 formula or calculations from given values for SV and ejection fraction. The values given for total peripheral resistance are approximations calculated by dividing the mean values for mean arterial blood pressure and CO. Not tested for statistical significance.

Clinical Implications

Reduction in LV Wall Thickness: All antihypertensive treatment is aimed at reducing afterload. In order to improve hemodynamics in those patients in whom hypertrophy has developed, therapy should also aim at improving preload, since LV end-diastolic volume is the main determinant of cardiac output during long-term antihypertensive treatment. This improvement in preload implies an increase in LV end-diastolic volume secondary to a decrease in LV wall thickness during long-term antihypertensive treatment. Further studies are needed to examine these mechanisms, necessitating repeated investigations over several years of antihypertensive treatment.

Antihypertensive treatment that reduces LV wall thickness without improving diastolic function, LV filling, and hence CO would seem to be of limited clinical value from a hemodynamic point of view.

Aging and LV Diastolic Filling: With increasing age from 50 to 70 years, there is an increase in LV relaxation time index of about 20% and in total electromechanical systole of about 10% (unpublished data). This means that the time available for LV filling at a heart rate of 60 beats/minute decreases from about 470 to 400 ms. When heart rate increases to 100 beats/minute, the time available for LV filling decreases to only 25% of this, that is, about 110 ms (Fig. 4). If LV hypertrophy or fibrosis is present, this will not only shorten this period still more, but also reduce LV distensibility. This unfortunately places the patient in a vicious circle. Even at heart rates as low as 100 to 120 beats/minute, the filling time becomes critical for the aged, hypertrophied left ventricle.

In many elderly hypertensive patients with symptoms of heart failure, therefore, this might not be due to poor systolic contraction, but to poor filling in stiff hearts.[30,31]

The situation is analogous to that in mitral stenosis in which SV and CO decreases with increasing heart rate because the degree of filling of the left ventricle is more time dependent than under normal conditions at a younger age.

In this situation, a reduction in preload may deteriorate LV function and decrease the physical capacity. If, instead, heart rate during physical exertion can be lowered with antiadrenergic therapy from, for example, 100 to 80 beats/minute, the diastolic filling time will increase by nearly 100% (Fig. 4), thereby increasing LV end-diastolic volume, SV, and CO and improve the physical capacity of the patient.[30] This, then, is due to prolonged time for LV diastolic filling.

Traditionally, heart failure has been associated with a decreased systolic inotropy in the left ventricle and therapeutic measures have been directed toward this (digitalis and other inotropic drugs and diuretics). By studying the relationship between ejection fraction and end-systolic wall stress, it should be possible to differentiate between heart failure due to deficient preload (mainly due to decreased distensibility in a hypertrophied left ventricle) and heart failure due to decreased systolic inotropy (classic heart failure).[18]

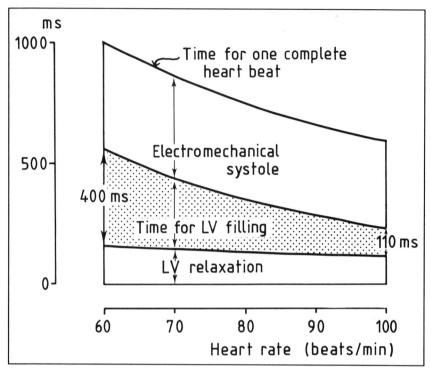

Figure 4. *Time available for LV diastolic filling at different heart rates at age 70 years (unpublished data). Note that when heart rate is lowered from 100 to 80 beats/minute, the time available for filling increases two fold.*

Further studies are needed in this field to define in a more precise manner the pathophysiologic consequences of LV hypertrophy, especially in regard to LV diastolic function in elderly patients with symptoms of heart failure. The time factor regarding LV diastolic filling is probably of increasing importance with increasing age and LV hypertrophy.

References

1. DUNN FB, CHANDRARATNA P, DECARVALHO JGR, BASTA LL, FROHLICH ED: Pathophysiologic assessment of hypertensive heart disease with echocardiography. Am J Cardiol 1977; 39: 789–795.
2. GUAZZI M, FIORENTINI C, OLIVARI MT, POLESE A: Cardiac load and function in hypertension. Am J Cardiol 1979; 44: 1007–1014.
3. SAVAGE DD, DRAYER JIM, HENRY WL, et al: Echocardiographic assessment of cardiac anatomy and function in hypertensive subjects. Circulation 1979; 59: 623–632.
4. FOUAD FM, TARAZI RC, GALLAGHER JH, MACINTYRE WJ, COOK SA: Abnormal left

ventricular relaxation in hypertensive patients. Clin Sci 1980; 59 (suppl 6): 411s–414.

5. DRESLINSKI GR, FROHLICH ED, DUNN FG, MESSERLI FH, SUAREZ DH, REISIN E: Echocardiographic diastolic ventricular abnormality in hypertensive heart disease: atrial emptying index. Am J Cardiol 1981; 47: 1087–1090.

6. DRESLINSKI GR, MESSERLI FH, DUNN FG, FROHLICH ED: Early hypertension and cardiac work. Am J Cardiol 1982; 50: 149–151.

7. DEVEREUX RB, SAVAGE DD, SACHS I, LARAGH JH: Relation of hemodynamic load to left ventricular hypertrophy and performance in hypertension. Am J Cardiol 1983; 51: 171–176.

8. JOHNSSON GL, KOTCHEN JM, MCKEAN HE, COTTRILL CM, KOTCHEN TA: Blood pressure related echocardiographic changes in adolescents and young adults. Am Heart J 1983; 105: 113–118.

9. WIKSTRAND J, BERGLUND G, WILHELMSEN L, WALLENTIN I: Orthogonal electrocardiogram, apex cardiogram, and atrial sound in normotensive and hypertensive 50-year-old men. Br Heart J 1976; 38: 779–789.

10. WIKSTRAND J, BERGLUND G, WILHELMSEN L, WALLENTIN I: Value of systolic and diastolic time intervals. Studies in normotensive and hypertensive 50-year-old men and in patients after myocardial infarction. Br Heart J 1978; 40: 256–267.

11. HARTFORD M: WIKSTRAND J, WALLENTIN I, LJUNGMAN S, WILHELMSEN L, BERGLUND G: Non-invasive signs of cardiac involvement in essential hypertension. Eur Heart J 1982; 3: 75–87.

12. HARTFORD M. Left ventricular function in primary hypertension. Thesis. Göteborg: University of Göteborg, 1983.

13. HARTFORD M, WIKSTRAND J, WALLENTIN I, LJUNGMAN S, WILHELMSEN L, BERGLUND G: Diastolic function of the heart in untreated primary hypertension. Hypertension 1984; 6: 329–338.

14. HARTFORD M, WIKSTRAND J, WALLENTIN I, LJUNGMAN S, BERGLUND G: Left ventricular wall stress, wall thickness and systolic function in untreated primary hypertension. Hypertension.

15. TARAZI RC, SEN S, SARAGOCA M, KHAIRALLAH P: The multifactorial role of catecholamines in hypertensive cardiac hypertrophy. Eur Heart J 1982; 3 (suppl A): 103–110.

16. HARTFORD M, WIKSTRAND J, WALLENTIN I, LJUNGMAN S, WILHELMSEN L, BERGLUND G: Left ventricular mass in middle-aged men. Relationship to blood pressure, sympathetic nervous activity, hormonal and metabolic factors. Clin Exp Hypertens 1983; A5: 1429–1451.

17. ROWLANDS DB, GLOVER DR, IRELAND MA, et al: Assessment of left-ventricular mass and its response to antihypertensive treatment. Lancet 1982; 1: 467–470.

18. WIKSTRAND J: Left ventricular function in early primary hypertension. Functional consequences of cardiovascular structural changes. Review. Hypertension 1984; 6: 108–116.

19. PAULUS WJ, BRUTSAERT DL: Relaxation abnormalities in cardiac hypertrophy. Eur Heart J 1982; 3 (suppl A): 133–137.

20. NAYLER WG, WILLIAMS A: Relaxation in heart muscle: some morphological and biochemical considerations. Eur J Cardiol 1978; 7 (suppl): 35–50.

21. NAGGAR CZ, STANLEY K, DOWNING LL: Effects of amyl nitrate on left ventricular

relaxation in patients with borderline hypertension. Am J Cardiol 1982; 50: 979–984.

22. HANRATH P, MATHEY DG, SIEGERT R, BLEIFIELD W: Left ventricular relaxation and filling pattern in different forms of left ventricular hypertrophy: an echocardiographic study. Am J Cardiol 1980; 45: 15–23.

23. IBRAHIM MM, TARAZI RC, DUSTAN HP, BRAVO EL, GIFFORD RW JR: Hyperkinetic heart in severe hypertension: a separate clinical hemodynamic entity. Am J Cardiol 1975; 35: 667–674.

24. TAKESHITA A, MARK AL: Decreased venous distensibility in borderline hypertension. Hypertension 1979; 1: 202–206.

25. LONDON GM, SAFAR ME, PAYEN DM, GITELMAN RC, GUERIN AM: Total, peripheral and intrathoracic effective compliance of the vascular bed in normotensive and hypertensive patients. Contrib Nephrol 1982; 30: 144–153.

26. TRIMARCO B, WIKSTRAND J: Regression of cardiovascular structural changes during antihypertensive treatment. Functional consequences and time course of reversal as judged from clinical studies. Review. Hypertension 1984; 6: 150–157.

27. WIKSTRAND J, TRIMARCO B, BUZZETTI G, et al: Increased cardiac output and lowered peripheral resistance during metoprolol treatment. Acta Med Scand 1983; 672: 105–110.

28. SCHLANT RC, FELNER JM, HEYMSFIELD SB, et al: Echocardiographic studies of left ventricular anatomy and function in essential hypertension. Cardiovasc Med 1977; 2: 477–491.

29. SCHLANT RC, FELNER JM, BLUMENSTEIN BA, et al: Echocardiographic documentation of regression of left ventricular hypertrophy in patients treated for essential hypertension. Eur Heart J 1982; 3 (suppl A): 171–175.

30. VEDIN A, WIKSTRAND J, WILHELMSSON C, WALLENTIN I: Left ventricular function and beta-blockade in chronic ischaemic heart failure. Double-blind, cross-over study of propranolol and penbutolol using non-invasive techniques. Br Heart J 1980; 44: 101–107.

31. WIKSTRAND J, BERGLUND G: Antihypertensive treatment with beta-blockers in patients aged over 65. Br Med J 1982; 285: 850–851.

15

Left Ventricular Relaxation in Hypertension

VIVIENNE-ELIZABETH SMITH, M.D.
ARNOLD M. KATZ, M.D.

Chronic pressure overloading of the heart, such as occurs with arterial hypertension, is commonly associated with concentric left ventricular hypertrophy (LVH).[1] Abnormalities of contractile (inotropic) reserve in this form of chronic pressure load hypertrophy are suggested by a number of studies,[2,3] but this finding is not constant.[4,5] Although diversity of methods and models probably accounts for some of the variability, the stage of hypertrophy is apparently an important factor as well.[6]

Abnormalities of diastolic function have also been demonstrated in this condition.[7-10] Since invasive studies in mildly symptomatic patients are not generally justified on clinical grounds, the results of these earlier reports tend to reflect the abnormalities characteristic of more marked hypertrophy. Developments in noninvasive methodologies, both echo and nuclear, have now made it possible to study diastolic function in patients with less advanced disease. As a consequence, recent experience suggests that abnormalities of diastolic function (lusitropic abnormalities) may be more frequent than those of systolic function in hypertensive cardiac hypertrophy at any stage.

Diastolic events can be analyzed in several ways. The phases of diastole are descriptively referred to as rapid filling, diastasis, and atrial systole. These designations, however, say little about the biochemical and mechanical correlates of ventricular relaxation that lead to the dissipation of systolic tension, and augmentation of diastolic volume (filling).

The precise determinants and especially the biochemical correlates of ventricular relaxation and filling are poorly understood. Isovolumic relaxation takes place at a time when the activator Ca^{2+} released into the cytosol of the myocardial cell at the onset of systole is being pumped back into the sarcoplasmic reticulum. It is therefore likely that the calcium cycle plays a key role in this phase of the diastolic performance of the heart. It is not known, however, the extent to which the myocardium is still actively dissipating tension during the early phases of ventricular filling. By whatever mechanism, impairment of this aspect of relaxation would delay the phase of rapid filling. The late diastolic phases of diastasis and ventricular filling from atrial systole may be governed less by ventricular energetics than by viscoelastic and inertial properties of the walls of the ventricle; their nature has been reviewed extensively elsewhere[11] and will not be discussed here.

An important study by Hanrath et al.[12] using echo methods has related relaxation and filling in chronic pressure overload. Prolongation of the relaxation time index (the time between minimal LV dimension and mitral valve opening), and a reduced rate of LV dimensional increase was found in patients with hypertrophy due to hypertension. Fouad and colleagues[13] reported abnormal ventricular filling in hypertensive subjects using isotope techniques, and Inouye et al[14] also noted that abnormal first third filling fraction and peak filling rate parameters correlated with ventricular wall thickness.

Impairment of relaxation has several important hemodynamic and clinical consequences. When relaxation abnormalities result in decreased compliance (the relationship between pressure and volume during the later phases of diastole), the diminished ventricular volume at end-diastole may reduce stroke volume and thus cardiac output. If, on the other hand, filling is normal or near normal, impaired relaxation will cause the ventricle to fill at an increased end-diastolic pressure, which can result in pulmonary vascular congestion and the clinical syndrome of LV failure. A dramatic example of this pathophysiologic abnormality is seen in hypertrophic cardiomyopathy, where the massively hypertrophied left ventricle leads to the symptoms of both "forward" and "backward" failure.

Besides the consequences of increased diastolic pressures and decreased filling volumes, there is increased reliance on the atrium to supply an adequate end-diastolic volume when the ventricle hypertrophies and becomes more "resistant" to filling.[12] In this setting, atrial arrhythmias are more frequent;[15] by preventing effective mechanical atrial systole, atrial fibrillation could compromise cardiac output by yet another mechanism.

In the preliminary study described in this chapter, additional evidence is presented that the lusitropic function of the ventricle is frequently abnormal in hypertension. Furthermore, this abnormality may be a general finding in patients with concentric LVH, but it can occur without an obvious increase in LV mass.

Methods

We selected a group of patients with mild to moderate essential hypertension (diastolic blood pressure 90 to 115 mmHg). Subjects with electrocardiographic evidence of LVH were excluded in order to restrict this study to patients with only mild disease of the left ventricle. Furthermore, in order to qualify for study, patients had to be without clinical or radionuclide exercise evidence of coronary artery disease, since this condition is well-known to be associated with abnormal patterns of ventricular filling.[16] Control subjects were chosen for comparability of age, sex, and heart rate, since both age[17,18] and heart rate[18] appear to influence ventricular filling rates.

Left ventricular mass was calculated from M-mode echo dimensions according to methods of Devereux and Reichek.[19] Radionuclide LV time-activity curves of a technetium-99m (^{99m}Tc) labeled blood pool were generated from a computerized nuclear probe. The average rapid left ventricular filling rate (LVFR$_{av}$) was taken as the difference between counts measured at the time of end-systole (ESC) and the end of rapid filling (RFC), divided by the time interval (T3 − T2) of rapid filling. The rate was normalized for end-diastolic (EDC) activity according to the following (Fig. 1):

$$LVFR_{av} = \frac{\dfrac{RFC - ESC}{T3 - T2}}{EDC}$$

Results and Discussion

Ejection fractions in the two groups of subjects were comparable, but the hypertensive patients had a prolonged LVFR$_{av}$ when compared with the controls (1.92 ± 0.28 versus 2.80 ± 0.42 end-diastolic counts per second; Fig. 2). The LVFR correlated significantly with LV mass index (r = −0.59; Fig. 3).

The relationship between relative wall thickness, (2 h/r, where h = posterior wall thickness and r = LV diastolic dimension) and LVFR$_{av}$ was examined in an effort to determine the effect of geometry on filling. In the subset of patients with increased relative wall thickness (more than 0.3), there was a significant negative correlation between relative wall thickness and LVFR$_{av}$ (r = −0.69), although there was no significant correlation for the entire group of hypertensive patients. This finding suggests that geometry has some influence on filling, although the negative correlation between relative wall thickness and filling could simply be a reflection of increased mass.

The lusitropic abnormalities accompanying mild hypertension may have appeared before LV mass had increased significantly, since 6 of 16 patients had normal mass but abnormal filling (Fig. 3). Although additional data, and especially serial studies in individual patients, will be needed to define the sequence at which these abnormalities develop in the hypertensive patient, our findings suggest that delayed rapid filling may be one of the first abnormalities to affect the left ventricle in hypertension.

The exquisite sensitivity of relaxation to chronic pressure overload may reflect the vulnerability of early phases of diastole to abnormalities in the biochemistry of active muscle relaxation, the effects of altered passive elastic properties of myocardium in chronic pressure load, or both.

Abnormal coronary flow reserve and reduced capillary luminal volume have been described in the hypertrophied ventricle,[20] so that the slowing of the rapid filling phase may arise from an imbalance between the rates of energy production and energy utilization in the overloaded myocardium. The precise biochemical mechanism by which such an energy deficiency might produce the lusitropic abnormality in the hypertensive heart is not yet established, but the slowing of relaxation may be related to a decrease in the myocardial content of adenosine triphosphate (ATP). It is well established

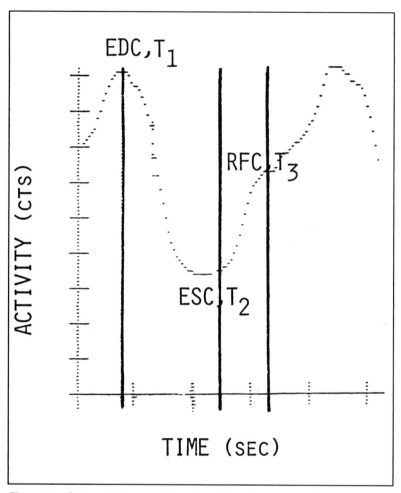

Figure 1: *Schematic time-activity curve of the left ventricle. Cursors are positioned at end-diastole (T_1), end-systole (T_2), and the end of rapid filling (T_3). EDC = end-diastolic counts; ESC = end-systolic counts; RFC = rapid filling counts*

that mitochondrial volume percent of myocardium[21,22] is reduced in hearts subjected to chronic pressure overload and that ATP content and high-energy phosphate levels are reduced when LV ejection pressure is increased.[23] The reduction in high-energy phosphate levels that occurs in the setting of mild hypertension is probably small and would be unlikely to influence the ability of ATP to interact with the high-affinity substrate binding sites of energy-consuming systems, such as the sarcoplasmic reticulum. However, even a slight decrease in ATP concentrations can inhibit calcium uptake by this intracellular membrane system.[24,25] The resulting decrease in

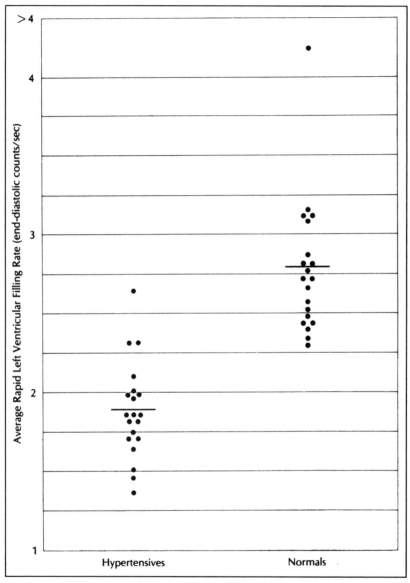

Figure 2: *Average rapid left ventricular filling rate in hypertensive patients (1.92 ± 0.28 EDC/sec) and normal control subjects (2.80 ± 0.42 EDC/sec). (Reprinted with permission from Hospital Practice 1984;19.)*

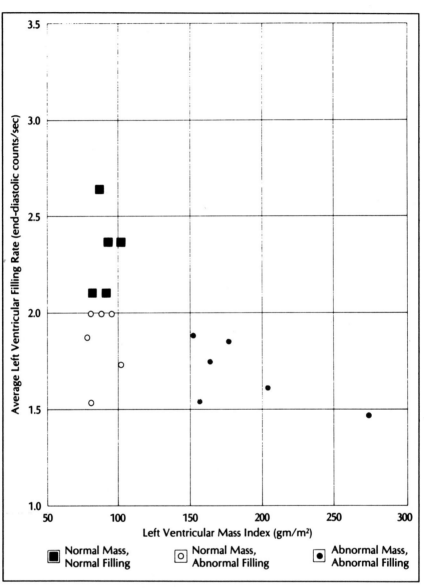

Figure 3: *Average rapid left ventricular filling rate as a function of LV mass index in hypertensive patients (r = −0.60, p < 0.01). (Modified with permission from Hospital Practice 1984;19.)*

the rate of active Ca^{2+} uptake into the sarcoplasmic reticulum, which is responsible for relaxation, could contribute to the observed lusitropic abnormalities even in the absence of frank hypertrophy. Chronic hemodynamic overloading may also affect the sarcoplasmic reticulum directly.[26]

Another possible explanation for the lusitropic abnormality described in this chapter is suggested by the now classic "plasticizing" effect of ATP on the contractile proteins.[27] Since ATP, at concentrations well above those necessary to saturate the myosin-ATPase enzyme, maintains the contractile proteins in a "plastic" state by dissociating actin and myosin, a slight decrease in myocardial ATP levels might also account for a decline in compliance of the chronically pressure overloaded heart.

The role of increased connective tissue content in determining passive properties of the hypertensive heart in diastole is not yet clear. Caulfield[28] has pointed out that collagen deposition is a dynamic process, and myocardial collagen content has been shown to increase almost immediately following imposition of an acute pressure load in animals.[29] Thus, the potential exists for an increased collagen content to play a role in altering diastolic properties even in apparently nonhypertrophied hearts. However, Schwarz et al[30] examined myocardial biopsy samples from patients with aortic valvular disease and found that myocyte volume, but not the extent of fibrosis, correlated with several parameters of diastolic function (end-diastolic pressure, stiffness, mean left atrial pressure). The failure to find correlations between one variable (fibrosis) and these parameters may only reflect the complex interplay of the structural elements that affect diastolic function; the pattern of collagen increase varies even in hearts with the same hypertrophic disease[28] and so could be expected to modify the effect of a given degree of fibrosis. Thus, although increased connective tissue deposition in hypertrophy is a potentially important determinant of diastolic function, the precise nature of the role of fibrosis remains uncertain.

Increased coronary artery turgor due to the elevated aortic pressure or intrinsic coronary arterial elastic changes[31] in hypertensive patients represents another factor that could impede ventricular filling, as has been suggested by Brutsaert et al,[32] but direct evidence for this explanation of either impaired relaxation or impaired filling is not yet available.

Thus, abnormalities of lusitropic function may be commonly found in hypertension, with or without increases in LV mass, and appear to indicate early effects of hypertension on the heart. However, further work is needed to elucidate their precise mechanisms and ultimate clinical significance.

Summary

Rapid LV filling, a noninvasively determined parameter of ventricular diastolic function, can be abnormal in hypertension and may reflect very early effects of the hypertensive state on the heart. Hypertrophy in the hypertensive heart develops in several stages; from minimal increases in mitochondrial content to replacement of myocytes by fibrosis, and may be preceded by this functional disorder. Understanding the mechanism for the lusitropic abnormalities seen in the hypertensive heart must therefore incorporate the effects of diverse biochemical and structural changes that occur in response to the chronic pressure overload.

References

1. LYNCH RP, EDWARDS JE: Pathology of systemic hypertension including background and complications. In: Hurst JW, ed. The heart. New York: McGraw-Hill, 1978; 1380–1390.
2. DEVEREUX RB, SAVAGE DD, SACHS I, LARAGH JH: Relation of hemodynamic load to left ventricular hypertrophy and performance in hypertension. Am J Cardiol 1983; 51: 171–176.
3. BORER JS, JASON M, DEVEREUX RB, et al: Function of the hypertrophied left ventricle at rest and during exercise: hypertension and aortic stenosis. Am J Med 1983; 75 (suppl): 34–39.
4. FRANCIS CK, CLEMAN M, BERGER HJ, et al: Left ventricular systolic performance during upright bicycle exercise in patients with essential hypertension. Am J Med 1983; 75 (suppl): 40–46.
5. BING OHL, BROOKS WW, WIEGNER AW: Myocardial mechanics in two models of pressure overload hypertrophy. In: Tarazi RC, Dunbar JB, eds. Cardiac hypertrophy in hypertension. New York: Raven Press, 1983; 167–177.
6. MIRSKY I, LAKS MM: Time course of changes in the mechanical properties of the canine right and left ventricles during hypertrophy caused by pressure overload. Circ Res 1980; 46: 530–542.
7. GAASCH WH, LEVINE HJ, QUINONES MA, ALEXANDER JK: Left ventricular compliance mechanisms and clinical implications. Am J Cardiol 1976; 38: 645–653.
8. HIROTA Y: A clinical study of left ventricular relaxation. Circulation 1980; 62: 756–763.
9. PETERSON KL, TSUJI J, JOHNSON A, DIDONNA J, LEWINTER M: Diastolic left ventricular pressure-volume and stress-strain relations in patients with valvular aortic stenosis and left ventricular hypertrophy. Circulation 1978; 58: 77–89.
10. GROSSMAN W, McLAURIN LP: Diastolic properties of the left ventricle. Ann Intern Med 1976; 84: 316–326.
11. GROSSMAN W, BARRY WH: Diastolic pressure volume relations in the diseased heart. Fed Proc 1980; 39: 148–155.
12. HANRATH P, MATHEY DG, SIEGERT R, BLEIFELD W: Left ventricular relaxation and filling pattern in different forms of left ventricular hypertrophy: an echocardiographic study. Am J Cardiol 1980; 45: 15–23.
13. FOUAD FM, TARAZI RC, GALLAGHER JH, MacINLYRE WJ, COOK SA: Abnormal left ventricular relaxation in hypertensive subjects. Clin Sci 1980; 59 (suppl 6): 411S–414S.
14. INOUYE I, MASSIE B, LOJE D, et al: Abnormal left ventricular filling: an early finding in mild to moderate systemic hypertension. Am J Cardiol 1983; 53: 120–126.
15. LOALDI A, PEPI M, AGOSTONI AG, et al: Cardiac rhythm in hypertension assessed through 24 hour ambulatory electrocardiographic monitoring. Br Heart J 1983; 50: 120–126.

16. BONOW, RD, BACHARACH SL, GREEN MV, et al: Impaired left ventricular diastolic filling in patients with coronary artery disease: assessment with radionuclide angiography. Circulation 1981; 315–323.

17. GERSTENBLITH G, FLEG JL, BECKER LC, et al: Maximum left ventricular filling rate in healthy individuals measured by gated blood pool scans: effect of age (abstr). Circulation 1983; 68 (suppl III): 101.

18. FIFER MA, BOROW KM, COLAN S, LORELL B: Left ventricular diastolic filling rate: contributions of heart rate, age and extent of systolic shortening (abstr). Circulation 1983; 68 (suppl III): 101.

19. DEVEREUX RB, REICHEK N: Echocardiographic determination of left ventricular mass in man: anatomic validation of the method. Circulation 1977; 55: 613–618.

20. ARAI S, MACHIDA A, NAKAMURA T: Myocardial structure and vascularization of hypertrophied hearts. J Exp Med 1968; 95: 35–54.

21. KAWAMURA K, KASHII C, IMAMURA K: Ultrastructural changes in hypertrophied myocardium of spontaneously hypertensive rats. Jpn Circ J 1976; 40: 1119–1145.

22. PAGE E, POLIMENI PI, ZAK R, EARLY J, JOHNSON M: Myofibrillar mass in rat and rabbit heart muscle, correlation of microchemical and stereological measurements in normal and hypertrophic hearts. Circ Res 1972; 30: 430–439.

23. HOCHREIN H, DORING HJ: Die energiereichen phosphate des myokards bei variation der Belastungbeidingungen. Pfluegers Arch 1960; 271: 548–563.

24. SHIGAKAWA M, DOUGHERTY JP, KATZ AM: Reaction mechanism of Ca^{2+}-dependent ATP hydrolysis by skeletal muscle sarcoplasmic reticulum in the absence of added alkali metal salts. I. Characterization of steady state ATP hydrolysis and comparison with that in the presence of KCl. J Biol Chem 1978; 253: 1442–1450.

25. NAKAMURA Y, TONOMURA Y: The binding of ATP to the catalytic and the regulatory site of Ca^{2+}, Mg^{2+}-dependent ATPase of the sarcoplasmic reticulum. J Bioenerg Biomembr 1982; 14: 307–318.

26. SCHEUER J: Alteration in sarcoplasmic reticulum in cardiac hypertrophy. In: Tarazi RC, Dunbar JB, eds. Cardiac hypertrophy in hypertension. New York: Raven Press, 1983; 111–122.

27. KATZ AM: Contractile proteins of the heart. Physiol Rev 1970; 50: 63–158.

28. CAULFIED J: Alterations in cardiac collagen with hypertrophy. In: Tarazi RC, Dunbar JB, eds. Cardiac hypertrophy in hypertension. New York: Raven Press, 1983; 167–175.

29. TURTO H, LUNDY S: Collagen metabolism of the rat heart during experimental cardiac hypertrophy and the effect of digitoxin treatment. Adv Cardiol 1976; 18: 41–45.

30. SCHWARZ F, FLAMENG W, SCHAPER J, HEHRLEIN F: Correlation between myocardial structure and diastolic properties of the heart in chronic aortic valve disease: effects of corrective surgery. Am J Cardiol 1978; 42: 895–903.

31. BEVAN RD: Adaptation of arterial vasculature to increased pressure and factors modifying the response. In: Tarazi RC, Dunbar, JB, eds. Cardiac hypertrophy in hypertension. New York: Raven Press, 1983; 319–335.

32. BRUTSAERT DL, RADEMAKERS FE, SYS SV: Triple control of relaxation implications in cardiac disease. Circulation 1984; 69: 190–196.

16

Left Ventricular Wall Stress and Hypertrophy

B. E. STRAUER, M.D.

Chronic hypertrophic heart disease is one of the most common cardiac diseases in man. It represents the consequence of primary myocardial mass augmentation, such as in hypertrophic obstructive cardiomyopathy, or secondarily of abnormal ventricular load, as in pressure and volume overload, in high output, and in metabolic disorders. From the functional point of view, ventricular hypertrophy provides one of the basic mechanisms that permits the heart to maintain normal cardiac pump function despite abnormal pressure or stress or volume load. On the other hand, cardiac hypertrophy is a significant precursor of cardiac enlargement and failure.

Cardiac Hypertrophy

During the development of hypertrophy, wall mass increases. This may have at least three consequences with regard to intraventricular volume, wall thickness, and wall mass[1-8] (Fig. 1).

1. In compensated pressure overload, as in arterial hypertension and in aortic stenosis, the ventricular wall becomes thickened and the mass is augmented, whereas end-diastolic volume remains normal or mildly increases. This leads to an increase in mass to volume ratio and is termed "concentric" hypertrophy. Here the ventricular response is appropriate to the pressure load burden on the ventricular wall.[9-14]

2. In decompensated pressure overload as well as in volume overload, both ventricular mass and volume increase, whereas wall thickness may remain unchanged or only moderately increased. This leads to ventricular dilation with constancy or even decrease in the mass to volume ratio and is termed "eccentric" hypertrophy. Here, ventricular response is inappropriate, since the heart dilates out of proportion to wall thickness changes.

3. In normally shaped pressure overload and also in hypertrophic obstructive cardiomyopathy, excess increase in wall thickness and mass may occur, thereby narrowing the intraventricular hole. Consequently, the mass to volume ratio increases. This type of excess hypertrophy is inappropriate and is termed "irregular," inappropriate hypertrophy.[13-15] Here, the ventricular response is also inappropriate, since the wall thickness in proportion to intraventricular volume changes.

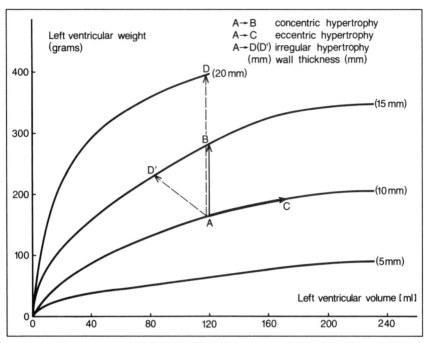

Figure 1. *Relationship between left ventricular (LV) volume, LV mass, and wall thickness.*

These three types of hypertrophy occur in experimental and in clinical hypertrophy and are associated with different cardiac dimensions, wall stress, ventricular function, and myocardial oxygen consumption (MVO_2).

Wall Stress (Afterload)

Stress represents the force per unit of cross-sectional area of the ventricular wall and is expressed in dynes per square centimeter (dynes/cm^2). Stress, in accordance with the modified Laplace equation, is directly related to pressure (p) and radius (r) and is inversely related to wall thickness (d). There are at least three types of stress acting at the ventricular wall: radial stress acts perpendicular to the endocardial surface. Longitudinal stress acts within the wall parallel to the long axis of the heart, and circumferential wall stress which, in a quantitative sense is the most important,[2-4, 16-21] acts within the wall parallel to the short axis of the ventricule. If wall hypertrophy is adequate with regard to the ventricular load, then the stress remains normal. If hypertrophy is inadequate, for the pressure and volume demand, then stress increases. If the wall thickens out of proportion to pressure and volume load, then stress is reduced. This behavior of pressure, mass to volume ratio, and

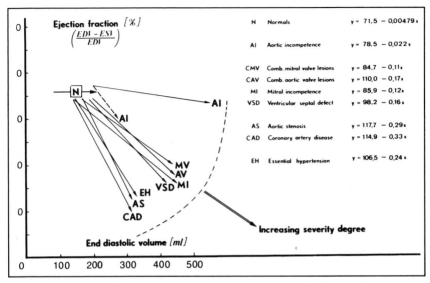

Figure 2. Relationship between end-diastolic volume and ejection fraction.

hence systolic wall stress therefore elucidates the importance of stress as a fundamental parameter for the assessment of the degree and appropriateness of cardiac hypertrophy.

Wall Stress and Function

Left ventricular (LV) size as represented by the end-diastolic volume shows an inverse relationship with LV function, as is evident from the ejection fraction (Fig. 2). With increase in end-diastolic volume, the ejection fraction decreases. However, steepness of this characteristic for different load conditions is quite variable: lowest decrease in function with increase in end-diastolic volume is present for volume overload, such as aortic incompetence, whereas the largest decrease in function is found for chronic pressure overload due to aortic stenosis and essential hypertension as well as for coronary artery diseases.

The different course of these characteristics most probably may be related to different contractile states or to different loading conditions of the left ventricle. Except for changes in contractility, the typical alterations in LV afterloading conditions may decrease LV function with increase in heart size.

Accordingly, the relationship between wall stress and function can be determined (Fig. 3). With increase in systolic wall stress, the LV function, as is evident from the ventricular ejection fraction, decreases. Doubling of stress leads to reduction in the ejection fraction by approximately 50%. Since systolic wall stress results from systolic pressure and from the mass to volume

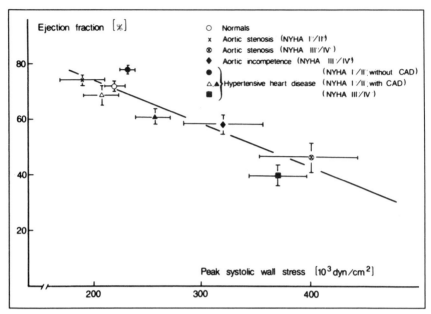

Figure 3. Relationship between systolic wall stress and ejection fraction. Note the decrease in ejection fraction with increase in wall stress (afterload).

ratio, it is comparable to the ventricular afterload that is imposed on the LV wall. It is therefore reasonable to assume that LV size, that is, end-diastolic volume, and systolic wall stress are important determinants of ventricular performance.

Wall Stress and Energetics

Myocardial oxygen consumption per weight unit is quite different in clinical heart disease. It is lowest in normotensive patients with coronary artery disease, normal in concentric and clinically compensated LV hypertrophy, even in extreme pressure load, and increased in dilated hearts with aortic valve disease (Fig. 4). In hypertrophic heart disease an inverse, nonlinear relationship exists between the mass to volume ratio and peak systolic wall stress. Largest mass to volume ratio was found for hypertrophic obstructive cardiomyopathy, and lowest values were present for decompensated pressure and volume overload due to aortic valve disease. Concentric LV hypertrophy due to essential hypertension and aortic stenosis was within this correlation, whereas in normotensives subjects it was shifted to lower systolic stress at equal mass to volume ratio, that is, to a lower isobaric relationship.

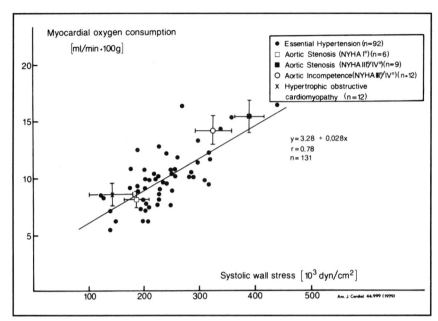

Figure 4. *Relationship between systolic wall stress and MVO₂.*

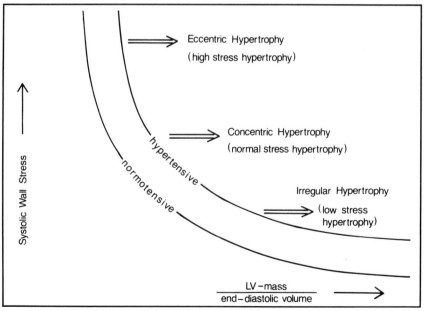

Figure 5. *Diagrammatic representation of the three possible kinds of left ventricular hypertrophy (LVH).*

With regard to these dynamic and metabolic characteristics, three types of LV hypertrophy may be classified (Fig. 5):

1. Appropriate hypertrophy that keeps systolic wall stress normal even at extreme pressure load, as a result of an appropriate increase in the mass to volume ratio parallel to pressure load

2. Inappropriate, or low-stress hypertrophy, which is associated with marked increase in LV mass out of proportion to intraventricular volume

3. Inappropriate, or high-stress hypertrophy, which is characterized by excess dilation out of proportion to ventricular mass development

Thus, at least two forms of inappropriate hypertrophy may occur in chronic hypertrophic heart disease.

From the metabolic point of view, high-stress hypertrophy has increased oxygen consumption per mass unit at an impairment of LV function. In contrast, low-stress hypertrophy may have normal or even decreased oxygen consumption per LV mass unit at normal LV function. This helps to explain, for example, the existence of normal, decreased, or increased oxygen consumption per LV mass unit in chronic pressure or volume overload. Despite large pressure load, the oxygen consumption may be normal or even decreased in aortic stenosis as long as heart and systolic wall stress are normal.

Wall Stress in Variations of Preload and Afterload

Reductions of both preload or afterload are therapeutically much more effective in dilated than in normally shaped hearts, as can be derived from the isobars of the mass to volume to stress relationships (Fig. 6):

With an increase in systolic pressure, at constant end-diastolic volume, systolic wall stress increases in all ventricles and at each comparable level of mass to volume ratio. However, the degree of pressure-induced wall stress alterations closely depends on the individual isobaric condition as well as on the initial mass to volume ratio. An equal increase in pressure, for example, from 120 to 200 mmHg (B→A), at a mass to volume ratio of 3.5 g/ml leads to a stress increase of only 70×10^3 dynes/cm^2, whereas the same increase in pressure (B'→A') at a mass to volume ratio of 1.5 is followed by a considerable increase in stress of 160×10^3 dynes/cm^2 (Fig. 6).

The same calculations and consequences as to systolic stress and, hence, MVO$_2$ are valid for therapeutically induced pressure reductions. This means that from a diagnostic and prognostic point of view, an increase in systolic pressure in a dilated hypertensive heart causes a greater increase in peak systolic wall stress and in MVO$_2$ than the same pressure increase in a nondilated, hypertensive heart. Because both stress and metabolic reserve are limited in man, the LV stress capacity is increasingly reduced with: an increase in initial systolic stress, a decrease in mass to volume ratio, and an increase in systolic pressure. However, a therapeutic reduction in systolic pressure will lead to greater reduction in both stress and oxygen consumption in patients with LV dilation than in patients with concentric hypertrophy. Thus, the relationship between mass to volume ratio and peak systolic wall stress eluci-

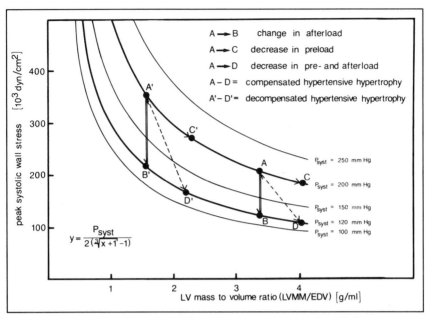

Figure 6. *Diagrammatic representation of concept of the relationship between mass to volume ratio and peak systolic wall stress for different isobaric conditions. Calculation of isobars was performed with use of the Laplace equation. The lack of parallelism and curvature of these isobaric relationships implies that systolic pressure (P_{syst}) changes occurring at points with a high mass to volume ratio lead to fewer stress changes than the same systolic pressure variations at a low mass to volume ratio. An equal increase in systolic pressure, for example, from 120 to 200 mmHg (that is, from B to A), at a mass to volume ratio of 3.5 leads to a stress increase of only 80 units (10^3 dynes/cm²). However, with the same increase in pressure (that is from B' to A') at a mass to volume ratio of 1.5, systolic wall stress is considerably increased by 160 units. The same consequences are valid for therapeutically induced pressure reductions (from A' to B', and from A to B, respectively). This means that the increase in systolic wall stress at a given increase in systolic pressure in hypertensive heart disease is greater in the dilated than in the nondilated heart. This relationship between mass to volume ratio and stress emphasizes the importance of heart size and systolic wall stress on changes in stress and, hence, in ventricular function and myocardial energy demand.*

dates the importance of pressure-dependent changes in systolic stress and, hence, in ventricular function and metabolic reserve.

Qualitatively similar relationships are valid for chronic alterations in end-diastolic volume (approximately "preload"). At constant systolic pressure, that is, in the course of each individual isobar, a decrease in end-diastolic volume and hence an increase in the mass to volume ratio are associated with a larger decrease in systolic wall stress when ventricular dilation is present. Accordingly, therapeutic reductions in preload are more effective

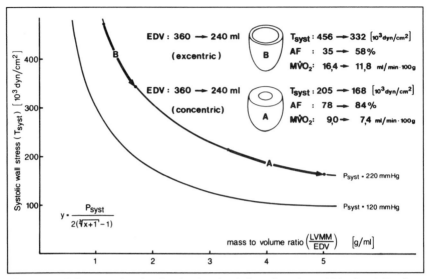

Figure 7. *Influence of preload reduction (end-diastolic volume 360 ml to 240 ml) on mass to volume ratio, systolic wall stress, ejection fraction, and MVO₂. Note, that only minor changes occur in a compensated, concentrically hypertrophied heart with regard to changes in the ejection fraction and in MVO₂, whereas in a dilated heart considerable increase in ventricular function and decrease in MVO₂ occur.*

with regard to LV unloading in a dilated than in a nondilated heart. The most pronounced decrease in systolic wall stress with consecutive improvement in LV function are found when both preload and afterload alterations occur, that is, when both blood pressure reduction and diminution in ventricular size are induced.

On the basis of the original values and isobar spectra, the functional and metabolic consequences may be derived for at least four types of preload and afterload alterations:

1. In compensated concentric hypertrophy (with large mass to volume ratio) reduction in end-diastolic volume, such as during hemofiltration in renal hypertensive heart disease, at constant systolic pressure leads to considerable increase in the mass to volume ratio and decrease in systolic wall stress (Fig. 7); however, ventricular function and MVO₂ remain almost unaltered. In contrast, the same preload reduction in a dilated heart may enhance ventricular function, as is evident from the LV ejection fraction, and may significantly lower MVO₂ (Fig. 7).

2. Reduction of systolic pressure, in concentric hypertrophy, for example, from 220 to 120 mmHg (as in the course of treatment of hypertensive crisis), has little or no direct effect on the mass to volume ratio (Fig. 8). Despite marked decrease in systolic wall stress, LV function, as the consequence of only small changes in the mass to volume to stress relationship, does not improve significantly, and MVO₂ is lowered by only 31%. In contrast, the

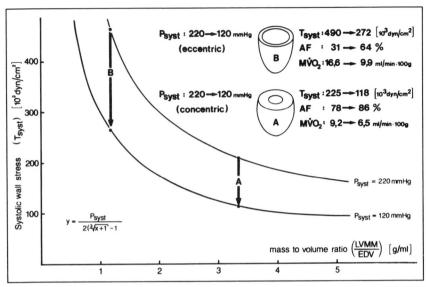

Figure 8. *Influence of systolic pressure reduction (from 220 to 120 mmHg) in the compensated, concentrically hypertrophied heart. Note that there are only minor changes in ventricular function and MVO₂, whereas in a dilated heart considerable increase in ejection fraction (from 31% to 64%) and marked decrease in MVO₂ (from 16.6 to 9.9. ml/min · 100 g) occur.*

same reduction of systolic blood pressure in a dilated heart with low ejection fraction leads to effective improvement in LV function and normalization of myocardial energy demand by alterations of these parameters (ejection fraction, MVO₂) by 94% and 40%, respectively (Fig. 8).

These data demonstrate that both preload and afterload reduction exert more beneficial effects with regard to LV function and myocardial energetics in decompensated, dilated hearts than in concentrically hypertrophied or nonhypertrophied ventricles with normal shape.

Wall Stress and Contractility

The inverse relationship between wall stress and function may be modified by inotropic interventions. This implies that, independent of changes in systolic wall stress, there may exist both increases and decreases in LV function at various contractile states.[10] In acute myocardial infarction considerable decrease in function at normal wall stress occurs due to a loss in contractile substance, that is, on the basis of myocardial necrosis. Similarly, in congestive cardiomyopathy, lower ejection fraction at equal systolic wall stress was found when compared with chronic pressure and volume load of the left ventricle. Conversely, in hyperthyroidism, an increase in LV ejection fraction

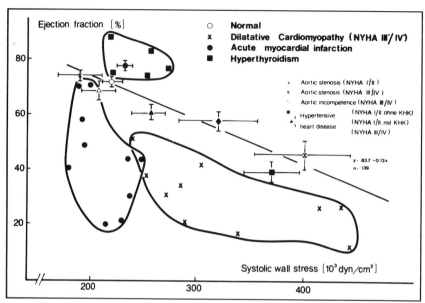

Figure 9. *Relationship between systolic wall stress and ejection fraction for chronic pressure and volume overload (regression line) as well as for acute myocardial infarction, for congestive cardiomyopathy and for hyperthyroidism. Note the increase to decrease in ejection fraction at comparable systolic wall stress when the contractile state of the heart is changed.*

is present (Fig. 9). Consequently, an improvement in ventricular function may be induced by changes in load, such as afterload reduction, according to the load-dependent and contractile-independent increase in ejection fraction, by positive inotropic interventions according to the contractile-dependent and load-independent upward shift of the stress-function relationship, and by a combination of both, that is, of unloading and contractile interventions.

Wall Stress in the Regression of Cardiac Hypertrophy

Regression of cardiac hypertrophy embraces a fascinating therapeutic concept, since, if possible, prevention or reversal of ventricular hypertrophy could contribute to prevention of cardiac failure. Experimental studies of our group have shown that long-term treatment of hypertensive heart disease with nifedipine may prevent LVH and LV failure. We therefore initiated a clinical study in patients with concentric hypertensive heart disease and with normotensive hypertrophic nonobstructive cardiomyopathy. The results for nine of these patients are shown in Table I and Figure 10.

TABLE I   **Left Ventricular Function and Geometry Following Chronic Nifedipine Treatment***

	Before	After	%
Systolic blood pressure (mmHg)	163 ± 44	146 ± 20	−11
LV muscle mass (g/m²; LVMM)	184 ± 38	159 ± 41	−15
End-diastolic volume (ml/m²; EDV)	63 ± 23	67 ± 24	+6
LVMM/EDV (g/ml)	2,91 ± 0,98	2,37 ± 0,77	−18
Systolic wall stress (10³ dynes/cm²)	199 ± 84	193 ± 44	−3
Ejection fraction (%)	69 ± 6	74 ± 9	+7

*Nine patients were analyzed, six with hypertensive hypertrophy and three with hypertrophic cardio-myopathy. Note the decrease in systolic pressure, LV muscle mass, and LV mass to volume ratio, and the increase in the ejection fraction of the left ventricle.

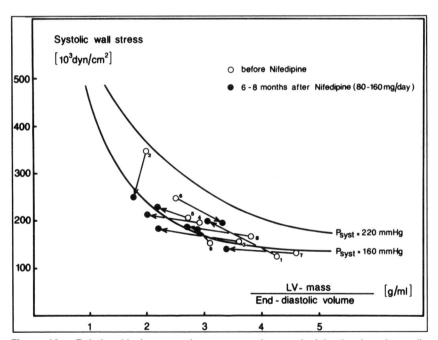

Figure 10. *Relationship between the mass to volume ratio (abscissa) and systolic wall stress (ordinate) before (○) and after (●) long-term treatment with nifedipine. Note that marked decrease in the LV mass to volume ratio occurs without significant increase in systolic wall stress.*

Following long-term treatment with nifedipine, a decrease in the abnormally increased mass to volume ratio could be achieved. Systolic wall stress was moderately and insignificantly increased. However, the decrease in the LV mass to volume ratio in these patients never exceeded values that were associated with an excess increase in systolic wall stress or in a depression of LV function. Therefore, pharmacologically induced hypertrophy regression may be realized, and the load potency of the left ventricle as well as the potency of the left ventricle to compensate for this overload represents a balanced steady state. This intervention seems to be safe, since inadequate ventricular hypertrophy (high-stress hypertrophy due to depressed mass to volume ratio) is not present.

Summary

Left ventricular function is inversely related to both LV volume (size) and systolic wall stress. Systolic wall stress represents the main determinant of the ventricular afterload. Systolic wall stress is directly correlated with MVO_2. Systolic stress is an important resultant of the appropriateness and degree of cardiac hypertrophy. In the course of chronic heart disease, at least two types of inappropriate hypertrophy may occur (low-stress and high-stress hypertrophy).

Preload and afterload are important determinants of LV function. Alterations in preload are regularly associated with alterations in afterload (wall stress), and chronic alterations in afterload usually induce alterations in preload. For the clinical evaluation of the chronically diseased heart, end-diastolic volume and end-diastolic wall stress are relevant equivalents of ventricular preload, whereas alterations of afterload may be quantified by the assessment of systolic wall stress. The functional and energetic consequences of chronic reduction of preload and afterload are more effective in a dilated heart with low ejection fraction than in a normally shaped heart with normal LV function. Best improvement in function and energetics is obtained by combined preload and afterload reduction.

Both afterload reduction and augmentation of myocardial contractility improve ventricular function. The underlying mechanisms are different. It is possible that the additive therapy with both inotropic and afterload-reduction drugs may be more useful for treatment of cardiac failure than one of the therapeutic principles alone.

Regression of LV hypertrophy may be safely realized by use of long-term treatment with calcium-antagonists in both hypertensive as well as in normotensive patients with hypertrophic cardiomyopathy.

References

1. ALPERT N, ed: Cardiac hypertrophy. New York: Academic Press, 1971.
2. BRETSCHNEIDER HJ, COTT L, HILGERT G, PROBST R, RAU G: Gaschromato-

graphische Trennung und Analyse von Argon als Basis einer neuen Fremd-gasmethode zur Durchblutungsmessung von Organen. Verh Dtsch Gest Kreislaufforsch 1960; 32: 267–273.

3. LINZBACH AJ: Heart failure from the point of view of quantitative anatomy. Am J Cardiol 1960; 5: 370.

4. LINZBACH AJ: Structural adaption of the heart in hypertension and the physical consequences. In: Strauer BE, ed. The heart in hypertension, Berlin: Springer-Verlag, 1981; 243–250.

5. MEERSON FS: Hyperfunktion, Hypertrophie und Insuffizienz des Herzens. Berlin: VEB Volk & Gesundheit, 1969.

6. BÜRGER S, STRAUER BE: Dynamics of left ventricular hypertrophy and contraction in spontaneously hypertensive rats. Circulation 1977; 56 (suppl II): III-910.

7. FORD LF: Heart size. Circ Res 1976; 39: 297.

8. HOOD WP: Dynamics of hypertrophy in left ventricular wall of man. In: Alpert NR ed. Cardiac hypertrophy. New York: Academic Press, 1971; 445.

9. HORT W: Morphologische und physiologische Untersuchungen an Ratten während eines Lauftrainings und nach dem Training. Virchows Arch. [Pathol. Anta] 1951; 320: 197.

10. JUST H, LIMBOURG P: Arterial hypertension: left ventricular function at rest and during exercise. In: Strauer BE, ed. The heart in hypertension. Springer-Verlag, 1981; 333–344.

11. BÜRGER S, MEINARDUS A, STRAUER BE: Hypertrophiegrad und Dynamik des linken Ventrikels bei der spontanen essentiellen Hypertonie der Ratte. Klin Wochenschr 1978; 56: 207.

12. LIMBOURG PH, JUST KF, LANG P, SCHÖLMERICH: Ventricular function at rest and during exercise in the hypertensive heart. In Roskamm H, Hahn C: Ventricular function at rest and during exercise. Berlin: Springer-Verlag, 1976.

13. STRAUER BE: Myocardial oxygen consumption in chronic heart disease: role of wall stress, hypertrophy and coronary reserve. Am J Cardiol 1979; 44: 730.

14. STRAUER BE: Ventricular function and coronary hemodynamics in hypertensive heart disease. Am J Cardio 1979; 44: 999.

15. KOCHSIEK K, HEISS HW, TAUCHERT M, STRAUER BE: Koronarreserve und Sauerstoffverbrauch bei hypertrophischer obstruktiver Cardiomyopathie. Verh Dtsch Ges Inn Med 1971; 77: 880.

16. STRAUER BE: Änderungen der Kontraktilität bei Druck- und Volumenbelastungen des Herzens. Verh Dtsch Ges Kreislaufforsch 1976; 42: 69.

17. STRAUER BE: Das hochdruckherz. Berlin: Springer-Verlag, 1979.

18. STRAUER BE: Hypertensive heart disease. Berlin: Springer-Verlag, 1980.

19. STRAUER BE: The heart in hypertension. Berlin: Springer-Verlag, 1981.

20. STRAUER BE: Ventrikelfunktion und koronare Hämodynamik bei der essentiellen Hypertonie, Verh Dtsch Ges Kreislaufforsch 1977; 43: 41.

21. WEBER KT, REICHEK, N., JANICKI, J.S., SHROFF, S.: The pressure overloaded heart: physiological and clinical correlates. In: Strauer BE, ed. The heart in hypertension. Berlin: Springer-Verlag, 1981; 287–306.

17

Disparate Hemodynamic Amplifying Capacities of the Heart and Arterial Resistance Vessels in Hypertension and Their Consequences

PAUL I. KORNER
ARCHER BROUGHTON
GARRY L. JENNINGS
MURRAY D. ESLER

One of the most important circulatory adaptations in hypertension is the hypertrophy that occurs in the muscles of the left ventricle and arterial resistance vessels in response to the increased arterial pressure load.[1–3] As a result, the left ventricle and vessels become amplifiers of inotropic and constrictor stimuli when compared with the properties of corresponding structures of the normotensive circulation.[4] This chapter considers the effects of these amplifying properties on the hemodynamics of hypertension at different stages of the disorder. In addition, it discusses the effects of prolonged control of blood pressure by treatment and the differential rates of regression of hypertrophy that they appear to induce in the left ventricle and resistance vessels. These have important implications for present-day treatment strategy in hypertension.

Cardiovascular Amplifiers in Established Hypertension

Arterial Resistance Vessels: Folkow[4] was the first to point out that the amplification of vascular resistance changes by a given constrictor stimulus in established hypertension was due to the increase in wall to lumen ratio. This occurs in all resistance vessels in the body.[5] Even after abolishing muscle tone by vasodilator drugs, resistance to blood flow in a given vascular bed is higher in the hypertensive than in the normotensive circulation,[6] due to encroachment by the media on the vessel lumen.[4] In hypertensive vessels, a given degree of muscle shortening produces greater narrowing of the vessel lumen than in normal vessels; hence, there is direct amplification of total peripheral resistance (TPR). This has been demonstrated in hypertension in the human and in many types of hypertension in experimental animals.

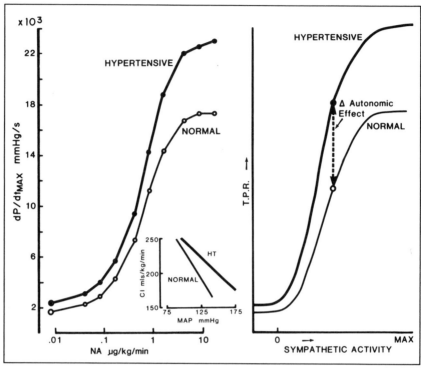

Figure 1. **Left:** *Relationship between norepinephrine infusion rate and LV $(dP/dt)_{max}$ in dogs with Goldblatt hypertension and in normal dogs; LAP controlled but heart rate and MAP allowed to increase.* **Insert:** *Relationship of MAP to cardiac index (CI); heart rate and LAP controlled.* **Right:** *Relationship between norepinephrine dose (sympathetic activity) and TPR in autonomically blocked rabbits.*

In rabbits with established renovascular hypertension in which the autonomic effectors had been blocked to avoid reflex effects, a given dose of norepinephrine, angiotensin II, and vasopressin produced about twice the increase in hind limb vascular resistance as in sham-operated control animals.[6,7] In these animals the increase in TPR was about 1.6 times the increase observed in sham-operated rabbits[8] (Fig. 1, right).

Left Ventricle: Myocardial contractile responses were studied in dogs after 2 to 4 months of renovascular hypertension and in a matched group of normal dogs. All animals were studied with the chest open, with left atrial and mean arterial pressures (LAP, MAP) independently controlled and with the autonomic effectors blocked.[9,10] The hypertensive dogs had well-developed concentric left ventricular (LV) hypertrophy without dilation.

Under identical loading conditions basal $(dP/dt)_{max}$ was about 35% greater in the hypertensive than in the normal dogs[10] (Fig. 2, left). Arterial pressure was allowed to increase in these experiments, to ensure adequate coronary

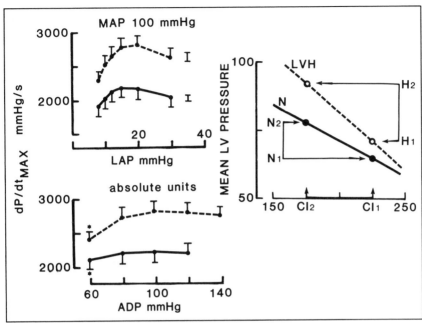

Figure 2. **Left:** *Top graphs show effects in autonomically blocked dogs on $(dP/dt)_{max}$ of varying left atrial pressure (LAP) in LV hypertrophy (interrupted lines) and in normal LV (solid lines); heart rate and MAP remained constant. Lower graphs show effects of altering aortic diastolic pressure (ADP); heart rate and LAP are constant.* **Right:** *Relationship of CI to mean LV pressure in autonomically blocked dogs during changes in MAP; LAP and heart rate remained constant (see insert, Fig. 1). A given change in CI is associated with a greater change in pressure in hypertensive than in normal LV: $(H_1 - H_2) > (N_2 - N_1)$.*

perfusion and oxygen delivery. This is important, since even under basal conditions reduction in perfusion pressure depresses myocardial contractility more readily in the hypertrophied left ventricular than in the normal heart[10,11] (Fig. 2, lower left).

Amplification of $(dP/dt)_{max}$ in the hypertensive left ventricle was strictly in proportion to the increased muscle mass. After dividing $(dP/dt)_{max}$ by wall thickness (or by the left ventricle to body weight ratio), the results were closely similar in the two groups.[10] Since $(dP/dt)_{max}$ is a measure of change in myocardial tension,[1,10], this indicates that the rate of development of active wall stress (tension to wall thickness) is the same in the hypertrophied and normal left ventricle.

We also studied the MAP-cardiac index (CI) relationship, with LAP and heart rate held constant.[1] The variables were linearly related over the range shown in Figure 1 (insert), but the slopes of the regression lines differed significantly.[1,12] Elzinga and Westerhof[13] have pointed out that mean LV pressure (MLVP) is a better measure of ventricular load than MAP, in view of the rectifier properties of the aortic valve. However, we found that the differences between hypertensive and normotensive groups in MLVP-CI relationship (Fig. 2, right) were similar to the differences in MAP-CI relationship (Fig. 1, insert; note variables are plotted on different axes in the two graphs). Both show that the hypertrophied left ventricle can maintain a given CI against a higher pressure load than the normal heart.

Under the conditions just discussed, MLVP is also an index of total LV tension. Figure 2 (right) shows that a given change in CI is associated with a greater change in MLVP in the hypertrophied than in the normal left ventricle. The ratio of the slopes of the regression lines is about 1.9, i.e., greater than the ratio of isovolumic $(dP/dt)_{max}$ (1.35) between the hypertrophied and normal hearts. This is due to greater systolic emptying, owing to the increase in wall/lumen ratio of the hypertensive left ventricle with concentric hypertrophy.

In man, experimental conditions cannot be as well controlled as in animals, so that intrinsic contractile performance has not been determined. Strauer[14] has observed enhancement of $(dP/dt)_{max}$ at a given filling pressure in patients with uncomplicated left ventricular hypertrophy (LVH) due to hypertension; wall stress and CI were similar to corresponding values in normotensive subjects, in agreement with the findings in dogs.

Changing Hemodynamics in the Course of Hypertension: The hemodynamic amplifying capacities of the left ventricle and vessels, respectively, change in the course of hypertension.[1,8] In mild hypertension, the hypertrophy of the left ventricle appears to be greater or equal to that of the vessels, accounting for the high CI-normal TPR pattern.[1,15] The difference between this pattern and the normal CI-high TPR index (TPRI) pattern of moderate to severe hypertension is not due to a difference in blood volume[15,16] or in venous compliance.[17,18] Echo evidence of LVH has been recently obtained in mild (borderline) hypertension in both adults and children[19-21] and in animals with genetic hypertension.[22]

That the hemodynamic patterns are due to differences in cardiac and vascular hypertrophy is also suggested by the recent study of Jennings et al.[23] After 1 year's normalization of the blood pressure by antihypertensive drugs, there was almost complete regression of the vascular hypertrophy. In a comparable echo study, Rowlands et al[24] have shown that regression of LVH was only partial. In the study of Jennings et al[16] the normal CI-high TPRI pattern reverted to the high CI-normal TPRI after 1 year's good control of blood pressure (Fig. 3). The nonautonomic component of TPRI was in the range previously found in normal subjects[25,26] and the elevation of CI was also not due to autonomic factors, since it was still present after autonomic block. The second study in Figure 3 was performed 4 weeks after stopping diuretics and several days after stopping the other drugs. This was to ensure that the observed effects were not due to residual effects of the drugs, but to the reversal of hypertension. At the time of the study, a small increase in pressure had again occurred.[16,26]

We have assumed that similar mechanisms are contributing to the hemodynamics of mild hypertension during the evolution of the disorder, as occur

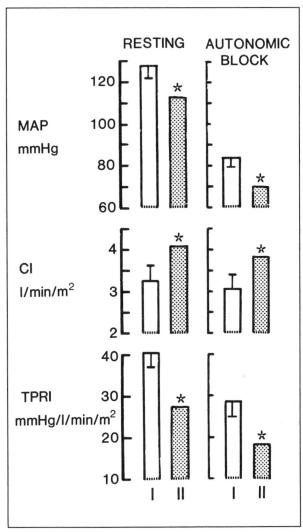

Figure 3. *Results obtained in 13 patients with essential hypertension showing mean arterial pressure (MAP), cardiac index (CI), and total peripheral resistance index (TPRI). Study I before the start of treatment; study II, after 1 year's antihypertensive therapy and a few days after cessation of all drugs. Resting values are shown on left; values obtained from total autonomic blockade are on right. Bar = 1 SED within subjects; *p < 0.05. (Based on data of Jennings et al.[23])*

in the mild hypertension that follows a prolonged period of effective therapy of patients with initially moderate/slope hypertension. One reason for the slightly greater left ventricle than vascular hypertrophy in mild hypertension could be the slightly greater workload due to the pulsatile component of cardiac work.[1]

In moderate to severe established hypertension, the hemodynamic amplifying capacity of the vessels exceeds that of the left ventricle, as discussed in the previous section. Once LV dilation occurs, the amplifying capacity of the left ventricle falls even further behind. At that time, in accordance with the Laplace relationship, more myocardial tension is necessary to develop a given LV pressure or $(dP/dt)_{max}$ than in uncomplicated concentric hypertrophy. In the dilated LV wall, stress increases,[1] which probably provides the major stimulus for the further increase in LV muscle mass that occurs in these patients.[14]

With LV dilation both $(dP/dt)_{max}$ and ejection fraction diminish, suggesting depression of myocardial contractility.[14] Maintenance of normal CI increasingly depends on support through the Frank-Starling mechanism and autonomic nervous system and there is the additional problem of maintaining adequate myocardial oxygen transport.[1,10] Eventually, resting CI becomes subnormal in this group of patients.[1,15] However, TPRI is elevated even further, indicating that there is no impairment of either the intrinsic amplifying capacity or the oxygen supply of the resistance vessels.

Rate of Redevelopment of Hypertension: After stopping antihypertensive drug treatment, the extent of the regression of the left ventricle and vascular hypertrophy (that is, of the gain of the cardiovascular amplifiers) appears to be a major determinant of the rate of redevelopment of hypertension. We found that in a group of previously untreated patients with uncomplicated essential hypertension, the supine systolic and diastolic pressures before treatment averaged 166/102 mmHg. After 5 weeks' treatment with timolol plus Moduretic, these pressures had decreased to 143/87 mmHg. Two weeks after cessation of treatment, the pressures had returned to the pretreatment values of 162/101 mmHg. This contrasts with the much smaller redevelopment of hypertension in the patients in Figure 3, whose pressures had been normalized by 1 year's antihypertensive therapy. The pretreatment pressures of 188/116 mmHg had decreased to 135/76 mmHg after 1 year, and had increased 2 weeks after stopping treatment to only 143/83 mmHg. At 10 weeks, pressures averaged 156/106 mmHg, still below pretreatment values in many of the patients. Blood pressure eventually returned to the pretreatment values in all patients, varying from 1 to 5 months in the different subjects.[8]

In the first group the period of treatment was short and the time to induce regression of cardiovascular hypertrophy was less than in the second group of patients, who had been treated for 1 year. Since then, we have observed even more gradual restoration of supine blood pressure in a third group of patients treated for a period of more than 2 years.[26,27] Preliminary echo studies suggest that it may take about 3 to 4 years of normalization of blood pressure to produce maximum regression of LV hypertrophy. Furthermore, the closer the LV mass has returned toward normal at the cessation of therapy, the more gradual is the subsequent redevelopment of hypertension.[27]

In a strategy of lifelong control of blood pressure of hypertensive patients, the reversal of the LVH and vascular muscle hypertrophy must be an important criterion of successful therapy. On present indications, regression of vascular hypertrophy by therapy appears to occur more readily and rapidly than regression of LVH. Inadequate regression of the latter thus appears to be an important factor influencing the rate of redevelopment of hypertension once treatment is stopped. This is particularly relevant when nonpharmacologic methods of treating hypertension are being considered. The effectiveness of these methods might be enhanced if their use were to follow an initial period of 2 to 3 years' drug treatment to bring about maximum regression of cardiovascular hypertrophy.

Conclusion

During the course of hypertension, there are changes in the capacity of the left ventricle and of the arterial resistance vessels to amplify CI and TPRI. In mild hypertension the capacity of the left ventricle to amplify CI somewhat exceeds the capacity of the vessels to amplify TPRI, probably because of the greater hypertrophy of the left ventricle and the greater systolic emptying at a given preload. In established moderate to severe hypertension, the hypertrophy of the vessels produces direct amplification of TPRI through greater narrowing of the vessel lumen. The hypertrophied left ventricle amplifies myocardial tension in proportion to the increase in muscle mass and this, together with the greater systolic emptying, allows it to maintain normal CI against a markedly increased MAP. With LV dilation, the hemodynamic amplifying capacity of the heart falls further behind that of the vessels, leading to the pattern of subnormal CI and high TPRI. Studies of the redevelopment of hypertension after cessation of therapy indicate that the rate of pressure increase is not merely related to the blood pressure levels achieved by the preceding treatment, but also to the latter's capacity to bring about regression of the hypertrophy of both the heart and vessels.

References

1. KORNER PI: The role of the heart in hypertension. In: Robertson JI, ed. Handbook of hypertension, vol 1. Amsterdam: Excerpta Medica, 1983; 97–132.
2. MESSERLI FH, DEVEREUX RB: Left ventricular hypertrophy—good or evil? Am J Med 1983; 75 (suppl 3A): 1–3.
3. TARAZI RC: The role of the heart in hypertension. Clin Sci 1982; 63: 347s–358s.
4. FOLKOW B: Physiological aspects of primary hypertension. Physiol Rev 1982; 62: 347–504.
5. SUWA N, TAKAHASHI T: Morphological and morphometrical analysis of circulation in hypertension and ischemic kidney. Munich: Urban & Schwarzenberg, 1971.

6. WEST MJ, ANGUS JA, KORNER PI: Estimation of nonautonomic and autonomic components of iliac bed vascular resistance in renal hypertensive rabbits. Cardiovasc Res 1975; 9: 697–706.

7. ANGUS JA, WEST MJ, KORNER PI: Assessment of autonomic and non-autonomic components of resting hindlimb vascular resistance and reactivity to pressor substances in renal hypertensive rabbits. Clin Sci Mol Med 1976; 51: 57s–59s.

8. KORNER PI: Causal and homeostatic factors in hypertension. Sixth Volhard Lecture. Clin Sci 1982; 63: 5s–26s.

9. BROUGHTON A, KORNER PI: Steady-state effects of preload and afterload on isovolumic indices of contractility in autonomically blocked dogs. Cardiovasc Res 1980; 14: 245–253.

10. BROUGHTON A, KORNER PI: Basal and maximal inotropic state in renal hypertensive dogs with cardiac hypertrophy. Am J Physiol 1983; 245: H33–H41.

11. BROUGHTON A, KORNER PI: Estimation of maximum left ventricular inotropic response from changes in isovolumic indices of contractility in the dog. Cardiovasc Res 1981; 15: 382–389.

12. KORNER PI: Circulatory regulation in hypertension. Br J Clin Pharmacol 1982; 13: 95–105.

13. ELZINGA G, WESTERHOF N: The pumping ability of the left heart and the effect of coronary occlusion. Circ Res 1976; 38: 297–302.

14. STRAUER BE: Hypertensive heart disease. Berlin: Springer-Verlag, 1980.

15. KORNER PI, FLETCHER PJ: Role of the heart in causing and maintaining hypertension. Cardiovasc Med 1977; 2: 139–155.

16. DUSTAN HP, TARAZI RC, BRAVO EL, DART RA: Plasma and extracellular fluid volumes in hypertension. Circ Res 1973; 32/33 (suppl I): 73–81.

17. WALSH JA, HYMAN C, MARONDE RF: Venous distensibility in essential hypertension. Cardiovasc Res 1969; 3: 338–349.

18. TAKESHITA A, MARK AL: Decreased venous distensibility in borderline hypertension. Hypertension 1979; 1: 202–206.

19. SAFAR ME, LEHNER JP, VINCENT M, PLAINFOSSE MT, SIMON AC: Echocardiographic dimensions in borderline and sustained hypertension. Am J Cardiol 1979; 44: 930–935.

20. CULPEPPER WS, SODT PC, MESSERLI FH, RUSCHHAUPT DG, ARCILLA RA: Cardiac status in juvenile borderline hypertension. Ann Intern Med 1983; 98: 1–7.

21. DEVEREUX RB, PICKERING TG, HARSHFIELD GA, et al: Left ventricular hypertrophy in patients with hypertension: importance of blood pressure response to regularly recurring stress. Circulation 1983; 68: 470–476.

22. YAMORI Y, MORI C, NISHIO T, et al: Cardiac hypertrophy in early hypertension. Am J Cardiol 1979; 44: 964–969.

23. JENNINGS GL, ESLER MD, KORNER PI: Effect of prolonged treatment on haemodynamics of essential hypertension before and after autonomic block. Lancet 1980; 2: 166–169.

24. ROWLANDS DB, GLOVER DR, IRELAND MA, et al: Assessment of left ventricular mass and its response to antihypertensive treatment. Lancet 1982; 1: 467–470.

25. KORNER PI, SHAW J, UTHER JB, WEST MJ, McRITCHIE RJ, RICHARDS JG: Autonomic and non-autonomic circulatory components in essential hypertension in man. Circulation 1973; 48: 107–117.

26. JENNINGS G, KORNER PI, ESLER M, RESTALL R: Redevelopment of essential hypertension after cessation of longterm therapy; preliminary findings. Clin Exp Hypertens 1984; A6: 493–505.

27. KORNER PI, JENNINGS GL, ESLER MD, BROUGHTON A: Role of cardiac and vascular amplifiers in the maintenance of hypertension and the effect of reversal of cardiovascular hypertrophy. Clin Exp Pharmacol Physiol 1985; 12: 205–209.

18

The Frank-Starling Mechanism in the Hypertrophied Heart at Various Levels of Afterload

MARGARETA NORDLANDER, Ph.D.
PETER FRIBERG, Ph.D.

In general, when an arterial pressure load is acutely imposed on the heart, the heart will counterbalance the enhanced load by increasing its contractility. By this type of autoregulation, which has been denoted "homeometric autoregulation,"[1] the heart will maintain stroke volume (SV), which otherwise would become reduced by the increase in arterial pressure.[1] When venous return to the heart is acutely enhanced, resulting in an increased volume load, the elevated diastolic distension will enhance the force of contraction according to the Frank-Starling mechanism. By this so-called heterometric autoregulation, excess blood delivered to the heart will also immediately be expelled.[1]

When a load is chronically imposed, the heart maintains pump function by means of cardiac luminal widening (or growth), wall hypertrophy (structural autoregulation) or both.[2] For example, in response to chronic pressure elevation, as during sustained hypertension or aortic stenosis, cardiac hypertrophy develops, characterized by wall thickening at a largely maintained intraventricular volume (concentric hypertrophy). During chronic volume overload, due to increased venous return, cardiac luminal widening occurs, which is usually associated with a corresponding increase in myocardial wall thickness (eccentric hypertrophy). Thus, such a type of luminal growth, often inappropriately called cardiac dilation, does by no means necessarily imply impeding cardiac failure, although this may often occur in the course of a severe long-standing pressure overload. The events leading to an increased myocardial wall thickness or to altered luminal dimensions illustrate a general pattern by which the left ventricular (LV) chamber and its myocardium tend to balance an increased workload by means of structural adaptation.

Definition of Afterload

The cardiac afterload is by definition the load that the myocardial fiber senses once it starts to contract, that is, the force opposing isotonic contraction.[1] As illustrated in experiments in vitro using papillary muscles, the greater the afterload, the more force the muscle will have to generate during isometric contraction. Arterial pressure is the primary determinant of afterload for the left ventricle as a whole, since the pressure it generates during isometric contraction has to exceed arterial pressure before any blood can be expelled. The situation for the individual myocardial cell is, however, also dependent on the geometric dimensions of the left ventricle. According to the law of Laplace, the wall tension per unit layer in a thick-walled sphere representing the left ventricle, that is, wall stress, is directly related to the transmural pressure and radius, but inversely related to the wall thickness. Therefore, for the individual contractile element, the wall stress during contraction is a more appropriate reflection of the afterload.[3] Thus, when evaluating cardiac performance in normotensive and hypertensive states, it is of great importance to consider the existing differences both in arterial pressure and in cardiac geometric dimensions, since hypertensive and normotensive hearts are likely to exhibit different levels of wall stress, even when exposed to equal arterial pressures. Hence, a maintained cardiac output, delivered against an increased arterial pressure implies an increased external cardiac work performance. This is made possible without any extra wall stress because of the previously mentioned structural autoregulation.

Different Forms of Hypertension

To study the functional, biochemical, and morphologic effects of left ventricular hypertrophy (LVH) in hypertension, spontaneously hypertensive rats (SHR) are often used in comparison with normotensive Wistar-Kyoto rats (WKY), since SHR are considered to be one of the most appropriate models of human primary hypertension.[4] In this model the hypertension develops fairly slowly, with a concomitantly slow increase in LVH.

A very different and far more rapid time course regarding the development of hypertension and left ventricular hypertrophy in rats is represented by the secondary renal hypertension that ensues when one renal artery is obstructed (2-kidney, 1-clip hypertension).[5] In this situation a more than 50% elevation of mean arterial pressure (MAP) can develop within a few days, and left ventricular hypertrophy is then fully developed within 2 to 3 weeks. Therefore, the SHR and renal forms of hypertension represent different kinds of pressure overloads due to the source and rate of pressure increase, and the ensuing structural cardiovascular adaptations will therefore most likely differ in important respects.[6]

In the intact individual many factors independently influence cardiac performance. For example, independent of neurohumoral influences on the heart, acute MAP increases will enhance cardiac contractility by way of homeometric autoregulation, thereby more or less balancing the reduction in SV, which otherwise would be induced by the increased resistance to ejection. Therefore, the Frank-Starling relationship reflecting the relation between SV and left ventricular end-diastolic pressure will become drastically influenced by the arterial pressure level. Furthermore, these relationships are fundamentally altered if the design of the left ventricle becomes changed. It is therefore not justifiable to compare maximal cardiac performance induced by volume overload at different arterial pressures in hypertensive and normotensive individuals, as has frequently been the case in studies performed in vivo.[7]

Frank-Starling Relationships in Primary Hypertension

Figure 1 illustrates the effects of rapid intravenous infusion of rat blood on mean arterial pressure of anesthetized SHR and WKY (left panel), on SV determined by a dye dilution technique in microscale (middle panel)[8] and on stroke work, which was calculated as the product of MAP-LV end-diastolic pressure and SV[9] (right panel). During this experimental procedure, MAP reached much higher levels in SHR than in WKY (Fig. 1, left panel) and, although SV was lower in SHR than in WKY at low LV end-diastolic pressure, this was not the case at high LV end-diastolic pressure (Fig. 1, middle panel). Furthermore, the stroke work of the heart was greatly enhanced in SHR (Fig. 1, right panel). Cardiac function curves were also performed in the anesthetized rat at various levels of arterial pressure, induced either by aortic clamping or systemic vasodilation by hydralazine infusion[9] in order to compare cardiac performance in SHR and WKY at equal MAP levels. At any MAP level between 100 and 215 mmHg, the maximally recorded SV, that is, peak SV obtained at LV end-diastolic pressure levels around 20 mmHg, was always higher in SHR than in WKY. This indicates a clearcut enhancement of maximal performance of the hypertrophied SHR left ventricle, which was particularly evident at high MAP levels. These results on fairly young SHR (4 months old) show that myocardial hypertrophy implies a most efficient adaptation of cardiac performance to balance the elevated pressure level. The situation can, of course, be a different one in case elements of relative myocardial ischemia or degeneration, or both, are added, such as found in aging man.

In order better to control the different parameters determining LV performance, we have also used an in vitro technique. Isolated hearts were perfused with Krebs-Henseleit bicarbonate buffer, electrically paced most frequently at 300 beats/minute, and their left ventricles were producing external work that was continuously recorded. Left atrial pressure (preload) and peak aortic pressure, which in the same heart determine afterload, could be changed independently. In this way cardiac function curves, reflecting the Frank-Starling relationships, could be obtained at any desired level of aortic pressure.[10] With this in vitro technique, left ventricular performance was analyzed both in 4- and 19-month old male SHR and in sex- and age-matched WKY (Fig. 2). The hearts of the 19-month-old SHR will here represent the

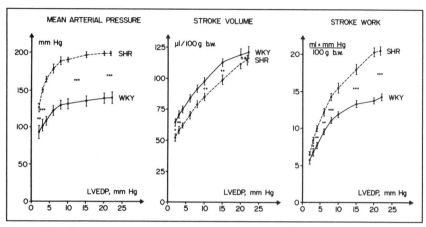

Figure 1. *Mean arterial pressure (MAP), stroke volume (SV), and stroke work (MAP-LVEDP × SV) when left ventricular end-diastolic pressure (LVEDP) was rapidly increased by rapid blood infusion in pentobarbital-anesthetized, closed chest SHR (n = 10) and WKY (n = 9). Note in the right panel, the leftward shift of the cardiac function curve in SHR, clearly illustrating an enhanced cardiac performance. Values are presented as means ± SE. *p < 0.05, **p < 0.01, ***p < 0.001. (Reprinted with permission from Lundin et al.[9])*

situation of a long-standing, severe pressure overload. As illustrated in Figure 2, the hypertrophied hearts of young SHR performed much better than those from age-matched WKY over the entire range of end-diastolic pressures at a hypertensive level of 130 mmHg in aortic pressure. When comparing the performance of the old SHR-WKY, this difference was less pronounced. At hypertensive aortic pressures, that is, 130 mmHg, young and old WKY had about equal maximal SV, indicating a well-maintained cardiac function at least up to the age of 19 months. However, with age, the initially enhanced performance of the SHR hearts gradually decreased toward that of a normotensive heart when working at hypertensive pressure levels (Fig. 2, lower right panel). When the Frank-Starling relations were instead determined at very low aortic pressure levels (50 mmHg; Fig. 2, upper left panel) cardiac performance in terms of peak SV was clearly lower both in young and old SHR than in the age-matched WKY. An explanation for this dramatic relative decline in SHR cardiac performance at subnormal afterloads is most likely that coronary flow at these low perfusion pressures is reduced beyond a critical level. The reason is that structural resistance vessel changes, which occur in all systemic circuits in hypertension, have also here caused a limitation of the maximal flow capacity.[11] In the normotensive situation, here represented by an afterload of 80 mmHg, there was no clear-cut difference between the Frank-Starling relationship between age-matched SHR and WKY.

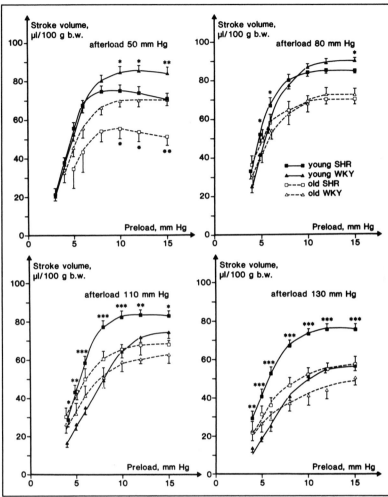

Figure 2. Stroke volume (SV) as a function of left atrial pressure (preload) that is Frank-Starling relationships at 4 different levels of peak aortic pressures (afterloads) in young, 4-month old, SHR (n = 10) and WKY (n = 10) and in old, 19-month old, SHR and WKY (n = 8, n = 11, respectively). At an afterload of 50 mmHg, reflecting a hypotensive level and also a lower degree of coronary flow, both young and old SHR left ventricles performed at reduced peak stroke volume versus their aged WKY controls. At an afterload of 130 mmHg, reflecting a hypertensive level and also an adequate coronary flow, young SHR performed a significantly higher peak SV compared with young WKY. With age, there was a reduction of the previously enhanced performance in young SHR toward the old WKY level, but still there was a tendency of higher SV in old SHR versus old WKY. No significant reduction of maximal myocardial performance (at afterload 130 mmHg) was observed from 4 to 19 months of age in WKY. Values are presented as means ± SE. *p < 0.05, **p < 0.01, ***p < 0.001 between young SHR and WKY. *p < 0.05, **p < 0.01 between old SHR and WKY. (Reprinted with permission from Friberg et al.[10])

Frank-Starling Relationships in Secondary Hypertension

Using the same perfusion system, the Frank-Starling relationships were also determined in hearts from rats with 2-kidney, 1-clip renal hypertension of 4 weeks' duration at various aortic pressures, to compare their maximal cardiac performance with those of normotensive rats. Such a comparison was also made with hearts from rats that had been renal hypertensive for 4 weeks but then had again become normotensive after removal of the renal clip for 1 week, although their left ventricles still displayed considerable hypertrophy.[12] Maximal cardiac performance was also evaluated in hearts from SHR and SHR with 2-kidney, 1-clip hypertension. Maximal cardiac performance or peak cardiac work was evaluated as the maximally obtained value of SV times paced heart rate times aortic pressure minus LV end-diastolic pressure, at any level of aortic pressure ranging from 50 to 130 mmHg.

As shown in Figure 3, peak cardiac work was increased in ordinary SHR, but decreased in 2-kidney, 1-clip rats compared with normotensive rats. However, in the previously renal hypertensive rats, which still had about the same LV weight to body weight ratio as the matched SHR, cardiac work performance was increased to about the same extent as in SHR. In contrast, in SHR made renal hypertensive, having an almost doubled LV weight to body weight ratio versus normotensive rats, maximal LV function was about equal to the normotensive controls, and hence clearly reduced compared with ordinary SHR. The implications of these findings are that the gradual LVH in primary hypertension proportionally improves cardiac function, but cardiac hypertrophy induced by renovascular hypertension does not. These data are in agreement with other investigations[6] reporting depressed contractility of papillary muscle preparations from renal hypertensive rats, a depression that was improved on removal of the affected kidney. It is therefore suggested that the renal hypertensive state may per se involve some negative inotropic influence of so far unknown nature, which evidently is dependent on the clamped, low-pressure kidney. This illustrates, as did the comparative study of Skelton and Sonnenblick,[13] that the alterations in contractility occurring in one form of cardiac hypertrophy cannot be directly applied to hypertrophy developed during another type of increased afterload.

Summary

The Frank-Starling relationship is dramatically influenced by the afterload level, and for a given heart, maximal SV declines with increases in arterial pressure. However, according to the law of Laplace, not only the arterial pressure level but also the cardiac wall to lumen dimensions will determine the afterload to which the individual contractile element is exposed. Therefore, an adequate increase in LV wall thickness, by myocardial hypertrophy,

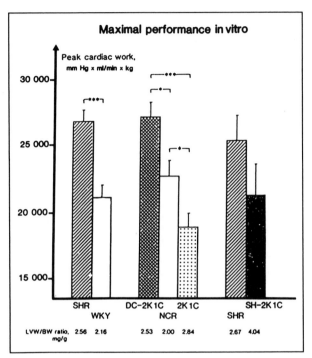

Figure 3. *Maximal performance expressed as peak cardiac work, calculated as a product of aortic pressure, left ventricular end-diastolic pressure (LVEDP), and heart rate and peak stroke volume, in various kinds of hypertension. SHR = spontaneously hypertensive rats (n = 10 left and n = 8 right); WKY = Wistar-Kyoto normotensive rats (n = 10), 2K1C = 4 week old 2-kidney, 1-clip renal hypertensive rats (n = 10), DC-2K1C = surgically 1 week declipped 2-kidney, 1-clip renal hypertensive rats (n = 11), NCR = normotensive Wistar control rats (n = 14), and SH-2K1C = spontaneously hypertensive rats superimposed with 2-kidney, 1-clip hypertension (n = 6). At the bottom of the figure are shown the left ventricular weight to body weight ratios (LVW/BW). Note the enhanced work produced by the SHR left ventricles compared with WKY ventricles. 2K1C as well as SH-2K1C showed a decreased performance. When the clip was removed for 1 week in the 2K1C group, maximal performance increased. Indeed, it increased above the control level (NCR) to about the same extent as SHR. Note the very close similarities in LVW/BW ratios between SHR and DC-2K1C. Values are presented as means ± SE. *p < 0.05, ***p < 0.001. (Reprinted with permission from Friberg et al.[12])*

will enable the hypertrophied heart to maintain a normal Frank-Starling relationship and maximal SV also at hypertensive levels. In SHR such an adequate hypertrophy seems to take place, since the adapted cardiac performance well matches the enhanced arterial pressure, as long as no degenerative phenomena are superimposed, as in the old SHR heart.[14] Also, in the renal hypertensive rat the LVH per se seems adequately to balance the enhanced arterial pressure, but in this hypertensive model some evidently extrinsic negative inotropic influence that directly or indirectly depends on the clamped kidney seems to be involved, masking the effect of hypertrophy on cardiac performance.

Thus, as long as the hypertrophied hearts from hypertensive persons work at hypertensive levels, their function is well maintained because of the structural myocardial adaptation, at least as long as no negative inotropic or myocardial degenerative influences are superimposed. However, at clearly subnormal aortic pressure levels, the structural resistance vessel adaptation, which always accompanies hypertensive states,[2] will limit the maximal performance of the hypertrophied heart in hypertension as it reduces the maximal coronary flow capacity. In situations in which also atherosclerotic processes restrict the coronary flow reserves, as is often the case in advanced human hypertension, a limited coronary supply capacity often has decisive effects on myocardial performance.

References

1. SARNOFF SJ, MITCHELL JH: The control of the function of the heart. In: Handbook of Physiology. Bethesda, MD: American Physiological Society, 1962; 409.
2. FOLKOW B: Physiological aspects of primary hypertension. Physiol Rev 1982; 62: 347–503.
3. GROSSMAN W, JONES D, McLAURIN LP: Wall stress and patterns of hypertrophy in the human left ventricle. J Clin Invest 1975; 56: 56–64.
4. FOLKOW B, HALLBÄCK M: Physiopathology of spontaneous hypertension in rats. In: Genest G, Koiw E, Kuchel O, eds. Hypertension. New York: McGraw-Hill, 1977; 507–529.
5. LUNDGREN Y, HALLBÄCK M, WEISS L, FOLKOW B: Rate and extent of adaptive cardiovascular changes in rats during experimental renal hypertension. Acta Physiol Scand 1974; 91: 103–115.
6. CAPASSO JM, STROBECK JE, MALHOTRA A, SCHEUER J, SONNENBLICK EH: Contractile behavior of rat myocardium after reversal of hypertensive hypertrophy. Am J Physiol 1982; 242: H882–H889.
7. SPECH MM, FERRARIO CM, TARAZI RC: Cardiac pumping ability following reversal of hypertrophy and hypertension in spontaneously hypertensive rats. Hypertension 1980; 2: 75–82.
8. STAGE L: Rapid determination of cardiac output in small animals from dye dilution measurements. Acta Physiol Scand 1978; 102: 43A.
9. LUNDIN S, FRIBERG P, MALLBÄCK-NORDLANDER M: Left ventricular hypertrophy improves cardiac performance in spontaneously hypertensive rats. Acta Physiol Scand 1982; 114: 321–328.

10. FRIBERG P, HALLBÄCK-NORDLANDER M, LUNDIN S: Cardiac performance of isolated hearts from young and old normotensive (WKY) and spontaneously hypertensive rats (SHR). Acta Physiol Scand [suppl] 1982; 508: 94.

11. NORESSON E, HALLBÄCK M, HJALMARSSON Å: Structural "resetting" of the coronary vascular bed in spontaneously hypertensive rats. Acta Physiol Scand 1977; 101: 363–365.

12. FRIBERG P, LUNDIN S, FOLKOW B, HALLBÄCK-NORDLANDER M: Left ventricular function in spontaneous and renal hypertension in rats. J Hypertension 1983; 1 (suppl II): s 265–s 271.

13. SKELTON CL, SONNENBLICK EH: Heterogeneity of contractile function in cardiac hypertrophy. Circ Res 1974; 34–35 (suppl II): II–33.

14. PFEFFER JM, PFEFFER MA, FISHBEIN MC, FROHLICH ED: (1979). Cardiac function and morphology with aging in the spontaneously hypertensive rat. Am J Physiol 1979; 237: H461–H468.

19

Cardiac Hypertrophy Reflecting Structural Vascular Changes

YUKIO YAMORI, M.D.

Cardiac hypertrophy is the most common complication of hypertension both in humans[1] and animal models for hypertension.[2] Although this hypertrophy is often considered only a secondary effect of the increased pressure load, our findings in very young spontaneously hypertensive rats (SHR)[3] suggested a more complex picture[4] for several reasons:

First, in SHR, the enhancement of protein synthesis is noted both in the heart and blood vessels in the absence of significant differences in arterial pressure.[5–8] Second, in adult SHR with hypertension, cardiac hypertrophy was histometrically proved to be significantly related to the thickening of coronary blood vessels.[2] Third, cardiac and vascular hypertrophy were concomitantly noted in rats with catecholamine-induced hypertension.[9] Fourth, under in vivo tissue culture conditions, catecholamines effectively induced myocardial hypertrophy[10] and activated ornithine decarboxylase activity, the index of protein synthesis of smooth muscle cells.[11,12] Fifth, dissociation between blood pressure and protein synthesis in the heart and blood vessels was first noted in SHR under various antihypertensive treatments.[13] This indicated that cardiac and vascular hypertrophy were not always secondary to blood pressure increase, but rather concomitantly resulted from such common causes as increased sympathetic tone.

Therefore, the concomitant occurrence of cardiovascular hypertrophy is important not only in the pathogenesis of hypertension, but also in the therapy of hypertension and, furthermore, may be useful for the detection of genetic predisposition to hypertension in SHR and humans.[2]

Concomitant Evolution of Cardiovascular Hypertrophy in SHR and Other Rat Strains

Our previous studies showed an increased heart weight in SHR very early (4 weeks after birth) in comparison with normotensive Wistar-Kyoto rats (WKY), and the weight of the precisely extirpated aorta also proved to be increased in SHR at the age of 4 weeks,[2,5] when no definite increase in blood pressure was noted. Since norepinephrine turnover of the heart was accelerated at this stage, catecholamine or increased sympathetic drive may be in-

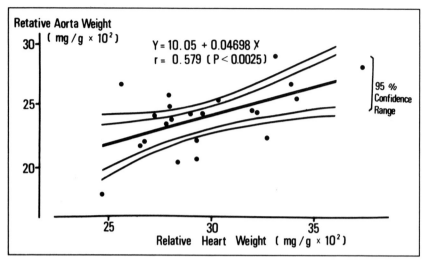

Figure 1. *Correlation between relative heart and aorta weight in 23 inbred rat strains.*

volved in the early development of hypertension as well as in structural cardiovascular changes;[2,5,14] norepinephrine turnover was significantly faster at the age of 60 days, but no longer significant at 90 days. This finding is consistent with the importance of the sympathetic nervous system in the early development of spontaneous hypertension.

As the biochemical index of cardiovascular hypertrophy, amino acid incorporation as well as protein/DNA ratios were examined in SHR and stroke-prone SHR (SHRSP).[15,16] The amino acid incorporation was already increased both in the heart and blood vessels (aorta and mesenteric arteries) as early as 4 weeks after birth. The increased protein to DNA ratios were noted not only in the left ventricle but also in the right ventricle and the aorta. Furthermore, significant positive correlation between relative heart weight and aorta weight was observed in 23 inbred rat strains, including SHR and SHRSP (Fig. 1). Genetic analysis of the heart and aorta weight from these 23 rat strains disclosed that the degrees of genetic determination were 0.739 ± 0.044 and 0.627 ± 0.054 in the heart and aorta weights, respectively.[17]

Hypertrophic Coronary Vessels in Hypertrophied Heart

Histologic studies further demonstrated that thickening of small coronary arteries due to medial hypertrophy or hyperplasia and occlusive arterial changes with thrombosis were often observed in the hypertrophied hearts of adult spontaneously hypertensive rats.[2] In the advanced stage, intraluminal proliferative changes are so marked that the arterial lumen is almost occluded, and such arterial hyperplasia coexists with myocardial hypertrophy. The ratio of the lumen to the transectional area of small coronary arteries (diameter of less than 100 and between 100 and 150 μ) in SHR, SHRSP, and WKY was determined histometrically using a quantitative picture analysis from 1 to 12 months of age. The normal ratio was clearly and significantly reduced even in young 1-month-old SHR compared with their age-matched WKY counterparts. Furthermore, there seemed to be an inverse correlation between heart weight and the lumen to transectional area ratios of coronary arteries in SHR and WKY from 1 to 6 months of age. Again, cardiac weight hypertrophy seemed to be a good indicator of vascular hypertrophy or hyperplasia, that is, for those structural vascular changes that are important in the further development and maintenance of hypertension.

Catecholamine-Induced Cardiovascular Hypertrophy

The rate of neuronal stimulation or circulating catecholamines in the concomitant evolution of cardiovascular hypertrophy was clearly demonstrated by the following experimental results.[9] Continuous intravenous norepinephrine infusion for 1 week into rats by osmotic minipumps significantly increased blood pressure, left ventricular (LV) weight, and the aortic weight. Concomitant alpha-receptor blockade infusion significantly lowered blood pressure and the aortic weight without significant reduction in LV weight. However, two beta-receptor blocking agents in norepinephrine-infused rats normalized LV weight and significantly reduced the aortic weight, although blood pressure was still higher than control noninfused rats.

These results suggest that beta-receptors play a modulating role in the structural cardiovascular response to blood pressure, and their stimulation or blocking is, therefore, supposed to induce the concomitant evolution or reduction of heart and aorta weights in hypertension.

Hypertrophy of Cultured Vascular Smooth Muscle Cells and Myocytes

The mechanisms involved in cardiovascular hypertrophy were further analyzed in vascular smooth muscle cells and myocytes under tissue culture condition free from the effect of blood pressure or undefined humoral factors.

Cultured smooth-muscle cells were obtained by an explant method from the thoracic aorta from the age-matched stroke resistant SHR (SHRSR), SHRSP, and WKY.[11,12] During repeated explant experiments, migration of cells from the aortic explants was more active in SHRSR and SHRSP than in WKY. Smooth-muscle cells from hypertensive rats proliferated significantly faster under subculture than those from the age-matched WKY, even at the age of 12 weeks. The mean doubling times were nearly 50 hours in WKY, but they were clearly shortened in SHRSP and SHR, 24 to 31 hours respectively. ^{3}H-thymidine and ^{14}C-leucine incorporations into DNA and protein were significantly greater in the cultured smooth muscle cells from SHR or SHRSP than in those from WKY.[11] Ornithine decarboxylase activity is the rate-limiting step for the biosynthesis of polyamine and is thus regarded as a good indicator of cellular hypertrophy or hyperplasia. The ornithine decarboxylase activity after the growth stimulation by fetal calf serum was greater in the smooth muscle cells from SHRSP and SHRSR than in those from WKY.[12] This finding again confirms the activated protein synthesis in the smooth muscle cells from hypertensive rats.

Although these culture experiments indicated that smooth-muscle cells from hypertensive rats were themselves different, several humoral factors affecting the growth of smooth muscle cells have been observed. To test the trophic effect of catecholamines from nerve endings or adrenal medulla on the vascular smooth muscle cells, isoproterenol or norepinephrine was added to the culture medium. The ornithine decarboxylase activity of the cultured smooth muscle cells was clearly increased after exposure to isoproterenol (9.5 μmol/liter) and reached the maximum, three fold increase 3 hours after exposure, whereas it was only slightly increased after exposure to norepinephrine (11.8 μmol/liter).[12] Although the beta blocker propranolol (19.3 μmol/liter) itself did not affect the basal activity, it completely blocked isoproterenol-induced activation of ornithine decarboxylase activity. We may conclude, therefore, that beta stimulation activates vascular protein synthesis independently of blood pressure, as suggested by our previous observation in vivo.[11]

Since culture myocytes are not a homogeneous cell population, they are not appropriate materials for biochemical studies. Thus, norepinephrine was applied to culture media repeatedly for 1 week and was confirmed to increase the nuclear size of cultured myocytes.

Concomitant Cardiac and Vascular Hypertrophy under Antihypertensive Treatment

Our earlier studies indicated the importance of activated vascular protein synthesis of the cardiovascular system in the establishment of hypertension,[2,5,14] and the effect of various antihypertensive agents was examined on the vascular protein synthesis, a sensitive index of cardiovascular structural changes existing in SHR (Fig. 2). The effect differed according to the mechanism of antihypertensive agents: hydralazine treatment effectively lowered blood pressure in SHRSP, but did not reduce LV weight so effectively or significantly decrease noncollagen protein synthesis in the left ventricle and the aorta during the acute to subacute stage of the treatment.[13] Contrary to the hydralazine treatment, the beta blocker propranolol did not reduce blood pressure so effectively in SHRSP, but decreased noncollagen and collagen protein synthesis in the heart and aorta.[9] Hence the blocking of neuronal input to arterial smooth muscle cells seemed to be important in the attenuation of vascular protein synthesis, that is, the prevention of structural

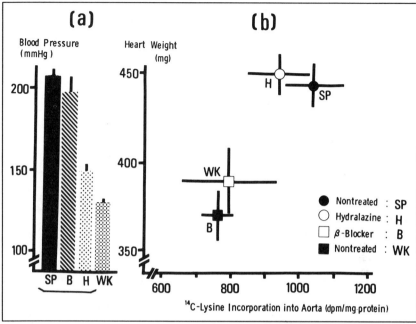

Figure 2. **a:** *Antihypertensive effect of beta blocker (propranolol; B) and hydralazine (H) in SHRSP (SP) compared with WKY (WK).* **b:** *Correlation between heart weight and vascular protein synthesis in SHRSP (SP) treated with hydralazine (H), beta blocker (B) compared with WKY (WK).*

vascular changes. These in vivo studies, therefore, indicate that in addition to the blood pressure itself, other factors, such as neurohumoral factors or genetic predisposition, also contribute to the structural changes in hypertension.

Clinical Detection of Incipient Cardiac Hypertrophy for Preventing Evolution of Vascular Hypertrophy in Hypertension

These experimental observations in SHR suggested that cardiac hypertrophy might develop early in life in persons with borderline elevations in arterial pressure or some predisposition to hypertension. If documented, this early incidence of cardiac hypertrophy could prove of major significance in our understanding of the disease and approach to its control. An extensive survey of schoolchildren in Japan was therefore undertaken involving more than 350 children aged 6 to 15 years (Shimane Heart Study).[1,18,19] The extensive analysis of echo in more than 1,000 normotensive children allowed the development of normal values for different age groups. Viewed against this background, some subjects with borderline hypertension had an LV mass clearly greater than 2 SD of normal for their age. The blood pressure in these subjects ranged from 126/80 to 134/86 mmHg, and they showed no other evidence of cardiovascular diseases. Similar results in juvenile hypertension were also reported by Culpepper et al.[20] More studies are obviously needed, particularly with long-term follow-up and correlation with personal and family history for complete correlation of the significance of early increases in LV mass. If documented in man, cardiac hypertrophy, especially in prehypertension, would have more important diagnostic and prognostic implications than vascular hypertrophy that is clinically undetectable.

Summary

Coexistence of cardiac and vascular hypertrophy in hypertension does not simply indicate that both are adaptive changes secondary to hypertension, but accumulating evidence obtained by in vivo and in vitro studies in SHR and other rat strains indicates the possibility that there should be common genetic predisposition to cardiac and vascular hypertrophy as well as common causative factors, such as sympathetic innervation and circulating catecholamines. Therefore, cardiac hypertrophy, which can be clinically detected more easily than vascular hypertrophy, may be used as the indicator for the evaluation and regression of vascular hypertrophy in hypertensive patients under antihypertensive therapy, and early detection of cardiac hypertrophy even in the young may be a useful indicator of the incipient stage of structural vascular changes in genetic hypertension.

References

1. TARAZI RC, DUNBAR JB: Cardiac hypertrophy in hypertension. In: Katz AM, ed. Perspectives in cardiovascular research, vol 8. New York: Raven Press, 1983.
2. YAMORI Y, MORI C, NISHIO T, et al: Cardiac hypertrophy in early hypertension. Am J Cardiol 1979; 44: 964–969.
3. OKAMOTO K, AOKI K: Development of a strain of spontaneously hypertensive rats. Jpn Circ J 1963; 27: 282–293.
4. FOLKOW B, HALLBACK M, LUNDGREN Y, SIVERTSSON R, WEISS L: Importance of adaptive changes in vascular design for establishment of primary hypertension studied in man and in spontaneously hypertensive rats. Circ Res 1973; 32, 33: (suppl I): I-2–I-16.
5. YAMORI Y: Contribution of cardiovascular factors to the development of hypertension in spontaneously hypertensive rats. Jpn Heart J 1974; 15: 194–196.
6. SEN S, TARAZI RC, KHAIRALLAH PA, BUMPUS M: Cardiac hypertrophy in spontaneously hypertensive rats. Circ Res 1974; 35: 775–781.
7. SEN S, TARAZI RC, BUMPUS FM: Age, hypertension and protein synthesis in SHR. In: Spontaneous hypertension: its pathogenesis and complications. Washington, DC: DHEW Publication no. (NIH) 77-1179, 1979; 59–63.

8. Cutilletta AF, Erinoff L, Heller A, Low J, Oparil A: Development of left ventricular hypertrophy in young spontaneously hypertensive rats after peripheral sympathectomy. Circ Res 1977; 40: 428–434.

9. Yamori Y, Tarazi RC, Ooshima A: Effect of β-receptor-blocking agents on cardiovascular structural changes in spontaneous and noradrenaline-induced hypertension in rats. Clin Sci 1980; 59: 4575–4605.

10. Igawa T, Yamori Y, Lewis LJ, Tarazi RC: Norepinephrine-induced hypertrophy of cultured myocytes. Submitted for publication.

11. Yamori Y, Igawa T, Kanbe T, Kihara M, Nara Y, Horie R: Mechanisms of structural vascular changes in genetic hypertension: analyses on cultured vascular smooth muscle cells from spontaneously hypertensive rats. Clin Sci 1981; 61 (suppl 7): 121s–123s.

12. Kanbe T, Nara Y, Tagami M, Yamori Y: Studies on hypertension-induced vascular hypertrophy in cultured smooth muscle cells from spontaneously hypertensive rats. Hypertension 1983; 5: 887–892.

13. Yamori Y, Nakada T, Lovenberg W: Effect of antihypertensive therapy on lysine incorporation into vascular protein of the spontaneously hypertensive rats. Eur J Pharmacol 1976; 38: 349–355.

14. Yamori Y: Neural and nonneural mechanisms in spontaneous hypertension. Clin Sci Mol Med 1976; 51: 431s–434s.

15. Yamori Y, Nagaoka A, Okamoto K: Importance of genetic factors in hypertensive cerebrovascular lesions: evidence obtained by successive selective breeding of stroke-prone and -resistant SHR. Jpn Circ J 1974; 38: 1095–1100.

16. Okamoto K, Yamori Y, Nagaoka A: Establishment of the stroke-prone spontaneously hypertensive rats (SHR). Circ Res 1974; 34, 35 (suppl I): I-143–I-153.

17. Tanase H, Yamori Y, Hamen C, Lovenberg W: Heart size in inbred strains of rats. Part 1. Genetic determination of the development of cardiovascular enlargement in rats. Hypertension 1982; 4: 864–872.

18. Saito M, Mori C, Nishio T, Soeda T, Abe K: Normal values of echocardiology in pediatrics. I. Left ventricular muscle volume (LVMV). Shimane Heart Study. Shimane J Med Sci 1978; 2: 63–69.

19. Nishio T, Mori C, Saito M, Soeda T, Abe K, Nakao Y: Left ventricular hypertrophy in early hypertensive children: its importance as a risk factor for hypertension. Shimane J Med Sci 1978; 3: 71–79.

20. Culpepper W, Hutcheon N, Arcilla R, Cutilletta A: Left ventricular hypertrophy in juvenile hypertension. Circulation 1979; (suppl II): 11–51.

PART V
CLINICAL ASPECTS

20

Left Ventricular Hypertrophy: Identification and Implications

RICHARD B. DEVEREUX, M.D.
JEFFREY S. BORER, M.D.
ELIZABETH M. LUTAS, M.D.
JOHN H. LARAGH, M.D.

The heart plays a central role in arterial hypertension, both generating the force required to elevate blood pressure and paying the consequences of hypertension as a target organ. At first, the heart's increased workload is paralleled by modest degrees of compensatory left ventricular hypertrophy (LVH).[1-3] At this stage, cardiac function remains normal. In some patients, however, particularly those whose hypertension becomes severe, the heart's adaptive capacity is eventually exceeded, which can lead to depressed cardiac function[4-6] and the onset of clinical congestive heart failure.[7,8]

In recent years, noninvasive methods have been developed that allow evaluation of cardiac anatomy and function. These methods include echo, which is safe, easily repeated, and relatively accurate in assessment of cardiac anatomy and function, and radionuclide cineangiography, which allows precise measurement of left ventricular (LV) function at rest and during exercise. In this review, we will consider the role of these methods in the evaluation of LVH in hypertension (Table I).

Echo

Echo measures directly the thickness of the LV walls as well as the chamber's internal diameter throughout the cardiac cycle. This attractive feature has made possible accurate noninvasive measurement of LV function and mass.[9,10] Echo methods have been discussed in recent reviews,[11,12] to which the reader is referred for technical details.

The initial echo methods for measuring LV mass were validated indirectly by comparison with quantitative angiography[13] or by using assumed geometric models of the left ventricle.[14] To determine whether the echo could be used for accurate measurements of LV mass, we initially compared postmortem LV weight in 34 patients with estimates derived from antemortem echoes using several geometric formulas.[10] We also tested an alternative "Penn convention," which excludes the thickness of endocardial interfaces

TABLE I   **Noninvasive Assessment of the Heart in Patients with Hypertension**

	Normal Values
Anatomy	
Echo	
Septal thickness	≤ 1.2 cm
Posterior left ventricular wall thickness	≤ 1.1 cm
Relative wall thickness	≤ 0.48
Left ventricular mass	≤ 215 grams
Left ventricular mass index	< 120 g/m^2 or ≤ 134 g/m^2 in males and ≤ 110 g/m^2 in females
Function	
Echo	
Fractional systolic shortening of left ventricular internal dimension	$\geq 26\%$
Ejection fraction	$> 55\%$
Estimated wall stresses	
End-systolic stress	20 to 115×10^3 dyne^5/cm^2
Radionuclide angiography	
Ejection fraction	
Rest	$\geq 45\%$
Exercise	$\geq 54\%$ and 5% above resting ejection fraction
Segmental wall motion abnormalities	Absent

from measurements of septal and posterior wall thickness (IVST and PWT) and includes them in the LV internal dimension (LVID). Highly accurate estimates of LV mass were obtained (Fig. 1) by using Penn convention measurements in the following regression equation:

$$LV\ mass = 1.04\ [(LVID + PWT + IVST)^3 - (LVID)^3] - 13.6\ g$$

We subsequently observed a similarly close correlation between echo LV mass by the Penn method and autopsy LV weight in a second series of 24 patients.[15] Other published echo methods correlated less accurately with autopsy LV weight in both autopsy series[10,15] but still yielded useful estimates of LV mass.

Echo measurements can also be used to assess left ventricular function. The most direct echo functional index is LV systolic fractional shortening (FS) in which the percent shortening of the LV minor axis between end-diastole and end-systole is calculated:

$$FS = \frac{LVIDd - LVIDs}{LVIDd}$$

Normal values are 26% or more. These same measurements may be used in the cube function formula to derive the LV ejection fraction (EF):

$$EF = \frac{(LVIDd)^3 - (LVIDs)^3}{(LVIDd)^3} \times 100$$

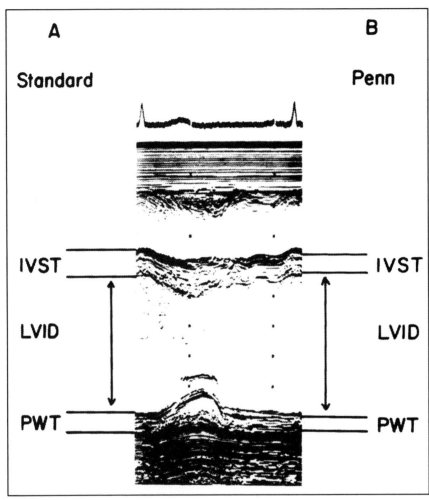

Figure 1. *Relationship between blood pressure measured by automatic portable recorder at work (horizontal axes) and indices of LVH (vertical axis).* **A:** *A highly significant relationship exists between workplace systolic blood pressure and LV mass index.* **B:** *An even closer relationship was observed between workplace diastolic blood pressure and end-diastolic relative wall thickness (Reprinted with permission from Devereux and Reichek.[10])*

The lower limit of normal for the ejection fraction in our laboratory is 56%.

In addition, LV wall stress may be calculated from LV measurements on high-quality echoes and simultaneous cuff blood pressure. Echo methods for estimation of peak systolic, mean systolic, and end-systolic wall stress have been validated by comparison with invasive measurements.[16,17] Our studies suggest that LV end-systolic stress (ESS) is the most useful of these measurements. It can be calculated from cuff systolic blood pressure (SBP) and end-systolic echo dimensions by the following formula:[16]

$$ESS = \frac{0.334 \times SBP \times LVIDs}{\left(PWTs \times \left(1 + \frac{PWTs}{LVIDs}\right)\right)}$$

Two-Dimensional Echo: Two-dimensional echo visualizes the heart in tomographic "slices." This facilitates measurement of the long axis of the left ventricle, an important element in calculation of LV volumes and myocardial mass, which is not directly measured by one-dimensional echo. Although two-dimensional echo techniques and measurement conventions have not yet been as well standardized as those for M-mode technique, initial results are promising. Thus, LV volume estimates appear to be sufficiently reproducible that small changes in ventricular size and ejection fraction can be detected.[18] Methods of determining LV mass have also been reported that were highly accurate in initial autopsy comparison studies.[19,20]

Normal Left Ventricular Anatomy: Following circulatory adjustments at birth, the left ventricle bears the predominant circulatory load. Accordingly, LV muscle makes up nearly half the weight of the heart. From the age of 2 years, heart weight and LV volume increase proportionally to body weight.[21,22] Interestingly, Rogé and colleagues[22] showed that LV wall thickness increases more rapidly during maturation than LVID. Therefore, relative wall thickness (twice wall thickness to chamber diameter) increases with age, parallel with the normal increase in arterial pressure. St. John Sutton and associates[23] extended this finding by showing that the increases in LV wall thickness and relative wall thickness that occur with age in normal adults are directly related to increases in arterial blood pressure within the normal range.

Left ventricular relative wall thickness in 79 normal subjects studied in our laboratory was 0.34 ± 0.05.[24] Similar findings have been reported in other studies[4,25,26] (Table II). Thus, a relative wall thickness of 0.48 or greater exceeds the 97th percentile of normal. The hemodynamic load in hypertension is not solely determined by the level of arterial pressure, however, since cardiac output may vary widely. The resultant differences in LV chamber size have at least as great an effect as the level of blood pressure on the degree of LVH in patients with hypertension.[27] Therefore, estimation of LV mass is needed in addition to calculation of relative wall thickness to provide a complete description of LVH in patients with hypertension. Penn method LV mass in our 79 normal subjects was 70 ± 25 g/m^2, which is similar to findings in previous echo series[4,25] (Table II) and in autopsy and angiographic studies.[1] Thus, an LV mass of 120 g/m^2 approximates the upper 95% confidence limit of normal. Since normal men have greater LV mass than normal women, it may prove to be preferable to use separate sex-specific normal limits (134 g/m^2 and 110 g/m^2, respectively, in 225 normal subjects studied at Cornell).

TABLE II   Echo Measurements in Normal Subjects and in Patients with Hypertension*

Study	No.	Mean Blood Pressure (mmHg)	Relative Wall Thickness	Left Ventricular Mass Index (g/m²)	Left Ventricular Fractional Shortening (%)
Normal subjects					
Devereux et al[24]	79	88 ± 9	0.34 ± 0.05	70 ± 25	35 ± 5
Reichek and Devereux[25]	17	92 ± 6	0.34 ± 0.04	62 ± 16	37 ± 6
Karliner et al[26]	29	—	0.34 ± 0.11	—	—
Dunn et al[4]	14	93 ± 4	0.33	87 ± 22	38 ± 4
Lutas et al[38]	87	99 ± 11	0.36 ± 0.07	81 ± 22	35 ± 6
Patients with hypertension					
Lutas et al[38]	81	112 ± 16	0.40 ± 0.10	103 ± 33	36 ± 7
Devereux et al[24]	118	116 ± 14	0.42 ± 0.08	114 ± 27	38 ± 7
Dunn et al[4]	13	123 ± 22	0.38	97 ± 25	39 ± 7
Karliner et al[26]	18	126	0.56 ± 0.14	—	37 ± 8
Reichek and Devereux[25]	17	129 ± 14	0.53 ± 0.11	137 ± 41	38 ± 6
Dunn et al[4]	8	139 ± 14	0.51	137 ± 39	33 ± 6
Dunn et al[4]	10	155 ± 16	0.60	209 ± 58	31 ± 3

*Mean (±SD where available).

Hypertensive Cardiac Adaptation and Disease

Anatomic Changes: Echo demonstrates LVH in a large number of patients with hypertension. The proportion of hypertensive patients who have LVH and the degree of LVH are both related to the severity of hypertension. Among 234 patients with mild to moderate hypertension (average blood pressure, 147/94 mmHg) studied at Cornell,[6] 108 showed LVH by an abnormally increased posterior LV wall thickness or LV mass, or both. Electrocardiographic and chest radiographic evidence of LVH was present in only 3% to 5% of these patients. In another study from this laboratory,[24] 51 of 118 patients (43%) with slightly higher levels of blood pressure (average 157/97 mmHg) had an LV mass above the 97th percentile of normal. With greater severity and duration of hypertension, the frequency of LVH increases further: 15 of 17 patients (88%) with moderate to severe hypertension (average blood pressure on treatment, 170/108 mmHg) had an abnormally increased LV mass or relative wall thickness.[26] Table II summarizes the results of echo studies that demonstrate that the degree of increase in relative wall thickness and LV mass is broadly proportional to the level of blood pressure.

Despite this broad proportionality, widely varying degrees of LVH are found in patients with similar levels of blood pressure.[27] Among many factors that may explain this, the most important may be that blood pressure during normal activity, not in the physician's office, is the true load imposed on the heart. In a recent study of 19 normotensive subjects and 81 patients with mild hypertension,[28] we showed that LVH was most closely related to blood pressure during occupational work, a major recurring stress in the lives of most adults. Left ventricular mass index was most closely related to workplace systolic blood pressure (r = 0.50, p < 0.001), whereas relative wall thickness was most closely related to workplace diastolic blood pressure (r = 0.59, p < 0.001). This difference suggests that these two major indices of LVH are related to different aspects of the hemodynamic load in hypertension.

Although most patients respond to systemic hypertension with concentric LVH, in which the LVPWT and IVST are similarly increased, a few patients develop asymmetric hypertrophy. At Cornell, in the studies of a large group of patients with mild to moderate hypertension[6,24] roughly 4% demonstrated disproportionate septal thickening with a septal to free wall thickness ratio of more than 1.3 using the National Institutes of Health measurement convention.[29] None of these subjects had mitral or aortic valve motion abnormalities suggestive of substantial outflow obstruction. Other investigators have found a similar[30] or higher[31] prevalence of disproportionate septal thickening in patients with hypertension. Current evidence suggests that this form of asymmetric ventricular hypertrophy differs from familial hypertrophic cardiomyopathy (hypertrophic obstructive cardiomyopathy or idiopathic hypertrophic subaortic stenosis). Although the reason why some but not all patients with hypertension develop disproportionate septal thickening remains uncertain, our own studies of the families of hypertensive patients with disproportionate septal thickness[32] suggest that this variant of hypertrophic cardiomyopathy may result from the interaction of a genetic predisposition to develop asymmetric hypertrophy with LV pressure overload as the necessary stimulus for myocardial hypertrophy.

The Effects of Hypertension on Left Ventricular Function: If cardiac hypertrophy is a successful adaptation to the increased cardiac work load of hypertension, then most patients with mild or even moderate hypertension should have normal LV function.[33–35] This hypothesis is supported by the results of echo studies of patients with hypertension which show that the LV ejection fraction decreased below a very stringent lower limit of normal (67%) in only 29 of 234 (12%) patients in one series[6] and 3 of 18 (17%) in another.[22] In two recent studies from our laboratory, left ventricular systolic FS was seriously depressed in only 2 of 118 patients,[24] and none of 60 patients[27] (2% and 0%, respectively).

Only in the presence of more severe hypertension does left ventricular systolic performance decline appreciably (Table II). In the study by Dunn and associates[4] left ventricular FS was similar to normal (38 ± 4%) in patients with mild hypertension (mean blood pressure, 123 ± 2; 39 ± 7%), whereas it fell modestly to 33 ± 6% (p < 0.05 versus normal) in a group of patients with mean blood pressure 139 ± 14 and 31 ± 3% (p < 0.01) in a group of patients with mean blood pressure of 155 ± 16. This decline in LV function with mounting hypertension does not necessarily indicate that LV muscle contractility is impaired, since normal muscle will perform poorly if it is subjected to excessive wall stresses.[1,3,36] High wall stresses occur if blood pressure increases out of proportion to the degree of LVH. As has been shown by Strauer[5,36] and confirmed by studies from the Cornell laboratory,[28] LV systolic function declines in patients with hypertension who have high wall stresses and may even be supernormal in patients in whom exuberant hypertrophy creates a low-stress ventricle.

Left Ventricular Mechanics and Functional Reserve in Hypertension: In the absence of coronary arterial disease, hypertension affects the left ventricle primarily by systolic overloading. When myocardium is functionally normal, LV performance is inversely related to the degree of loading stresses. To assess the degree to which LV performance in hypertensive patients is related to loading stresses imposed by high blood pressure, we recently compared echo left ventricular FS to ESS, a measure of afterload. The FS/ESS relationship has been previously shown in our laboratory to demonstrate a highly significant, inverse linear correlation between these variables in both normotensive and hypertensive subjects.[26,37]

In a group of 60 asymptomatic hypertensive patients we recently studied with both echoes and radionuclide cineangiograms,[38] FS/ESS relationships in most patients were within normal limits. However, 2 of these patients had intrinsic myocardial dysfunction (low FS in relation to ESS) apparent even at rest. Further assessment of the relationship between arterial pressure and radionuclide LV ejection fraction produced somewhat unexpected results. Thus, in these 60 patients, LV ejection fraction at rest was directly related to systolic arterial pressure (r = 0.33, p < 0.01) and inversely related to resting end-systolic wall stress.[38] These data are concordant with the tendency of patients with early hypertension to exhibit slightly supernormal resting LV function in the echo studies listed in Table II. In contrast, an inverse relationship was observed between the level of arterial blood pressure at rest and LV functional reserve, measured by the change in ejection fraction from rest to exercise (r = −0.35, p < 0.01). Of note, 19 of 60 patients (32%) manifested a subnormal radionuclide cineangiographic ejection fraction response during exercise (that is, either less than 5% change from rest to exercise, or maximal exercise ejection fraction less than 54%) although the change in ejection fraction was unrelated to ESS and most of these patients showed a normal FS/ESS relationship at rest.

Finally, we have observed that the increment in ejection fraction during exercise tends to decline with increasing LV mass,[40] suggesting that progressive hypertrophy involves production of functionally subnormal myocardium. Assessment of LV function at rest by either echo[26] or radionuclide cineangiography[38] has not been sensitive enough to detect this abnormality.

Evolution of Hypertensive Heart Disease

Recent studies using echo have begun to define the evolution of cardiac changes in uncontrolled hypertension and the response of the heart to various forms of treatment. Left ventricular hypertrophy progresses and systolic function tends to decrease in patients whose blood pressure is not controlled, whereas effective antihypertensive therapy has the opposite effect.[40]

Our preliminary results obtained by combined study with radionuclide cineangiography and echo suggest the possibility that hypertensive patients may be classified into three groups according to LV functional characteristics.[38,41] The first and least affected group lacks evidence of myocardial dysfunction by echo and radionuclide cineangiography, both at rest and during exercise. The second and more affected group manifests dysfunction only during exercise, and the third and most severely affected group manifests load independent LV dysfunction at rest, as well as subnormal functional response during exercise. Further studies assessing the interrelationship of cardiac structural and functional abnormalities and their natural history will be needed to delineate accurately the progression from hypertensive cardiac adaptation to reversible and finally irreversible stages of hypertensive heart disease.

Preliminary evidence suggests that specific types of antihypertensive medications may differ qualitatively in their effects on the heart. For example, propranolol and other sympatholytic drugs cause regression of LVH in patients with hypertension even when the degree of blood pressure reduction is small,[40,42] which is similar to findings in spontaneously hypertensive rats. Other types of antihypertensive medication seem to affect LVH only when blood pressure is dramatically reduced.[40,43,44]

Clinical Implications

Echo measurements of LV dimensions provide much more accurate information about LV anatomy and function than previously available noninvasive methods, such as electrocardiography and chest radiographs.[45–47] These techniques continue to be actively investigated in patients with hypertension, hence their clinical uses are still evolving. Echo cannot yet be recommended as a routine test for every patient with hypertension. However, current studies indicate that the echo yields especially important information in several groups of patients with hypertension.

First, the echo is a powerful tool for elucidation of the causes of apparent cardiac enlargement on physical examination or chest radiographs. These include increased ventricular wall thickness, chamber enlargement, pericardial effusion, and noncardiac causes, such as atypical chest configuration or poor inspiration. A finding of severe LVH, for example, might influence the physician toward aggressive antihypertensive therapy, since evidence of LVH has been repeatedly shown to predict increased morbidity and mortality in patients with hypertension.[48-51]

Second, echo is the most accurate available method for the diagnosis of hypertrophic cardiomyopathy or mitral valve prolapse, which may be suspected on the basis of murmurs and other physical findings. It is often difficult to differentiate between these diagnoses and nonspecific findings in some patients with essential hypertension.

Third, accurate exclusion of ventricular hypertrophy or dysfunction would add evidence in support of a suspected diagnosis of "white coat hypertension" (occurring only in the physician's presence) in certain patients with no apparent end-organ damage. To make this diagnosis definitively, direct proof of the usual normality of blood pressure is needed and can be obtained from 24-hour blood pressure recordings. Conversely, some patients with mild hypertension but with a greater than average elevation in blood pressure while at work have been shown to have a greater degree of LVH,[52] indicating the complementary nature of echo and of 24-hour blood pressure recording.

Acknowledgment

Supported in part by grant HL-18323 from the National Heart, Lung, and Blood Institute. Dr. Borer is an Established Investigator of the American Heart Association, Dallas, Texas.

References

1. DEVEREUX RB, REICHEK N: Left ventricular hypertrophy. Cardiovasc Rev Rep 1980; 1: 55–68.

2. WIKMAN-COFFELT J, PARMLEY WW, MASON DT: The cardiac hypertrophy process: analyses of factors determining pathological vs. physiological development. Cir Res 1979; 45: 697–707.

3. GROSSMAN W: Cardiac hypertrophy: useful adaptation or pathologic process? Am J Med 1980; 69: 576–584.

4. DUNN FG, CHANDRARATNA P, DE CARVALHO JGR, BASTA LL, FROHLICH ED: Pathophysiologic assessment of hypertensive heart disease with echocardiography. Am J Cardiol 1977; 39: 789–795.

5. STRAUER BE: Ventricular function and coronary hemodynamics in hypertensive heart disease. Am J Cardiol 1979; 44: 999–1006.

6. SAVAGE DD, DRAYER JIM, HENRY WL, et al: Echocardiographic assessment of cardiac anatomy and function in hypertensive patients. Circulation 1979; 59: 623–632.

7. KANNEL WB, CASTELLI WP, McNAMARA PM, McKEE PA, FEINLEIB M: Role of blood pressure in the development of congestive heart failure. N Engl J Med 1972; 287: 781–787.

8. JONES RS: The weight of the heart and its chambers in hypertensive cardiovascular disease with and without failure. Circulation 1953; 7: 357–369.

9. POMBO JF, TROY BL, RUSSELL RO Jr: Left ventricular volumes and ejection fraction by echocardiography. Circulation 1971; 43: 480–490.

10. DEVEREUX RB, REICHEK N: Echocardiographic determination of left ventricular mass in man. Anatomic validation of the method. Circulation 1977; 55: 613–618.

11. DEVEREUX RB: Cardiovascular evaluation of the hypertensive patient. In: Hunt JC, ed. Hypertension update II: mechanisms, diagnosis, treatment. Lyndhurst, NJ: Health Learning Systems, 1984; 27–42.

12. REICHEK N: Echocardiographic assessment of left ventricular structure and function in hypertension: methodology. Am J Med 1983; 75(suppl 3A): 19–25.

13. MURRAY JA, JOHNSTON W, REID JM: Echocardiographic determination of left ventricular dimensions, volumes and performance. Am J Cardiol 1972; 30: 252–257.

14. BENNET DH, EVANS DW, RAJ MVJ: Echocardiographic left ventricular dimensions in pressure and volume overload. Br Heart J 1975; 37: 971–977.

15. DEVEREUX RB, ALONSO DR, LUTAS EM, PICKERING TG, HARSHFIELD GA, LARAGH JH: Sensitivity of echocardiography for detection of left ventricular hypertrophy. In ter Keurs HEDJ, Schippenheyn JJ, eds. Left ventricular hypertrophy. The Hague: Martinus Nijhoff, 1983; 16–37.

16. REICHEK N, WILSON J, ST. JOHN SUTTON M, PLAPPERT RA, GOLDBERG S, HIRSHFELD JW: Noninvasive determination of left ventricular end-systolic stress: validation of the method and initial application. Circulation 1982; 65: 99–108.

17. QUINONES MA, MOKOTOFF D, NOURI S, WINTERS WL Jr, MILLER RR: Noninvasive quantification of left ventricular wall stress: validation of method and application to assessment of chronic pressure overload. Am J Cardiol 1980; 45: 782–790.

18. GORDON EP, SCHNITTGER I, FITZGERALD PJ, WILLIAMS P, POPP RL: Reproducibility of left ventricular volumes by two-dimensional echocardiography. J Am Coll Cardiol 1983; 2: 506–513.

19. REICHEK N, HELAK J, PLAPPERT T, ST. JOHN SUTTON M, WEBER KT: Anatomic validation of left ventricular mass estimates from clinical two-dimensional echocardiography: initial results. Circulation 1983; 67: 348–352.

20. SCHILLER NB, SKIOLDEBRAND CG, SCHILLER EJ, et al: Canine left ventricular mass estimation by two-dimensional echocardiography. Circulation 1983; 68: 210–216.

21. HENRY WL, WARE J, GARDIN JM, HEPNER SI, McKAY J, WEINER M: Echocardiographic measurements in normal subjects: growth-related changes that occur between infancy and early childhood. Circulation 1978; 57: 278–284.

22. ROGÉ CLL, SILVERMAN NH, HART PA, RAY RM: Cardiac structure growth pattern determined by echocardiography. Circulation 1978; 57: 285–290.

23. ST. JOHN SUTTON M, REICHEK N, LOVETT J, KASTOR JA: Effects of age, body size and blood pressure on the normal human left ventricle. Circulation 1980; 62(suppl III): 305.

24. DEVEREUX RB, SAVAGE DD, DRAYER JIM, LARAGH JH: Left ventricular hypertro-

phy and function in high, normal and low-renin forms of essential hypertension. Hypertension 1982; 4: 524–531.

25. REICHEK N, DEVEREUX RB: Reliable estimation of peak left ventricular systolic pressure by M-mode echocardiographic determined end-diastolic relative wall thickness: identification of severe valvular aortic stenosis in adult patients. Am Heart J 1982; 103: 202–209.

26. KARLINER JS, WILLIAMS D, GORWIT J, CRAWFORD MH, O'ROURKE RA: Left ventricular performance in patients with left ventricular hypertrophy caused by systemic arterial hypertension. Br Heart J 1977; 39: 1239–1245.

27. DEVEREUX RB, SAVAGE DD, SACHS I, LARAGH JH: Relation of hemodynamic load to left ventricular hypertrophy and performance in hypertension. Am J Cardiol 1983; 51: 171–176.

28. DEVEREUX RB, PICKERING TG, HARSHFELD GA, et al: Left ventricular hypertrophy in patients with hypertension: importance of blood pressure response to regularly recurring stress. Circulation 1983; 68: 470–476.

29. MARON BJ, EPSTEIN SE: Hypertrophic cardiomyopathy: recent observations regarding the specificity of three hallmarks of the disease: asymmetric septal hypertrophy, septal disorganization and systolic anterior motion of the anterior mitral leaflet. Am J Cardiol 1980; 45: 141–154.

30. COHEN A, HAGAN AD, WATKINS J, et al: Clinical correlates in hypertensive patients with left ventricular hypertrophy diagnoses with echocardiography. Am J Cardiol 1981; 47: 335–341.

31. CRILEY JM, BLAUFUSS AH, ABBASI AS: Nonobstructive IHSS. Circulation 1975; 52: 963.

32. SAVAGE DD, DEVEREUX RB, SACHS I, LARAGH JH: Disproportionate ventricular septal thickness in hypertensive patients. J Cardiovasc Ultrasonogr 1982; 1: 79–85.

33. BADEER HS: Biological significance of cardiac hypertrophy. Am J Cardiol 1964; 14: 133–138.

34. MEERSON FZ: The failing heart: adaptation and deadaptation. New York: Raven Press, 1983.

35. LINZBACH AJ: Hypertrophy, hyperplasia and structural dilatation of the human heart. Adv Cardiol 1976; 18: 1–13.

36. STRAUER BE: Myocardial oxygen consumption in chronic heart disease: role of wall stress, hypertrophy and coronary reserve. Am J Cardiol 1979; 44: 730–740.

37. LUTAS EM, DEVEREUX RB, REIS G, et al: Increased cardiac performance in mild essential hypertension: left ventricular mechanics. Hypertension (in press).

38. BORER JS, JASON M, DEVEREUX RB, et al: Function of the hypertrophied left ventricle at rest and exercise: hypertension and aortic stenosis. Am J Med 1983; 75(suppl 3A): 34–39.

39. JASON M, HERROLD E, BORER JS, et al: Depressed left ventricular functional reserve in essential hypertension: pathophysiological implications. J Am Coll Cardiol 1984; 3: 591.

40. DEVEREUX RB, SAVAGE DD, SACHS I, LARAGH JH: Effect of blood pressure control on left ventricular hypertrophy and function in hypertension. Circulation 1980; 62(suppl III): 36.

41. BORER JS, JASON M, DEVEREUX RB, PICKERING T, ERLE S, LARAGH JH: Left ventric-

ular performance in the hypertensive patient. Exercise-mediated separation of loading influences from intrinsic muscle dysfunction. Chest 1983; 83: 314–316.

42. IBRAHIM MM, MADKOUR MA, MOSSALLAM R: Effect of beta blockade therapy on hypertensive cardiac hypertrophy. Am J Cardiol 1981; 47: 469.

43. DUNN FG, BASTAIN B, LAWRIE TDV, LORIMER AR: Effect of blood pressure control on left ventricular hypertrophy in patients with essential hypertension. Clin Sci 1980; 59: 441s–443s.

44. DRAYER JIM, GARDIN JM, WEBER MA: Echocardiographic left ventricular hypertrophy in hypertension. Chest 1983; 84: 217–221.

45. DEVEREUX RB, REICHEK N: Repolarization abnormalities of left ventricular hypertrophy: clinical, echocardiographic and hemodynamic correlates. J Electrocardiol 1982; 15: 47–54.

46. DEVEREUX RB, PHILLIPS MC, CASALE PN, EISENBERG RR, KLIGFIELD P: Geometric determinants of electrocardiographic left ventricular hypertrophy. Circulation 1983; 67: 907–911.

47. DEVEREUX RB, CASALE PN, EISENBERG RR, MILLER DH, KLIGFIELD P: Electrocardiographic detection of left ventricular hypertrophy using echocardiographic determination of left ventricular mass as the reference standard. Comparison of standard criteria, computer diagnosis and physician interpretation. J Am Coll Cardiol 1984; 3: 82–87.

48. BRESLIN DJ, GIFFORD RW JR, FAIRBAIRN JF II: Essential hypertension: a twenty-year follow-up study. Circulation 1966; 33: 87–97.

49. SOKOLOW M, PERLOFF D: The prognosis of essential hypertension treated conservatively. Circulation 1961; 23: 697–713.

50. KANNEL WB: Blood pressure and risk of coronary heart disease: the Framingham Study. Chest 1969; 56: 43–52.

51. CASALE PN, MILNER M, DEVEREUX RB, et al: Value of echocardiographic left ventricular mass in predicting cardiovascular morbid events in hypertensive men. Circulation 1985; 72 (suppl 3): 130.

52. DEVEREUX RB, LUTAS EM, CASALE PN, et al: Standardization of M-mode echocardiographic left ventricular anatomic measurements. J Am Coll Cardiol 1984; 4: 1222–1230.

21

Asymmetric Septal Hypertrophy and the Early Phase of Hypertension

M.E. SAFAR, M.D.
V.M. DIMITRIU, M.D.

In patients with sustained essential hypertension, symmetric cardiac hypertrophy is a characteristic feature that is often considered as a response to progressive increase in pressure load. During the last few years, cardiac hypertrophy has also been reported in the early phase of essential hypertension, in particular in children and in young men. Several studies indicated that the increase in cardiac mass was associated with a disproportionate septal hypertrophy. The present chapter is devoted to the analysis and the interpretation of this latter problem.

Incidence of Asymmetric Septal Hypertrophy in Hypertension

Disproportionate septal hypertrophy has been reported in 1% to 47% of subjects with chronic elevation of blood pressure.[1–8] The reasons for this wide range of incidence rate is difficult to explain, but there are several possibilities. First, echo studies were performed in persons with hypertension on the basis of different criteria, such as electrocardiographic findings or the severity of hypertension,[1,8] an approach that can modify the evaluation of the prevalence of septal hypertrophy. Second, most investigations included a large number of subjects on antihypertensive treatment, which is known to act on cardiac hypertrophy, particularly on the thickness of the septal wall.[9] In two reports involving more than 50 subjects, 207 patients took antihypertensive drugs, whereas 102 had no treatment.[3,4] Despite these difficulties, it is important to note that earlier assumptions regarding the rarity of asymmetric septal hypertrophy among hypertensive patients are being revised. Review of more than 1,368 hypertensive subjects in the Framingham Study[10] has shown an incidence of 10% of disproportionate septal hypertrophy among 190 patients with echo evidence of left ventricular hypertrophy (LVH).

One possible explanation for the difficulty in evaluating prevalence (1% to 47%) is that echo measurements of ventricular septal thickness are known to be more variable and artefacts more common than comparable measurements of left ventricular posterior wall thickness.[4–11] In particular, with

M-mode scan, the echo beam may be directed at a tangent through the septum, the resultant recording showing a falsely thick septum. On the other hand, the echo "dropout" may cause septal thickness to be underestimated. From this viewpoint, the two-dimensional echo may have the advantage of providing a more precise definition of the ventricular septal borders, thus allowing selection of the most optimal location and proper angulation at which to take the measurements.[4,5] However, in the case of the study of borderline hypertension, technical variations in the measurement of ventricular septal thickness have a unique practical interest: if the aim is to recognize asymmetric septal hypertrophy in patients with borderline hypertension, groups of controls and of patients with sustained hypertension should be statistically compared in a prospective study so that technical variations can be equally distributed among the studied populations.

Asymmetric Septal Hypertrophy and the Early Phase of Hypertension in Man

Asymmetric septal hypertrophy has been reported as a characteristic feature in young men (mean age, 27.3 ± 1.2 years; ± 1 SEM) with borderline hypertension, in comparison with normal subjects and with patients with sustained essential hypertension of the same age and sex.[12] Further studies indicated that the result was not dependent on sex and previous treatment.[13,14] Disproportionate septal thickening in patients with borderline hypertension was associated with an increase in cardiac output,[12,13] a reduction in preejection periods[12] and in peak velocity of left ventricular (LV) contraction,[13] and an increase in plasma norepinephrine.[14] Similar results, including hemodynamic and biochemical evidence of sympathetic overactivity, were also reported in older subjects with mild to moderate hypertension.[5,15,16] Mean age was 53.7 ± 1.6 years.[15,16]

Comparable findings have been observed in the Muscatine Study,[17] which involved 264 schoolchildren classified according to the level of systolic pressure in the lowest, middle, or highest quintile of the distribution for their age and sex. Children with blood pressures in the upper quintile had increased values for the interventricular septum and LV posterior wall before correction for age, sex, height, weight, and triceps skinfold thickness. After correction, only the increase in the interventricular septum was observed, suggesting the possible importance of this abnormality in the early phase of hypertension. However, in children with suspected hypertension, disproportionate septal hypertrophy has not always been observed, even when measurements of cardiac mass were taken into account.[18–22]

For a long time, an association between asymmetric septal hypertrophy and sustained hypertension has been reported in patients with muscular subaortic stenosis.[23] The lack of abnormal systolic anterior movement of the anterior mitral cusp cannot exclude completely this possibility in patients with borderline hypertension.[8,12] However, in these patients, the diagnosis of muscular stenosis does not fit with the negative response to amyl nitrite. Furthermore, the incidence rate of hypertension is extremely low in patients with hypertrophic cardiomyopathy, and autopsy studies have shown that the disproportionate septal thickening present in two patients with hypertension, did not have the features characteristic of genetic hypertrophic cardiomyopathy.[24]

Asymmetric Septal Hypertrophy and the Early Phase of Genetic Hypertension in Rats

Since cardiac hypertrophy has been universally reported in the early phase of several types of genetic hypertension in rats,[25] the relationship of this finding with disproportionate septal hypertrophy in patients with borderline hypertension is of interest. However, comparisons between the two observations have to be presented cautiously.

In most echo investigations in hypertensive men, cardiac hypertrophy has been demonstrated from the calculation of cardiac mass, a parameter evaluated from geometric models assuming a constant cardiac density.[26] Cardiac density is influenced by the degree of hyperplasia and hypertrophy of myocardial cells as well as by the myosin and collagen content of the heart.[27] Such components may be modified according to the severity of hypertension, the type of antihypertensive treatment, and also the age of patients,[28,29] a critical point in the case of early hypertension. Thus, the use of constant factors in the formulas used for the calculation of cardiac mass may minimize the validity of this index for the follow-up of patients with early hypertension.

On the other hand, important differences are to be noticed between echo findings in men and cardiac hypertrophy in rats. In spontaneous hypertension in rats, cardiac hypertrophy involves both the left and the right ventricle.[9,25] Furthermore, it is possible that hypertrophy is not always restricted to the heart, but involves other parts of the vascular system[25] and even the lungs and the kidneys.[28]

Early Cardiac Hypertrophy and the Pressure Load

At an early phase of spontaneous hypertension in rats, it has been shown that an increase in LV weight is found before arterial pressure has reached hypertensive levels.[29] From this finding, it is acknowledged that the role of pressure load in the mechanism of hypertrophy may be minimized.[9] However, such an assumption must be questioned on several grounds. First, intra-arterial blood pressure is difficult to measure in young rats, so that in most cases the indirect tail cuff method is used. Consequently, only systolic pressure is evaluated, a parameter that can also be considered an index of elevated mean arterial pressure or of reduced arterial distensibility, with resulting systolic hypertension.[30] Second, if the cause and effect relationship between pressure and cardiac hypertrophy is admitted, it is conceivable that the curve is not linear, with a reduced slope within the lower pressure ranges. Indeed, cardiac hypertrophy is associated very early with structural alterations of resistive vessels,[31] a fact that can modulate the pressure-heart weight curve.

Finally, there is little doubt that arterial pressure levels alone do not adequately reflect the cardiac pressure load. Cardiac hypertrophy is certainly more closely related to the systolic than to the diastolic pressure.[9,32,33] Indeed, systolic pressure is not the exclusive reflection of diastolic pressure but is also influenced by several independent factors, such as the LV ejection and the compliance of the aorta and large proximal arteries.[34] Thus, LV load is better assessed from calculations of peak systolic wall stress[35] and aortic impedance[34,36] than from the simple measurement of blood pressure. In men with sustained essential hypertension, the cardiac mass on volume ratio is strongly correlated with aortic compliance,[37] indicating that both the resistive and the elastic vessels are involved in the mechanism of the elevated postload.

In young patients with borderline hypertension, it is possible that the increased septal thickness represents the initial stage of hypertrophy due to pressure overload. Since the septum has a flatter aspect than the posterior wall, this would lead to higher local tension with subsequent hypertrophy.[38] Indeed, Drayer et al[39] have proposed that increases in ventricular septal thickness during antihypertensive treatment might be partly explained on the basis of anatomic adjustments to a decrease in LV internal diameter. However, in patients with borderline hypertension, explanations based exclusively on pressure do not appear to fit with the total absence of correlation between the degree of septal hypertrophy and the level of blood pressure.[12,13] There is some evidence that a better correlation with LV mass may be obtained with blood pressure monitoring.[32,33,40] However, this latter possibility already suggests that factors other than the pressure itself can modulate the septal response, in particular arterial compliance.[37]

Asymmetric Septal Hypertrophy and the Autonomic Nervous System

Several functional factors other than arterial pressure may influence cardiac hypertrophy in hypertensive disease. Angiotensin II might be involved either through its potentiation of sympathetic effects or by an independent stimulating action on myocardial protein synthesis.[9,41] However, in patients with borderline and sustained essential hypertension, plasma renin activity is not correlated with the degree of hypertrophy,[12,42] thus minimizing the role of the renin-angiotensin system. Prostaglandins (PG) may also be important since, in patients with borderline hypertension, plasma PGE_2 concentrations are positively correlated with cardiac output and negatively correlated with the ratio between preejection period and LV ejection time.[43]

However, of particular importance seems to be the role of the autonomic nervous system in the development of septal hypertrophy.

Many investigators have reported the trophic role of the sympathetic nervous system on cardiac muscle in animals.[41] Cardiac hypertrophy may be induced by norepinephrine infusions[44] and prevented when the pressor effects are blunted by concomitant alpha-adrenergic blockade.[45] Ostman-Smith[46] has recently reviewed the evidence showing involvement of the cardiac sympathetic nerves in the induction of adaptive cardiac hypertrophy and emphasized the selective sympathetic innervation of each individual heart chamber. In particular, the septum, at least in its base, seems to be rich in sympathetic nerve supply.

In young men with borderline hypertension, increased activity of the sympathetic nervous system is a characteristic feature.[47] For this reason, several studies have emphasized the possible links between ventricular septal thickness and indices of sympathetic tone. It has been reported that the ratio of ventricular septal thickness to LV posterior wall thickness was correlated with the duration of preejection periods, which is influenced by sympathetic tone.[12] Corea et al[14] found that the same ratio was positively correlated with plasma norepinephrine levels, whereas epinephrine and plasma renin activity were not. Indeed, in patients with sustained essential hypertension, the regression of cardiac hypertrophy after antiadrenergic agents often predominates on the septal wall.[48–50]

In this context, it is important to note that the relationship between the autonomic system and cardiac hypertrophy is bimodal and not restricted to the influence of the first on the latter.[46] Cardiac hypertrophy can lead to modifications in myocardial catecholamines[51] and diminished cardiac response to adrenergic stimuli.[52] In this view, it is important to notice that, in patients with borderline hypertension, septal hypertrophy is both positively correlated to preejection period and negatively correlated to cardiac index.[53] This observation suggested that, as in spontaneous hypertension in rats, the decrease in myocardial contractility was associated with an increase in septal hypertrophy.[54]

Conclusion

From the finding of asymmetrical septal hypertrophy in borderline hypertension, it could be considered that the heart plays a dominant role in the initiation of hypertension. Such an assumption is extremely important but should be tempered in several ways. First, concomitant alterations in the structure and the geometry of small and large arteries[30,31,37,54,55] may occur and have still been poorly evaluated, although they should be considered as active forces that can influence even the early evolution of the disease. Second, from a clinical viewpoint, it must be recalled that hypertension is a common disease and that a coincidental occurrence with asymmetric septal hypertrophy is not completely excluded. In this respect, the frequency of septal hypertrophy in athletes and in patients with genetic disorders must be taken into consideration.

Addendum

Since this paper was written, the prevalence of septal hypertrophy in borderline hypertension was further confirmed by Dr. R.B. Devereux (personal communication) in large populations.

References

1. DUNN FG, CHANDRARATNA P, deCARVALLO JGR, BASTA LL, FROHLICH EF: Pathophysiologic assessment of hypertensive heart disease with echocardiography. Am J Cardiol 1977; 39: 789–795.
2. SCHLANT RC, FELNER JM, HEYNSFIELD SB, et al: Echocardiographic studies of left ventricular anatomy and function in essential hypertension. Cardiovasc Med 1977; 2: 477–484.
3. SAVAGE DD, DRAYER JIM, WALTER LH, et al: Echocardiographic assessment of cardiac anatomy and function in hypertensive subjects. Circulation 1979; 59: 623–632.
4. COHEN A, HAGAN AD, WATKINS J, et al: Clinical correlates in hypertensive patients with left ventricular hypertrophy diagnosed with echocardiograpy. Am J Cardiol 1981; 47: 335–341.
5. WICKER P, ROUDAUT R, HAISSAGUERE M, VILLEGA-ARINO P, CLEMENTY J, DALLOCHIO M: Prevalence and significance of asymmetric septal hypertrophy in hypertension: an echocardiographic and clinical study. Eur Heart J 1983; 4 (suppl G): 1–5.
6. DRAYER JIM, SAVAGE DD, HENRY WL, MATHEWS EC JR, LARAGH JH, EPSTEIN SE: Incidence of echocardiographic left ventricular hypertrophy and left atrial enlargement in essential hypertension (abstr). Circulation 1976; 54 (suppl II): II-233.
7. KARLINER JS, WILLIAMS D, GORWIT W: Left ventricular hypertrophy caused by systemic hypertension. Br Heart J 1977; 39: 1239–1245.
8. ABI-SAMRA F, FOUAD FM, TARAZI RC: Determinants of left ventricular hypertrophy and function in hypertensive patients: an echocardiographic study. Am J Med 1983; 75 (suppl 3A): 26–33.
9. TARAZI RC: The role of the heart in hypertension. Clin Sci 1982; 63: 347s–358s.
10. SAVAGE DD, GARRISON RJ, KANNEL WB: Prevalence characteristics and correlates of echocardiographic left ventricular hypertrophy in a population-based sample-; preliminary findings: the Framingham study (abstr). Circulation 1982; 66 (suppl II): II-63.
11. BERNSTEIN RF, CHUWA TEI, CHILD JS, SHAH PM: Angled interventricular septum on echocardiography: anatomic anomaly or technical artifact. J Am Coll Cardiol 1983; 2: 297–304.
12. SAFAR ME, LEHNER JP, VINCENT MI, PLAINFOSSE MT, SIMON AC: Echocardiographic dimensions in borderline and sustained hypertension. Am J Cardiol 1979; 44: 930–935.

13. NIEDERLE P, WIDIMSKY J, JANDOVA R, RESSL J, GROSPIC A: Echocardiographic assessment of the left ventricle in juvenile hypertension. Int J Cardiol 1982; 2: 91–101.

14. COREA L, BENTIVOGLIO M, VERDECCHIA P, MOTOLESE M: Role of adrenergic over-activity and pressure overload in the pathogenesis of left ventricular hypertrophy in borderline and sustained essential hypertension in man. Clin Sci 1982; 63: 379s–381s.

15. TOSHIMA H, KOGA Y, YOSHIOKA H, AKIYOSHI T, KIMURA N: Echocardiographic classification of hypertensive heart disease. A correlative study with clinical features. Jpn Heart J 1975; 16: 377–393.

16. NOMURA G, KUMAGAI E, MIDORIKAWA K, et al: Asymmetric ventricular hypertrophy in patients with essential hypertension. Jpn Heart J 1982; 23: 181–190.

17. SCHIEKEN RM, CLARKE WR, LAUER RM: Left ventricular hypertrophy in children with blood pressure in the upper quintile of the distribution (the Muscatine Study). Hypertension 1981; 3: 669–675.

18. YAMORI Y, MORICHUZO M, NISHIO T: Cardiac hypertrophy in early hypertension. Am J Cardiol 1979; 44: 964–969.

19. CULPEPPER WAS, SODT PC, MESSERLI FH, RUSCHCHAUPT DC, ARCILLA RA: Cardiac status in juvenile borderline hypertension. Ann Intern Med 1983; 98: 1–7.

20. GOLDRING D, HERNANDEZ A, CHOI S: Blood pressure in a high school population: II. Clinical profile of the juvenile hypertensive. J Pediatr 1979; 95: 298–304.

21. LAIRD WP, FIXLER DE: Left ventricular hypertrophy in adolescents with elevated blood pressure assessment by chest roentgenography, electrocardiography, and echocardiography. Pediatrics 1981; 67: 255–259.

22. ZAHKA KG, NEILL CA, KIDD L, CUTILETTA MA, CUTILETTA AF: Cardiac involvement in adolescent hypertension. Hypertension 1981; 3: 664–668.

23. MARON BJ, EPSTEIN SE: Hypertrophic cardiomyopathy: recent observations regarding the specificity of three hallmarks of the disease: asymmetric septal hypertrophy, septal disorganization and systolic anterior motion of the anterior mitral leaflet. Am J Cardiol 1980; 45: 141–153.

24. MARON BJ, EDWARDS JE, EPSTEIN SE: Occurrence of disproportionate ventricular septal thickening in patients with systemic hypertension. Chest 1978; 73: 466–477.

25. VINCENT M, SACQUET J, SASSARD J: The Lyon strains of hypertensive, normotensive and low blood pressure rats. In: de Jong W, ed. Handbook of hypertension. Vol. III: Experimental and genetic models of hypertension. Amsterdam: Elsevier, 1984.

26. DEVEREUX RB, REICHEK N: Echocardiographic determination of left ventricular mass in man: anatomic validation of the method. Circulation 1977; 55: 613–618.

27. SEN S: Regression of cardiac hypertrophy: experimental animal model. Am J Med 1983; 75 (suppl 3A): 87–93.

28. SAFAR ME, BENESSIANO JR, HORNYCH AL: Asymmetric septal hypertrophy and borderline hypertension. Int J Cardiol 1982; 2: 103–108.

29. SEN S, TARAZI RC, KHAIRALLAH PA, BUMPUS FM: Cardiac hypertrophy in spontaneously hypertensive rats. Circ Res 1974; 35: 775–784.

30. SIMON AC, LAURENT S, LEVENSON J, BOUTHIER J, SAFAR M: Estimation of forearm arterial compliance in normal and hypertensive men from simultaneous pres-

sure and flow measurements in the brachial artery, using a pulsed Doppler device and a first-order arterial model during diastole. Cardiovasc Res 1983; 17: 331–338.

31. FOLKOW B: Physiological aspects of primary hypertension. Physiol Rev 1982; 62: 348–503.

32. DRAYER JIM, WEBER MA, DEYOUNG JL: BP as a determinant of cardiac left ventricular muscle mass. Arch Intern Med 1983; 143: 90–92.

33. DEVEREUX RB, PICKERING TG, HARSHFIELD GA, et al: Left ventricular hypertrophy in patients with hypertension: importance of blood pressure response to regularly recurring stress. Circulation 1983; 68: 470–476.

34. O'ROURKE MF: Arterial function in health and disease. Edinburgh: Churchill Livingstone, 1982; 67–184.

35. GROSSMAN W, JONES D, MCLAURIN LP: Wall stress and patterns of hypertrophy in human left ventricle. J Clin Invest 1975; 56: 56–64.

36. MILNOR WR: Arterial impedance as ventricular afterload. Circ Res 1975; 36: 565–569.

37. BOUTHIER JD, DELUCA N, SAFAR ME, SIMON ACH: Cardiac hypertrophy and arterial distensibility in essential hypertension. Am Heart J 1985; 109: 1345–1352.

38. BURTON AC: Transmural pressures, pressure gradients and resistance to flow in the vascular bed. In: Physiology and biophysics of the circulation. Chicago: Year Book Medical Publishers, 1965; 84.

39. DRAYER JIM, GARDIN JM, WEBER JA, ARONOW WS: Changes in ventricular septal thickness during diuretic therapy. Clin Pharmacol Ther 1982; 32: 283–288.

40. DIMITRIOU R, DEGAUDEMARIS R, DEBRU JL, et al: Données de l'echcardiogramme, du profil tensionnel d'effort et de la mesure de la tension artérielle limite. Arch Mal Coeur 1984; 77: 1162–1166.

41. TARAZI RC, SEN S: Catecholamines and cardiac hypertrophy. In: Hezzy RC, Caldwall ADS, eds. Catecholamines and the heart. London: Academic Press and Royal Society of Medicine, 1979; 47–57.

42. DEVEREUX RB, SAVAGE DD, DRAYER JIM, LARAGH JH: Left ventricular hypertrophy and function in high, normal and low-renin forms of essential hypertension. Hypertension 1982; 4: 524–531.

43. SAFAR ME, HORNYCH AF, LEVENSON JA, et al: Central haemodynamics and plasma prostaglandin E_2 in borderline and sustained essential hypertensive patients before and after indomethacin. Clin Sci 1981; 61: 323s–325s.

44. LAKS MM, MORADY F, SURANT HSC: Myocardial hypertrophy produced by chronic infusion of subhypertensive dose of norepinephrine in the dog. Chest 1973; 64: 75–80.

45. YAMORI Y, TARAZI RC, OOSHIMA A: Effect of β-receptor-blocking agents on cardiovascular structural changes in spontaneous and nonadrenaline-induced hypertension in rats. Clin Sci 1981; 59: 457s–460s.

46. OSTMAN-SMITH I: Cardiac sympathetic nerves as the final common pathway in the induction of adaptive cardiac hypertrophy. Clin Sci 1981; 61: 265–272.

47. SAFAR ME, WEISS YA: Borderline blood pressure elevation. In: Amery A, ed. Hypertensive cardiovascular disease: pathophysiology and treatment. The Hague: Martinus Nijhoff, 1982; 365–376.

48. FOUAD FM, NAKASKIMA Y, TARAZI RC, SALCEDO EE: Reversal of left ventricular

hypertrophy with methyldopa. Am J Cardiol 1982; 49: 795–801.

49. Von Bibra H, Richardson PJ: Left ventricular hypertrophy in patients with moderate essential hypertension, an echographic study. In: Robertson JIS, Caldwell ADS, eds. Left ventricular hypertrophy in hypertension. New-York: Grune & Stratton, 1979; 47–54.

50. Wollam GL, Hall WD, Porter VD, et al: Time course of regression of left ventricular hypertrophy in treated hypertensive patients. Am J Med 1983; 75 (suppl 3A): 100–110.

51. Fischer JE, Horst W, Kopin IJ: Norepinephrine metabolism in hypertrophied rat hearts. Nature 1965; 207: 951–953.

52. London GM, Safar ME, Weiss YA, Milliez PL: Isoproterenol sensitivity and total body clearance of propranol in hypertensive patients. J Clin Pharmacol 1976; 16: 174–182.

53. Lehner JP, Safar ME, Dimitriu VM, Simon AC, Carrez JP, Plainfosse MT: Systolic time intervals and echocardiographic findings in borderline hypertension. Eur J Cardiol 1979; 9/4: 319–331.

54. Folkow B: Neurotrophic effects on the vascular bed. Acta Med Scand 1983; [suppl] 672: 95–99.

55. Ventura H, Messerli FH, Oigman W, et al: Impaired systemic arterial compliance in borderline hypertension. Am Heart J 1984; 108: 132–136.

22

Clinical Determinants and Manifestations of Left Ventricular Hypertrophy

FRANZ H. MESSERLI, M.D.

Pathophysiologic Considerations

Left ventricular hypertrophy (LVH) can be defined as an increase in functioning myocardial mass that can be idiopathic in its origin or secondary to an increase in preload, an impairment of the pump function, an increased afterload, or the combination of two or more of these factors. An increase in preload (volume overload), defined by a high left ventricular (LV) end-diastolic pressure and volume, initially produces LV dilation, thereby elevating wall stress. Subsequently, an increase in muscle mass ensues, resulting in eccentric hypertrophy and bringing wall stress back to normal. An impairment of pump function by myocardial necrosis or infiltration will lead to a compensatory increase in the number of the remaining contractile elements, thus producing a pseudohypertrophy pattern: functioning LV mass remains unchanged but total mass will be increased because of nonfunctioning tissue. An increase in afterload produces predominantly concentric LVH, thus decreasing the LV radius to posterior wall thickness ratio.[1,2]

Although these mechanisms can be distinctly separated from a pathogenetic point of view, in clinical practice most often the combination of two or more will be encountered. For instance, coronary heart disease, obesity, and hypertension are frequently present in the same patient; each of these conditions, however, will affect LV structure and function in a different way. In the following review, the main physiologic and pathologic determinants of LV function and structure, such as level of arterial pressure, cardiac output (CO), body weight, age, exercise, race, and adrenergic factors, as well as the clinical manifestations of LVH, are considered.

Determinants of Left Ventricular Hypertrophy

Arterial Pressure: The connection between systolic pressure and cardiac mass was documented with autopsy findings by Evans[3] more than half a century ago. Subsequently, epidemiologic data have allowed arterial hy-

TABLE I   **Pathogenetic Factors in Left Ventricular Hypertrophy**

Concentric LVH	Eccentric LVH
Arterial hypertension	Increase in body mass (obesity)
Aging	High cardiac output states
Isometric exercise	Endurance exercise
Sympathetic stimulation (?)	Volume overload

pertension to be correlated with various cardiac complications.[4-7] The fundamental LV adaptation to a pressure overload has been documented to be concentric hypertrophy.[1,2] This can be demonstrated by echo by an increase in relative wall thickness (or a decrease in the radius to wall thickness ratio). Concentric hypertrophy has been found in essential hypertensive patients by a variety of investigators[8-14] (Table I). Rolands et al[14] showed that mean 24-hour systolic blood pressure was the most powerful determinant of LV mass as calculated from echo data. We recently performed a multiple stepwise regression analysis of data from 171 patients and found systolic pressure to be the best predictor of relative wall thickness (Table II).[15]

Obesity: High blood pressure and overweight go hand in hand, but the reason for their common association and whether or not it is causal remains unknown. Although both disorders increase LV stroke work and produce

TABLE II   **Multiple Stepwise Regression: Analysis Between Clinical, Hemodynamic, and Echo Findings in 171 Patients**

	Multiple Regression Analysis	β^*
Internal diastolic diameter ($F = 10.638$; $p < 0.05$)	Weight	0.261
	Diastolic pressure	−0.236
	Heart rate	−0.159
	Total blood volume	0.104
	Cardiac output	0.084
Posterior wall thickness ($F = 10.983$; $p < 0.05$)	Weight	0.302
	Systolic pressure	0.205
	Total blood volume	0.200
	Age	0.192
	Cardiac output	−0.075
Left ventricular mass ($F = 11.670$; $p < 0.05$)	Weight	0.255
	Total blood volume	0.248
	Age	0.161
	Heart rate	−0.084
	Diastolic pressure	0.074
Relative wall thickness ($F = 10.252$; $p < 0.05$)	Systolic pressure	0.390
	Weight	0.120
	Age	0.093
	Heart rate	0.081

*β = standardized regression coefficient.
Modified with permission from Messerli et al.[15]

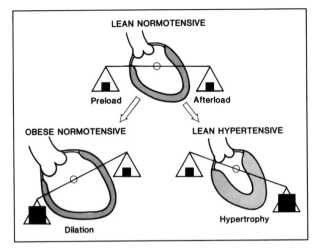

Figure 1. *Cardiac effects of obesity and hypertension. Obesity predominantly increases preload, whereas hypertension is associated with a high afterload. (Modified with permission from Messerli.[16])*

LVH, these occur because of different pathogenetic mechanisms.[16] Although the elevated systolic pressure is the incriminating hemodynamic variable in hypertension, an increase in stroke volume that increases LV stroke work is the predominant pathogenetic factor in obesity. A high increase in stroke volume (SV) produces an elevated end-diastolic pressure unless diastolic LV compliance decreases. An increment in preload results in a LV adaptation that initially consists of an increase in chamber volume. As a consequence of Laplace's law, LV wall tension increases in parallel with ventricular diameter, and eccentric LVH results (Fig. 1). A persistent increase in wall tension or systolic wall stress represents a stimulus to augment the number of contractile elements, and eccentric LVH results.

Clearly, both disorders, hypertension and obesity, synergistically burden the heart. Their combined presence in the same patient will heavily tax the left ventricle and herald premature congestive failure.[17,18]

Body weight was indeed the most powerful determinant of LV chamber size, wall thickness, and LV mass in our multiple stepwise regression analysis[15] (Table II, Fig. 2).

Aging: Aging has been documented specifically to affect cardiovascular function and structure.[19,20] Resting LV function is usually well maintained throughout senescence, although a slight decline of cardiac index (CI) of about 25 ml/min/m^2 per year with age has been found in various invasive studies.[21–25] An increase in arterial wall thickness was documented by Sjögren[26] and Gardin et al[27] who also demonstrated that LV diastolic diameter remained unchanged with age. Gerstenblith et al[28] reported a positive correlation between posterior wall thickness and age, but no decrease in CO

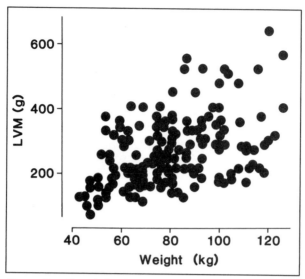

Figure 2. *Correlation between body weight and LV mass (LVM). (Reprinted with permission from Messerli et al.[15])*

in a population that was free of cardiovascular disease, in particular free of arterial hypertension. We recently reported a 24% increase in posterior wall thickness and a 40% increase in LV mass (as well as a decrease in CO) in elderly hypertensive patients who were matched with regard to mean arterial pressure with a group of hypertensive subjects who were more than 40 years younger.[29] In contrast to wall thickness, LV diastolic diameter was not affected by age. The increased afterload in arterial hypertension accelerates both the decline in CO and the increase in LV mass (Fig. 3).

What, then, in normal man stimulates the LV wall to thicken with age? Several factors come to mind that may be contributing to this physiologic "LVH" in the elderly. First, arterial pressure increases throughout life even within the normotensive range in a Westernized population and probably remains an important determinant of LV wall thickness. Second, peripheral resistance increases and arterial compliance decreases with progressing age; both factors are major determinants of aortic input impedance.[29] These changes occur irrespective of the level of arterial pressure. Third, as occurs in other organs, functioning muscle fibers are gradually replaced by inactive tissue, stimulating the remaining contractile elements to hypertrophy. Whatever the reason, the increase in LV wall thickness and mass in an otherwise normal elderly population has distinct implications on our assessment of what constitutes a "normal" cardiac structure (and function) throughout a lifespan.

Exercise: Isometric exercise, such as wrestling and weight lifting, is associated with an increased afterload to the left ventricle and often with a decreased venous return due to a concomitantly performed Valsalva maneu-

TABLE III   **Effects of Endurance Training on Left Ventricular Structure**

Author	Training	Number Age (yr)	Resting Heart Rate	Percent Change in VO₂ max	Posterior Wall Thickness	End-diastolic Diameter
DeMaria et al,[32] 1978	Running 11 weeks	24(26)	69 ± 3(−6)	9	9.1 ± 0.3(1.0)*	48.0 ± 1.0(2.0)*
Ehsani et al,[33] 1978	Swimming 9 weeks	8(25)	70 ± 5(−7)	15	9.4 ± 0.4(0.7)*	48.7 ± 1.7(3.3)*
Perronet et al,[34] 1980	Bicycling 20 weeks	20(40)	63 ± 3(+2)	20	10.0 ± 1.0(−0.3)	47.8 ± 3.3(0.3)
Adams et al,[35] 1981	Running 11 weeks	25(22)	63 ± 1.0(−9)	12	10.9 ± 1.9(−0.6)	45.7 ± 4.1(4.6)*

VO₂ = rate of oxygen consumption.
*p < 0.05; values in parentheses indicate change versus nontrained state.

ver. As a consequence, the left ventricle has been shown to respond to repeated isometric training with concentric hypertrophy. An increased wall thickness (septal more than free wall) without any change in the internal diameter has indeed been found in wrestlers and weight lifters.[30,31] This pattern may mimic hypertrophic cardiomyopathy, and in one study septal to posterior wall thickness ratio has been found to be consistently greater than 1.3 in weight lifters.[31]

Endurance exercise, such as running, bicycling, and swimming, is associated with an increased venous return, increased SV, and a relative decrease in peripheral resistance. Thus, LV preload becomes elevated, but afterload decreases. As a consequence, cardiac adaptation to prolonged daily endurance exercise consists primarily of LV enlargement. Accordingly, LV chamber volume has been found to be enlarged by about 10% in endurance athletes[30,32–35] (Table III). With prolonged training, LV wall thickness may also increase, although this increase rarely exceeds 1 to 2 mm and has been less consistently documented in the published series.[32,33] An increase in LV volume can be found after only 3 months of regular aerobic exercise, such as 50-minute jogging sessions 5 days a week at 80% of maximal heart rate.[35] Regular endurance training decreases resting heart rate and this effect by itself may change LV chamber size. Nevertheless, DeMaria et al[36] concluded that a 10 beat/minute change in heart rate would only be associated with a 2.7% change in end-diastolic dimensions. Accordingly, sinus bradycardia and an increased SV cannot account for structural changes of the athlete's heart.

Ballet dancers, whose art demands the combination of vigorous isometric and endurance exercise, have been shown to exhibit a particular form of cardiac adaptation consisting of LVH and chamber enlargement.[37] Perhaps frequent exposure to stage fright associated with a high sympathetic outflow may be an additional factor in the pathogenesis of "ballet dancer's heart."

Race: The Evans County Georgia Study has demonstrated that black patients exhibit increased voltages on the electrocardiogram and greater cardiac

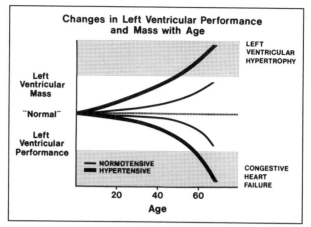

Figure 3. *Effects of aging and progressing severity of hypertension on cardiac performance (cardiac output) and left ventricular mass.*[60]

enlargement on chest roentgenogram than white patients despite having similar levels of arterial pressure.[38] Moreover, the Hypertension Detection and Follow-up Program documented a higher prevalence of LVH in blacks than in whites after adjustment for age and arterial pressure.[39] Recent data from our laboratory have demonstrated a greater increase in LV mass in black patients than in white patients despite the fact that arterial pressure was held equal in both groups.[40] Thus, although wall thickness changes were similar in black patients and white patients, qualitative differences can be found in the adaptive process to arterial hypertension.

High Cardiac Output States and Volume Overload: States with high CO and volume overload, such as pregnancy, renal failure, anemia, and arteriovenous fistulas, also affect LV dimensions, wall thickness, and mass. In pregnancy the radius to wall thickness ratio augments disproportionately, indicating predominant LV dilation.[41,42] When pregnancy is associated with hypertension, however, an exaggerated increase in LV mass can be found.[43] For more than half a century, patients with sickle cell anemia have been known to have cardiac enlargement.[44] Echo evaluation revealed left atrial and ventricular enlargement, increased myocardial mass, and hemodynamic changes that were similar to those in other forms of anemia.[45] Similarly, chronic renal failure has been shown to enlarge LV chamber (by about 20%) and to thicken ventricular walls,[46] changes that reverted toward normal after successful transplantation.[47]

Adrenergic Influences and Mitral Prolapse: A majority of patients with mitral prolapse have been shown to have elevated circulating and urinary catecholamine levels, a hyperdynamic circulatory state, or both.[48,49] Since myocardial dyskinesias, arrhythmias, and nonspecific disturbances of ventricular repolarization are commonly associated with the mitral valve prolapse syndrome, it is tempting to speculate that these patient groups are at a greater risk for the development of LVH in the future. In this regard, it must be remembered that prolonged exposure to high circulating norepinephrine levels can produce "norepinephrine myocarditis" in experimental studies.[50,51] Such experimental evidence corroborates a common clinical contention that cardiomyopathy and congestive heart failure are common sequelae in patients with pheochromocytoma.[52–55] A persistent excessive bombardment of cardiac adrenergic receptors with catecholamines could conceivably facilitate the development of myocardial hypertrophy.[56] Septal hypertrophy in particular has been reported to be influenced by sympathetic activity.[57]

Manifestation of Left Ventricular Hypertrophy

Ectopic Impulse Generation: Although LV adaptation occurs at a very early stage in hypertension, it remains clinically silent and has been considered to represent a beneficial response to an increased afterload.[58] In a recent report, no difference with regard to arrhythmias was demonstrated by Holter monitoring of normotensive patients and those with borderline and established essential hypertension.[59] However, in patients who have LVH by electrocardiographic criteria and more severe hypertension, a distinct increase in ventricular (but not atrial) premature contractions was found.[60] Of 16 patients with LVH, five had episodes of more than 30 premature ventricular contractions per minute. Higher grade ventricular ectopic activity, such as coupled premature ventricular contractions, was seen in two, and multifocal premature ventricular contractions were seen in three in the group with LVH (Table IV). Hence, whenever LVH reaches a certain critical mass, ectopic impulse generation seems to become more prevalent, thereby predisposing these patients to ventricular arrhythmias. Although the connection between an increased prevalence of ventricular premature beats and sudden death remains controversial, patients with LVH have been documented to be at a greater risk of sudden death than those with a normal myocardium.[61] Electrocardiographic monitoring of patients with LVH allows identification of those who have the highest risk and, therefore, require the most aggressive therapeutic intervention.

TABLE IV   Classification of Patients with Regard to Lown's Criteria

| | | Hypertensive | |
Maximal Lown Class	Normotensive	Without LVH	With LVH*
0	10	6	2
I	4	4	4
II	0	0	5
III	0	0	3
IV	0	0	2

LVH = left ventricular hypertrophy.
*p < 0.04 versus both other groups.

Myocardial Ischemia: Left ventricular mass and myocardial wall tension are major determinants of myocardial oxygen consumption (MVO_2). Accordingly, myocardial oxygen requirements augment in LVH, and coronary reserve becomes impaired. Strauer[62] reported a decrease in coronary reserve by one third (from normal) in patients with compensated essential hypertension and normal coronary arteries despite an increase in coronary blood flow, possibly resulting from an imbalance between muscle growth and vascular proliferation.[63] In addition, any increase in arterial pressure by itself interferes with MVO_2 by increasing the double product and LV stroke work and, on a long-term basis, by promoting coronary atheromatosis. Thus, the hypertensive patient with a hypertrophied left ventricle must be regarded as being at a high risk for ischemia, even in the absence of coronary atheromatosis. The impairment of coronary reserve in LV hypertension corroborates clinical experience that patients with accelerated hypertension often exhibit classic symptoms of angina pectoris without significant coronary artery stenosis on the angiogram.

Neither increased ventricular ectopic activity nor impaired coronary reserve is always clinically significant, especially in the early stage of LVH. However, their presence in a later phase of the disease clearly argues against the concept of LVH being merely a beneficial adaptive or compensatory process to the high pressure load.

Summary

The left ventricle adapts to an increased afterload such as that produced by arterial hypertension with concentric LVH. However, this adaptive process can be modified by a variety of physiologic and pathophysiologic states. Progressive aging, black race, and perhaps disorders with an increased sympathetic outflow seem to accelerate LVH. Obesity, volume overload, and other high CO states predominantly produce dilation of the left ventricle, and their combination with arterial hypertension results in eccentric LVH. Similarly, endurance exercise increases LV volume more than wall thickness, whereas isometric exercise produces an increase in wall thickness only. The presence or absence of some physiologic and pathogenetic factors has direct implication on the assessment of what constitutes a "normal" LV structure and function. Left ventricular hypertrophy has been shown to increase ventricular ectopic impulse generation and to put patients at a high risk of sudden death. Moreover, the increase in myocardial mass lowers coronary reserve and enhances cardiac oxygen requirements. Thus, the presence of LVH has to be considered as an ominous sign rather than as a benign adaptive process.

References

1. GAASCH WH: Left ventricular radius to wall thickness ratio. Am J Cardiol 1979; 43: 1189–1194.

2. DEVEREUX RB, REICHEK N: Left ventricular hypertrophy. Cardiovasc Rev Rep 1980; 1: 55–68.

3. EVANS G: A contribution to the study of arteriosclerosis, with special reference to its relation to chronic renal disease. Q J Med 1921; 14: 215–282.

4. BRESLIN DJ, GIFFORD RW JR, FAIRBAIRN JF II: Essential hypertension: a twenty-year follow-up study. Circulation 1966; 33: 87–97.

5. KANNEL WB: Blood pressure and risk of coronary heart disease: the Framingham Study. Chest 1969; 56: 43–52.

6. Hypertension Detection and Follow-up Program Cooperative Group: Five-year findings of the hypertension detection and follow-up program: I. Reduction in mortality of persons with high blood pressure, including mild hypertension. JAMA 1979; 242: 2562–2577.

7. TARAZI RC: Longterm effective antihypertensive therapy. Ann Intern Med 1980; 93: 771–772.

8. DUNN FG, CHANDRARATNA P, deCARVALHO JGR, BASTA LL, FROHLICH ED: Pathophysiologic assessment of hypertensive heart disease with echocardiography. Am J Cardiol 1977; 39: 789–795.

9. SAVAGE DD, DRAYER JIM, HENRY WL, et al: Echocardiographic assessment of cardiac anatomy and function in hypertensive patients. Circulation 1979; 59: 623–632.

10. COHEN A, HAGAN AD, WATKINS J, et al: Clinical correlates in hypertensive patients with left ventricular hypertrophy disguised with echocardiography. Am J Cardiol 1981; 47: 335–341.

11. SCHLANT RC, FELNER JM, BLUMENSTEIN BA, et al: Echocardiographic studies of left ventricular anatomy and function before and after treatment of essential hypertension (abstr). Am J Cardiol 1977; 39: 296.

12. DEVEREUX RB, PICKERING TG, HARSHFIELD GA, et al: Relation of hypertensive left ventricular hypertrophy to 24-hour blood pressure (abstr). Circulation 1981; 64: 321.

13. LOGAN AL, GILBERT BW, HAYNES RB, MILNE BJ, FLANAGAN PT: Early effects of mild hypertension on the heart. Hypertension 1981; 3 (suppl II): 187–190.

14. ROWLANDS DB, GLOVER DR, IRELAND MA, et al: Assessment of left ventricular mass and its response to antihypertensive treatment. Lancet 1982; 1: 467–470.

15. MESSERLI FH, SUNDGAARD-RIISE K, VENTURA HO, DUNN FG, OIGMAN W, FROHLICH ED: Clinical and hemodynamic determinants of left ventricular dimensions. Arch Intern Med 1984; 144: 477–481.

16. MESSERLI FH: Cardiovascular effects of obesity and hypertension. Lancet 1982; 1: 1165–1168.

17. GORDON T, KANNEL WB: Obesity and cardiovascular disease: the Framingham study. Clin Endocrinol Metab 1976; 5: 367–374.

18. ALEXANDER J, PETTIGROVE JR: Obesity and congestive heart failure. Geriatrics 1967; 22: 101–106.

19. LAKATTA EG: Alterations in the cardiovascular system that occur in advanced age. Fed Proc 1979; 38: 163–167.

20. GERSTENBLITH G, WEISFELDT ML, LAKATTA EG: Age changes in myocardial function and exercise response. Prog Cardiovasc Dis 1976; 19: 1–21.

21. BRANDFONBRENER M, LANDOWNE M, SHOCK NW: Changes in cardiac output with

age. Circulation 1955; 12: 557–566.

22. STRANDELL T: Circulatory studies on healthy old men. Acta Med Scand 1964; 175 (suppl 414): 1–44.

23. CONWAY J, WHEELER R, SANNERSTEDT R: Sympathetic nervous activity during exercise in relation to age. Cardiovasc Res 1971; 5: 577–581.

24. JULIUS S, ANTOON A, WHITLOCK LS, CONWAY J: Influence of age on the hemodynamic response to exercise. Circulation 1967; 36: 222–230.

25. MESSERLI FH, FROHLICH ED, SUAREZ DH, et al: Borderline hypertension: relationship between age, hemodynamics and circulating catecholamines. Circulation 1981; 64: 760–764.

26. SJÖGREN AL: Left ventricular wall thickness determined by ultrasound in 100 subjects without heart disease. Chest 1971; 60: 341–346.

27. GARDIN JM, HENRY WL, SAVAGE DP, EPSTEIN SE: Echocardiographic evaluation of an older population without clinically apparent heart disease (abstr). Am J Cardiol 1977; 39: 277.

28. GERSTENBLITH G, FREDERIKSEN J, YIN FCP, FORTUIN NJ, LAKATTA EG, WEISFELDT MI: Echocardiographic assessment of a normal adult aging population. Circulation 1977; 56: 273–278.

29. MESSERLI FH, GLADE LB, DRESLINSKI GR, et al: Hypertension in the elderly: haemodynamic, fluid volume, and endocrine findings. Lancet 1983; 2: 893–986.

30. MORGANROTH J, MARON BJ, HENRY WL, EPSTEIN SE: Comparative left ventricular dimensions in trained athletes. Ann Intern Med 1975; 82: 521–524.

31. MENAPACE FJ, HAMMER WJ, RITZER TF, et al: Left ventricular size in competitive weight lifters: an echocardiographic study. Med Sci Sports Exerc 1982; 14: 72–75.

32. DeMARIA AN, NEUMANN A, LEE G, FOWLER W, MASON DT: Alterations in ventricular mass and performance induced by exercise training in man evaluated by echocardiography. Circulation 1978; 57: 237–244.

33. EHSANI AA, HAGBERG JM, HICKSON RC: Rapid changes in left ventricular dimensions and mass in response to physical conditioning and deconditioning. Am J Cardiol 1978; 42: 52–56.

34. PERONNET F, PERRAULT H, CLEROUX J, et al: Electro- and echocardiographic study of the left ventricle in man after training. Eur J Appl Physiol 1980; 45: 125–130.

35. ADAMS TD, YANOWITZ FG, FISHER AG, RIDGES JD, LOVELL K, PRYOR TA: Noninvasive evaluation of exercise training on college-age men. Circulation 1981; 64: 958–965.

36. DeMARIA AN, NEUMANN A, SCHUBART PJ, LEE G, MASON DT: Systemic correlation of cardiac chamber size and ventricular performance determined with echocardiography and alterations in heart role in normal persons. Am J Cardiol 1979; 43: 1.

37. COHEN JL, GUPTA PK, LICHSTEIN E, CHADDA KD: The heart of a dancer: noninvasive cardiac evaluation of professional ballet dancers. Am J Cardiol 1980; 45: 959–978.

38. McDONOUGH JR, GARRISON GE, HAMES CG: Blood pressure and hypertensive disease among negroes and whites. Ann Intern Med 1964; 61: 208–228.

39. Hypertension Detection and Follow-up Program Cooperative Group: Race, edu-

cation, and prevalence of hypertension. Am J Epidemiol 1977; 106: 351–361.

40. DUNN FG, OIGMAN W, SUNDGAARD-RIISE K, et al: Racial differences in cardiac adaptation to essential hypertension determined by echocardiographic indices. J Am Coll Cardiol 1983; 1: 1348–1351.

41. RUBLER S, DAMANI PM, PINTO ER: Cardiac size and performance during pregnancy estimated with echocardiography. Am J Cardiol 1977; 40: 534–540.

42. KATZ R, KARLINER JS, RESNIK R: Effects of a natural volume overload state (pregnancy) on left ventricular performance in normal human subjects. Circulation 1978; 58: 434–441.

43. LARKIN H, GALLERY EDM, HUNYOR SN, GYORY AZ, BOYCE ES: Haemodynamics of hypertension in pregnancy assessed by M-mode echocardiography. Clin Exp Pharmacol 1980; 7: 463–468.

44. HERRICK JB: Peculiar elongated and sickle shaped red blood corpuscles in a case of severe anemia. Arch Intern Med 1910; 6: 517–521.

45. GERRY JL, BAIRD MG, FORTUIN NJ: Evaluation of left ventricular function in patients with sickle cell anemia. Am J Med 1976; 60: 968–972.

46. SCHARF S, WEXLER J, LONGNECKER RE, BLAUFOX MD: Cardiovascular disease in patients on chronic hemodialytic therapy. Prog Cardiovasc Dis 1980; 22: 343–356.

47. IKAHEIMO M, LINNALUOTO M, HUTTUNEN K, TAKKUNEN J: Effects of renal transplantation on left ventricular size and function. Br Heart J 1982; 47: 155–160.

48. DECARVALHO JGR, MESSERLI FH, FROHLICH ED: Mitral valve prolapse and borderline hypertension. Hypertension 1979; 1: 518–522.

49. BOUDOULAS H, REYNOLDS JC, MAZZAFERRI E, WOOLEY CF: Metabolic studies in mitral valve prolapse syndrome. A neuroendocrine-cardiovascular process. Circulation 1980; 61: 1200–1205.

50. GORDON AL, INCHIOSA MA JR, LEHR D: Isoproterenol-induced cardiomegaly: assessment of myocardial protein content, actomyosin ATPase and heart rate. J Mol Cell Cardiol 1972; 4: 543–557.

51. SZAKAS JE, MEHLMAN B: Pathologic changes induced by 1-norepinephrine: quantitative aspects. Am J Cardiol 1960; 5: 619–627.

52. YANKOPOULAS N, MONTERO A, CURD WG JR, KAHIL ME, CONDON REJ: Observations on myocardial function during chronic catecholamine oversecretion. Chest 1979; 66: 585–587.

53. RADTKE W, KAZMIER F, RUTHERFORD B, SHEPS SG: Cardiovascular complications of pheochromocytoma crisis. Am J Cardiol 1975; 35: 701–705.

54. BAKER G, ZELLER N, WEITZNER S, LEACH JK: Pheochromocytoma without hypertension presenting as cardiomyopathy. Am Heart J 1971; 83: 688–693.

55. GARCIA R, JENNINGS J: Pheochromocytoma masquerading as a cardiomyopathy. Am J Cardiol 1972; 29: 568–571.

56. RAAB W, LEPESCHKIN E: Biochemical versus haemodynamic factors in the origin of hypertensive heart disease. Acta Med Scand 1950; 138: 81–93.

57. COREA L, BENTIVOGLIO M, VERDECCHIA P, MOTOLESE M: Left ventricular wall thickness and plasma catecholamines in borderline and stable essential hypertension. Eur Heart J 1982; 3: 164–170.

58. LUNDIN S, FRIBERG P, HALLBACK-NORDLANDER M: Left ventricular hypertrophy improves cardiac function in spontaneously hypertensive rats. Clin Sci 1981;

61 (suppl 7): 109s–111s.

59. MESSERLI FH, GLADE LB, VENTURA HO, et al: Diurnal variations of cardiac rhythm, arterial pressure, and urinary catecholamines in borderline and established essential hypertension. Am Heart J 1982; 104: 109–114.

60. MESSERLI FH, VENTURA HO, ELIZARDI EG, DRESLINSKI GR, DUNN FG, FROHLICH ED: Hypertension and sudden death: increased ventricular ectopic activity in left ventricular hypertrophy. Am J Med 1984; 77: 18–22.

61. KANNEL WB: Prevalence and natural history of left ventricular hypertrophy. Am J Med 1983; 75 (suppl 3A): 4–11.

62. STRAUER BF: Hypertensive heart disease. New York: Springer-Verlag, 1980.

63. MARCUS ML, KOYANAGI S, HARRISON DG, DOTY DB, HIRATZKA LF, EASTHAM CL: Abnormalities in the coronary circulation that occur as a consequence of cardiac hypertrophy. Am J Med 1983; 75 (suppl 3A): 62–66.

23

Abnormalities in the Coronary Circulation that Occur as a Consequence of Cardiac Hypertrophy

MELVIN L. MARCUS, M.D.
SAMON KOYANAGI, M.D.
DAVID G. HARRISON, M.D.
DONALD B. DOTY, M.D.
LOREN F. HIRATZKA, M.D.
CHARLES L. EASTHAM, B.A.

Patients with hypertrophied ventricles often exhibit manifestations of myocardial ischemia, such as ST segment depression and angina with exercise. In addition, in patients with hypertrophied hearts cardiac failure eventually develops. Even though the complications associated with cardiac hypertrophy have been observed for decades, their pathogenesis has been difficult to elucidate. It has often been hypothesized that abnormalities in myocardial perfusion may be responsible for the complications associated with cardiac hypertrophy, but convincing data to support this hypothesis have been lacking until recently.[1,2] Early studies of resting coronary blood flow in patients with cardiac hypertrophy did not reveal any abnormalities.[3,4]

In studies concerning myocardial perfusion in hypertrophied ventricles, substantial progress has been made in the past decade, primarily because practical methods of measuring regional myocardial perfusion in animals became available[5] and several approaches to measuring coronary reserve in human subjects were introduced.[6–8] It is now generally acknowledged that certain types of cardiac hypertrophy are associated with major abnormalities in coronary reserve.[1,2]

A conceptual diagram that relates changes in cardiac muscle mass to alterations in coronary microcirculation is shown in Figure 1. The size of the box refers to the size of the heart, and the circles in the box represent the total cross-sectional area of the coronary resistance vessels. The normal relationship between the cardiac mass and the coronary circulation is illustrated by the center box.

When the heart enlarges, the coronary circulation could enlarge commensurately (left upper box). This type of relationship exists when volume-induced left ventricular hypertrophy (LVH) occurs in mature animals,[9,10] or

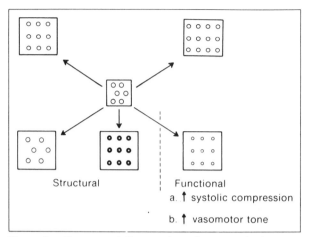

Figure 1. *Conceptual diagram that relates ventricular mass to the cross-sectional area of the coronary resistance vessels. The center box reflects the normal situation, that is, the ratio of ventricular mass (size of the box) to size of the vascular bed (total area of the circles within the box) is normal. See text for further explanation.*

when moderate LVH secondary to hypertension persists over a long segment of an animal's life span.[11] Alternatively, with hypertrophy, the relative growth of the coronary circulation could surpass that of the muscle mass (right upper box). Animal experiments suggest that this occurs when cardiac hypertrophy is secondary to thyrotoxicosis[12] or when pressure-induced hypertrophy is produced in utero.[13] Thus, in some animal models of disease, coronary reserve is well preserved in the presence of cardiac hypertrophy.

The three boxes at the bottom of Figure 1 illustrate three mechanisms by which coronary reserve in hypertrophied ventricles could be compromised. First, there could be inadequate growth of new vessels (bottom left box). This almost certainly occurs in dogs with pressure-induced right ventricular (RV) hypertrophy.[14] In this animal model, coronary perfusion pressure is normal and minimal coronary vascular resistance is significantly increased.[14] Inadequate growth of new vessels might also be responsible for decreases in coronary reserve that have been noted in animals with aortic obstruction.[15–19] Studies that have demonstrated impaired coronary reserve in patients with various types of valvular or congenital heart disease can best be explained by postulating inadequate growth of the coronary bed.[6,7,20–24] Vascular hypertrophy in coronary resistance vessels (center bottom box) could theoretically limit maximal coronary dilator capacity. This process narrows the lumen of the coronary resistance vessels and in the aggregate decreases the total cross-sectional area of the coronary bed. Vascular hypertrophy has been shown to occur in coronary resistance vessels of rats with spontaneous hypertension.[25] Thus, systemic hypertension is a stimulus that promotes vascular hypertrophy in coronary resistance vessels. The decreased coronary reserve that has been documented in animals[11,26,27] and in patients[6] with systemic hypertension may reflect this type of abnormality in vascular geometry. Third, it is possible that extravascular compressive forces could compromise coronary reserve (right bottom box). Because the heart impedes its own blood supply during systole, it is conceivable that marked increases in wall tension or contraction could increase minimal coronary resistance. Although such an effect has been postulated, studies that have addressed this question have not shown that increases in extravascular compressive forces are responsible for a significant decrease in coronary reserve in hypertrophied ventricles.[26] It is important to emphasize that the three mechanisms alluded to in the bottom three boxes of Figure 1 are not mutually exclusive. They could occur simultaneously.

In this brief review it will not be possible to describe in detail the many studies that support the hypothesis that coronary reserve is impaired in hypertrophied ventricles. However, two recent studies that may be of interest to internists will be briefly discussed. These studies are related to effects of hypertension and LVH on infarct size, and direct measurements of coronary reserve in patients with severe LVH secondary to aortic stenosis.

Two Recent Studies

Effects of Hypertension and Left Ventricular Hypertrophy on Infarct Size: Epidemiologic studies have shown that acute myocardial infarction (MI) is poorly tolerated by patients with hypertension and LVH.[28] In this patient group, acute MI is associated with a threefold increase in the incidence of sudden cardiac death, and post-infarction complications, such as heart failure, occur much more frequently than one might expect.[28] One explanation for these observations is that coronary obstructive disease is more severe in patients with increased systemic pressure because hypertension accelerates coronary atherosclerosis.[29,30] This factor almost certainly contributes to the clinical manifestations of myocardial ischemia in patients with hypertension.

We postulated that other abnormalities intrinsic of pressure-hypertrophied muscle (decreased coronary reserve,[1,2] decreased capillary density,[31] and abnormal electrophysiologic characteristics)[32,33] might also contribute to the adverse effects of coronary occlusion in hypertrophied hearts. To gain insight into the pathophysiology of acute MI when it occurs in a hypertrophied heart, we produced sudden coronary occlusion in awake, chronically instrumented dogs with renal hypertension and moderate LVH.[34,35] Similar studies were performed in control dogs. Two observations from these studies are of clinical interest. First, sudden cardiac death following coronary occlusion occurred more frequently in dogs with hypertension and LVH[34] (Fig. 2). Second, infarct size, expressed as a function of the area at risk (three-dimensional perfusion field of the occluded coronary vessel) was signifi-

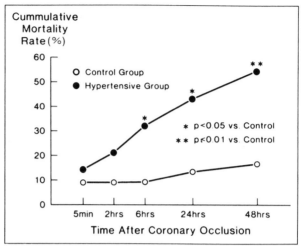

Figure 2. *Effects of sudden coronary occlusion on mortality in control dogs (control group) and hypertensive dogs with left ventricular hypertrophy (hypertensive group). Mortality was much higher in the hypertensive group. The cause of death was primarily ventricular fibrillation. The data suggest that chronic hypertension and left ventricular hypertrophy adversely affect the consequences of sudden coronary occlusion in dogs. (Data reproduced with permission from Koyanagi et al.[34])*

cantly increased in dogs with hypertension and LVH[35] (Fig. 3). Since the site of coronary occlusion and the size of the risk areas in the dogs with hypertension and LVH were similar to those in the controls, the differences observed cannot be related to more extensive coronary disease or more proximal coronary occlusion. Rather, the data suggest that intrinsic abnormalities in hypertrophied cardiac muscle, hemodynamic effects of hypertension, or both, must adversely affect the outcome of coronary occlusion when it occurs in the setting of hypertension and LVH.

Measurements of Coronary Reserve in Patients with Aortic Stenosis: Patients with aortic stenosis that is severe enough to require aortic valvular replacement frequently complain of exertional angina. In most clinical series, a substantial percentage of adult patients with aortic stenosis and exertional angina have significant coronary obstructive disease.[36] In this subgroup, obstructive coronary disease could certainly be responsible for the pathogenesis of angina. In the patients with aortic stenosis and angina, in whom the conduit coronary vessels are free of atherosclerotic lesions, the pathophysiology of myocardial ischemia is less certain.

We postulated that angina in patients with aortic stenosis and normal coronary vessels might occur if the intense LVH that accompanies severe aortic

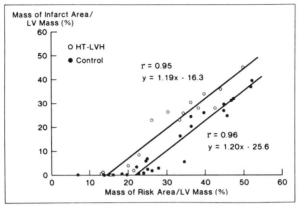

Figure 3. *Effects of chronic hypertension and left ventricular hypertrophy (HT-LVH) on the infarct—to—risk relationship. In this study, dogs were subjected to sudden coronary occlusion in the awake state. Forty-eight hours later, infarct size was determined by pathologic techniques and the risk area was defined by postmortem coronary angiography. Over the entire range of risk areas examined, infarcts were larger in dogs with chronic hypertension and left ventricular hypertrophy than in controls. (Data reproduced with permission from Moraski et al.[36])*

stenosis was associated with inadequate growth of the coronary vascular bed. This would result in a decrease in coronary reserve. To test this hypothesis, we developed a method of assessing coronary reserve in patients.[8] Our approach involves placing a Doppler probe on a coronary vessel at the time of open-heart surgery. The probe permits us to measure phasic coronary blood flow velocity in individual coronary vessels, such as the left anterior descending coronary artery. To produce maximal coronary dilation, the coronary vessel being examined is occluded for 20 seconds. This brief coronary occlusion produces severe myocardial ischemia in the perfusion field of the occluded vessel. As a consequence, the downstream coronary vessels dilate maximally. When the coronary occlusion is released and normal perfusion pressure is restored to the maximally dilated coronary bed, coronary blood flow velocity increases markedly and then returns toward control in the following 60 seconds[8] (Fig. 4). This vascular response to transient myocardial ischemia is called coronary reactive hyperemia. The magnitude of the coronary reactive hyperemic response is an excellent index of coronary reserve. When we studied coronary reactive hyperemic responses in patients with normal coronary vessels perfusing a normal ventricle, the peak to resting velocity ratio following release of a 20-second coronary occlusion was about 6:1.[8] Thus, the coronary circulation in human subjects can increase its flow about 600% in response to 20 seconds of intense myocardial ischemia.[8] We

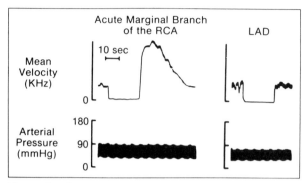

Figure 4. *Coronary reactive hyperemia responses in a patient with severe aortic stenosis. These studies were made at the time of open-heart surgery before cardiopulmonary bypass. The patient's right ventricle was of normal size; the left ventricle was severely hypertrophied; the coronary reactive hyperemia response obtained from the acute marginal branch of the coronary artery (RCA) was normal; the coronary reactive hyperemia response obtained from the left anterior descending (LAD) coronary artery was strikingly attenuated. The data suggest that severe left ventricular hypertrophy in patients with aortic stenosis markedly limits coronary reserve. (Adapted with permission from Marcus et al.[21])*

have also shown that measurements of coronary reactive hyperemia with the Doppler probe can be accomplished safely (no significant complications in more than 500 occlusions in 200 patients).

In patients with aortic stenosis and angiographically normal coronary vessels, coronary reactive hyperemia in the left anterior descending coronary artery is markedly impaired[21] (Fig. 4). Furthermore, the impairment is selective. Coronary reactive hyperemia in vessels that perfuse the non-hypertrophied right ventricle, in patients with aortic stenosis, are nearly normal.[2,21]

These studies demonstrate that coronary reserve is profoundly depressed in patients with aortic stenosis and intense LVH. This abnormality is of sufficient magnitude to explain the development of angina in these patients in the absence of coronary obstructive disease. Furthermore, it is possible that repeated episodes of ischemia may provoke subendocardial fibrosis and thereby contribute to the development of heart failure.

Summary

This review has emphasized the potential clinical importance of inadequate growth of the coronary bed that sometimes accompanies cardiac hypertrophy. The impairment in coronary reserve that results from this abnormality may well contribute to the pathogenesis of myocardial ischemia and heart failure in patients with hypertrophied hearts. Furthermore, cardiac hypertrophy may adversely affect the response of the myocardium to ischemia when this results from coexistant coronary obstructive disease. As a consequence, the complications of occlusive coronary disease (sudden death and heart failure) may be exaggerated when patients with hypertrophied hearts experience coronary occlusion.

Acknowledgment

This study was supported in part by National Institutes of Health (National Heart, Lung, and Blood Institute), Grants HL 14388 and HL 20827, by research funds from the Iowa Heart Association, and by the Veterans Administration.

References

1. MARCUS ML, MUELLER TM, GASCHO JA, KERBER RE: Effects of cardiac hypertrophy secondary to hypertension on the coronary circulation. Am J Cardiol 1979; 44: 1023–1028.

2. MARCUS ML, GASCHO JA, MUELLER TM, ET AL: The effects of ventricular hypertrophy on the coronary circulation. Basic Res Cardiol 1981; 76: 575–581.

3. BING RJ, HAMMOND MM, HANDELSMAN JC, ET AL: The measurement of coronary blood flow, oxygen consumption, and efficiency of the left ventricle in man. Am Heart J 1949; 38: 1–24.

4. ROWE GG, CASTILLO CA, MAXWELL GM, CRUMPTON CW: A hemodynamic study of hypertension including observations on coronary blood flow. Ann Intern Med 1961; 54: 405–412.

5. HEYMANN MA, PAYNE BD, HOFFMAN JIE, RUDOLPH AM: Blood flow measurements with radionuclide-labeled particles. Prog Cardiovasc Dis 1977; 20: 55–79.

6. STRAUER BE: Hypertensive heart disease. New York: Springer-Verlag, 1980.

7. TAUCHERT M, HILGER HH: Application of the coronary reserve concept to the study of myocardial perfusion. In: Schaper W, ed. The pathophysiology of myocardial perfusion, 1st ed. Amsterdam: Elsevier/North-Holland Biomedical Press, 1979; 141–167.

8. MARCUS ML, WRIGHT C, DOTY D, ET AL: Measurements of coronary velocity and reactive hyperemia in the coronary circulation of humans. Circ Res 1981; 49: 877–891.

9. GASCHO J, MUELLER TM, EASTHAM CL, MARCUS ML: Abnormalities of the coronary circulation in normotensive dogs with volume-induced left ventricular hypertrophy. Cardiovas Res 1982; 16: 288–292.

10. HULTGREN PB, BOVE AA: Myocardial blood flow at rest and during exercise in dogs with volume overload induced left ventricular hypertrophy. Fed Proc 1978; 37: 647.

11. WRANGLER RD, PETERS KG, MARCUS ML, TOMANEK RJ: Effects of duration and severity of arterial hypertension and cardiac hypertrophy on coronary vasodilator reserve. Circ Res 1982; 51: 10–18.

12. MARCUS ML, CHILIAN WM, WANGLER RD, PETERS KG, TOMANEK RJ: Does the stimulus producing hypertrophy alter the interaction between the coronary vascular bed and myocardial mass? Fed Proc 1982; 41: 1097.

13. VLAHAKES GJ, TURLEY K, VERRIER ED, HOFFMAN JIE: Greater maximal coronary flow in conscious lambs with experimental congenital right ventricular hypertrophy. Circulation 1980; 62: 111.

14. MURRAY PA, VATNER SF: Reduction of maximal coronary vasodilator capacity in conscious dogs with severe right ventricular hypertrophy. Circ Res 1981; 48: 27–33.

15. HOLTZ J, RESTORFF WV, BARD P, BASSENGE E: Transmural distribution of myocardial blood flow of coronary reserve in canine left ventricular hypertrophy. Basic Res Cardiol 1977; 72: 286–292.

16. REMBERT JC, KLEINMAN LH, FEDOR JM, WECHSLER AS, GREENFIELD JC: Myocardial blood flow distribution in concentric left ventricular hypertrophy. J Clin Invest 1978; 62: 379–386.

17. BACHE RJ, VROBEL TR, RING WS, EMERY RW, ANDERSEN RW: Regional myocardial blood flow during exercise in dogs with chronic left ventricular hypertrophy. Circ Res 1981; 48: 76–87.

18. O'KEEFE DD, HOFFMAN JIE, CHEITLIN R, O'NEILL MJ, ALLARD JR, SHAPKIN E: Coronary blood flow in experimental canine left ventricular hypertrophy. Circ Res 1978; 43: 43–51.

19. WHITE FC, SANDERS M, PETERSON T, BLOOR CM: Ischemic myocardial injury after exercise stress in the pressure-overloaded heart. Am J Pathol 1979; 97: 473–486.

20. DOTY D, WRIGHT C, EASTHAM C, MARCUS ML: Coronary reserve in atrial septal defect. Circulation 1980; 62: III–115.

21. MARCUS ML, DOTY D, WRIGHT C, EASTHAM C: Mechanism of angina in patients with aortic stenosis and normal coronary arteries. Circulation 1980; 62: III–111.

22. DOTY D, EASTHAM C, HIRATZKA L, WRIGHT C, MARCUS M: Determinants of coronary reserve in patients with supravalvular aortic stenosis. Circulation 1982: 66 (suppl 1): 186–192.

23. MARCUS ML, DOTY D, HIRATZKA L, WRIGHT C, EASTHAM C: Impaired coronary reserve in children with cyanotic congenital heart disease. Circulation 1981; 64: 127.

24. EASTHAM CL, DOTY DB, HIRATZKA LF, WRIGHT CB, MARCUS ML: Volume-overload left ventricular hypertrophy impairs coronary reserve in humans. Circulation 1981; 64: 26.

25. YAMORI Y, MORI C, NISHIO T, ET AL: Cardiac hypertrophy in early hypertension. Am J Cardiol 1979; 44: 964–969.

26. MUELLER TM, MARCUS ML, KERBER RE, YOUNG JA, BARNES RW, ABBOUD FM: Effect of renal hypertension and left ventricular hypertrophy on the coronary circulation in dogs. Circ Res 1978; 42: 543–549.

27. MARCUS ML, MUELLER TM, EASTHAM CL: Effects of short- and long-term left ventricular hypertrophy on coronary circulation. Am J Physiol 1981; 241: H358–H362.

28. KANNEL WB: Role of blood pressure in cardiovascular morbidity and mortality. Prog Cardiovasc Dis 1974; 17: 5–24.

29. HOLLANDER W, PRUSTY S, KIRKPATRICK B, PADDOCK J, NAGRAJ S: Role of hypertension in ischemic heart disease and cerebral vascular disease in the cynomolgus monkey with coarctation of the aorta. Circ Res 1977; 40: 70–83.

30. PICK R, JOHNSON PJ, GLICK G: Deleterious effects of hypertension on the development of aortic and coronary atherosclerosis in stumptail macaques (Macaca speciosa) on an atherogenic diet. Circ Res 1974; 35: 472–482.

31. RAKUSAN K: Quantitative morphology of capillaries of the heart. Number of capillaries in animal and human hearts under normal and pathological conditions. Methods Achiev Exp Pathol 1971; 5: 272–286.

32. ARONSON RS: Characteristics of action potentials of hypertrophied myocardium from rats with renal hypertension. Circ Res 1980; 47: 443–454.

33. GELBAND H, BASSETT A: Depressed transmembrane potentials during experimentally induced ventricular failure in cats. Circ Res 1973; 32: 625–634.

34. KOYANAGI S, EASTHAM C, MARCUS ML: Effects of chronic hypertension and left ventricular hypertrophy on the incidence of sudden cardiac death following coronary occlusion in conscious dogs. Circulation 1982; 65: 1192–1197.

35. KOYANAGI S, EASTHAM CL, HARRISON DG, MARCUS ML: Increased size of myocardial infarction in dogs with chronic hypertension and left ventricular hypertrophy. Circ Res 1982; 50: 55–62.

36. MORASKI RE, RUSSEL RO JR, MANTLE JA, RACKLEY CE: Aortic stenosis, angina pectoris, coronary artery disease. Cathet Cardiovasc Diagn 1976; 2: 157–164.

24

Relationship Between the Rhythm and the Hemodynamic Load in the Hypertensive Heart

MAURIZIO D. GUAZZI, M.D.

Although pathophysiology of the hypertensive human heart and the influence of therapy have been investigated extensively over the years, one facet has remained almost entirely neglected, that is, cardiac rhythm in high blood pressure. The availability of methods for 24-hour ambulatory electrocardiographic (ECG) recording, through which cardiac arrhythmias can be reliably identified and quantitated,[1,2] made the approach to this aspect feasible. Data reported in the medical literature[3,4] indicate that atrial and ventricular ectopic activities are more frequent in hypertensive compared with normotensive subjects, and that prevalence and frequency of ventricular arrhythmias is higher in hypertensive patients with left ventricular hypertrophy (LVH) evaluated by ECG criteria than in patients with uncomplicated established hypertension.[5]

Enhancement of cardiac ectopic activity is considered one of the major cardiovascular risks associated with hypokalemia, and an increased susceptibility to digitalis-related arrhythmias in hypokalemic patients is well documented[6,7] and widely accepted. It has also been suggested that patients with hypokalemia without heart disease who do not take digitalis have an increased incidence of ectopic beats.[8] If it is considered that of all patients who receive a thiazide diuretic for the treatment of primary hypertension hypokalemia will develop in 20% to 40%,[9,10] the possibility should be taken into account that low serum potassium is involved in the elicitation of arrhythmias in a considerable portion of the hypertensive population. However, Papademetrion and collaborators[3] subjected a group of primary hypertensive subjects with diuretic-induced hypokalemia to 24-hour ambulatory ECG monitoring before and after correction of hypokalemia and proved that in uncomplicated hypertension correction of diuretic-induced hypokalemia does not significantly reduce the occurrence of spontaneous atrial or ventricular ectopic activity. Therefore, other possibilities should be examined.

In essence, hypertension is a circulatory disorder that alters the hemodynamics of the heart. In the natural history of high blood pressure the condition of the heart is subjected to a progression of interrelated anatomic and functional changes.[11,12] Schematically, three subsequent structural steps may be outlined: normal heart, concentric hypertrophy, and hypertrophy associated with left ventricular (LV) cavity enlargement. The influences that these three conditions exert on the load and on the function of the heart, both in systole[13,14] and diastole,[15,16] are different. It is validly established that the performance of the left and also of the right side of the human heart in hypertension is quite sensitive to the level of LV afterload,[17] that systolic cardiac function is generally maintained in the heart with normal structure, that it is possibly enhanced in the presence of concentric hypertrophy,[13,18] and that, in parallel with the increased afterload, it is depressed when the heart becomes enlarged.[18,19] Because of these reasons, it is conceivable that cardiac rhythm in hypertension may be somehow related to the structure and through this to the functional state of the heart; also, that influences of antihypertensive therapy on the rhythm of the heart may be, in part, related to the effects on ventricular afterload and function. These aspects were investigated in our laboratory[20] and will be discussed in this chapter.

Rate and Structure of the Heart in Hypertension

On the basis of echo measurements, 85 untreated, hospital—admitted patients with uncomplicated primary hypertension were divided into three groups. Group 1 (normal-sized heart) consisted of 24 patients in whom septal and posterior wall thickness and end-diastolic LV minor axis were within 1 SD of the normal control values (group 0 included 31 normal subjects); group 2 (concentric hypertrophy) included 33 patients with normal or reduced LV end-diastolic minor axis and both septal and posterior wall thickness exceeding mean plus 1 SD of control; group 3 (hypertrophy associated with LV cavity enlargement) consisted of 28 patients in whom wall thickness was within the same range as in group 2, but end-diastolic minor axis exceeded the mean plus 1 SD for this group. The latter patients generally exhibited variable degrees of repolarization abnormalities referable to a "strain" pattern.[21]

These four groups of patients were subjected to two subsequent 24-hour ambulatory ECG recordings, and the following data were quantified in each patient: the total number of heart beats for 24 hours, the highest and the lowest heart rate/minute, the number of any atrial premature contractions, of any ventricular premature contractions, and of any "complex" ventricular contractions. Under the term "complex" we included bigeminy, couplets, and salvos of unsustained ventricular tachycardia (defined as three or more ventricular depolarizations occurring in succession at a rate between 100 and 200 cycles/min). The upper limit of variability between the two measurements was 2% for the total number of beats/24 hours, 4% for the highest and the lowest rate/minute, and 10% for the number of arrhythmias. The averages were taken as the representative values for each patient.

The number of beats per 24 hours was significantly much higher than normal (group 0) in groups 1 and 3, and this difference was associated with

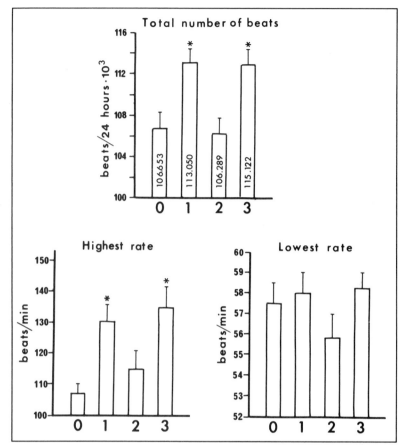

Figure 1. *Averages (SD) of the total number of heart beats and of the highest and lowest rate/minute recorded during 24 hours in the control (group 0) and in the three hypertensive groups. *Significant differences from group 0 (p < 0.01). (Reprinted with permission from Loaldi A et al.[20])*

higher averages of the maximal and minimal heart rate/minute recorded in the 24 hours. In group 2 these values were similar to normal (Fig. 1). That group differences in the 24-hour number of beats were not casual, but reflected a distinct feature, is supported by the observation that the highest and the lowest rates/minute varied from group to group in parallel with the total beats. The increased heart rate in 24 hours in group 1 may be related to younger age or to hyperdynamic activity of the heart, such as that characterizing the early phase of hypertension. In group 3 tachycardia might simply reflect a mechanism of compensation for the increased circulatory load and the impaired performance of the heart. In contrast, a normal or enhanced cardiac performance in group 2 may be the reason why the chronotropic activity of the heart was maintained within normal limits.

TABLE I   Types, Prevalence (%) and Frequency of Cardiac Arrhythmias During 24 hours in the Untreated Condition in the Normotensive and Hypertensive Groups*

Arrhythmias in the 24 Hours	Atrial Premature Contractions				Ventricular Premature Contractions				Bigeminy				Couplets				Salvos of Ventricular Tachycardia			
	0	1	2	3	0	1	2	3	0	1	2	3	0	1	2	3	0	1	2	3
251–300			3				8													
201–250			2				6													
151–200			5	2			3													
101–150			9	12			7													
51–100			7	9			3													
11–50	6	12	6	4	3	4	6	1				3				1				
1–10	7	12	1	1	6	14	20	0	1	3	5	5				5				6
0					4	6	8		12	21	28	20	13	24	33	22	13	24	33	22
Prevalence	100	100	100	100	75	75	75	100	8	13	17	28	0	0	0	22	0	0	0	22

*For details about groups, see text, p. 242.

Ectopic Activity and Structure of the Heart in Hypertension

Types, prevalence, and frequency of cardiac arrhythmias recorded in the control subjects and in the three groups are summarized in Table I. Atrial and ventricular premature contractions were observed in the majority of both normotensive and hypertensive subjects (prevalence ranging from 75% to 100% of cases); the frequency of atrial extrasystoles, however, was definitely higher in group 2 and that of ventricular extrasystoles was higher in group 3, compared with the other groups. Prevalence and frequency of bigeminy were low and were similar in all the groups. Couplets and short runs of ventricular tachycardia were recorded only in group 3, in 22% of the patients. The frequency of the salvos of ventricular tachycardia did not exceed 10 in the 24 hours. In the control and group 1 patients the averages of atrial and ventricular extrasystoles in 24 hours were comparable and both types of arrhythmias did not exceed 25 in either group. In group 2 the number of ventricular extrasystoles was also similar to normal, whereas that of atrial extrasystoles (128 in 24 hours) was significantly higher than in the control and hypertensive group 1 subjects. The average number of ventricular extrasystoles (214 in 24 hours) strongly differentiated group 3 from the other groups; the average of atrial extrasystoles (106 in 24 hours) was also larger than normal in this group.

Changes in Cardiac Arrhythmias and Left Ventricular Afterload with Treatment

Patients in groups 1 and 2 were divided into three subgroups that were treated, respectively, with atenolol (100 mg/day), verapamil (120 mg 3 times daily), and nifedipine (10 mg 4 times daily). Patients in group 3 were subdi-

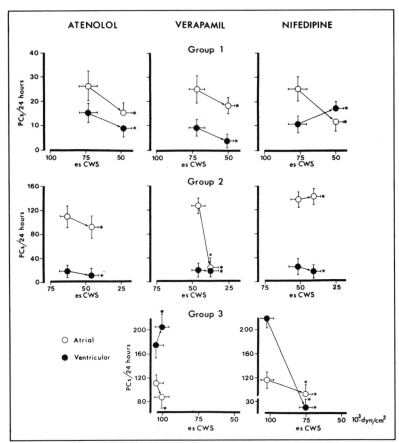

Figure 2. *Averages (SD) of atrial (○) and ventricular (●) premature contractions (PCs) per 24 hours at baseline and after atenolol, verapamil, and nifedipine, and corresponding values of left ventricular end-systolic circumferential wall stress (es CWS). *Significant differences from baseline (p < 0.01). (Reprinted with permission from Loaldi A et al.[20])*

vided into two groups that received, respectively, verapamil and nifedipine. For the purpose of manipulating LV afterload, the two calcium channel blockers, verapamil and nifedipine, were chosen because their potent vasodilating antihypertensive action[22] could be expected remarkably to unload the heart; the beta blocker atenolol was chosen as representative of a class of compounds having a predominant place in the treatment of high blood pressure (we decided not to test the beta blocker in group 3 because we were concerned about possible deterioration in cardiac function in the presence of left ventricular enlargement). A 24-hour ambulatory ECG monitoring was repeated after 7 days of treatment in each patient.

Figure 2 illustrates the averages of atrial and ventricular premature contractions recorded during 24-hour continuous monitoring in the pre- and post-treatment periods, and the corresponding values of end-systolic LV circumferential wall stress.[23] End-systolic stress reflects the maximal level of the instantaneous myocardial force for the existing instantaneous myocardial length or volume during the ejection phase. Thus, end-systolic stress is literally the afterload that limits the ejection, and we considered that it may have a special conceptual value as an afterload marker.

In group 1 atenolol, verapamil, and nifedipine showed a similar ventricular unloading efficacy and did not influence arrhythmias significantly. In group 2 the average number of atrial premature depolarizations was impressively increased in the baseline. If the number of heart beats in 24 hours and maximal and minimal heart rate/minute are interpreted as reflecting normal adrenergic activity in this group, then excessive neural influences could be ruled out as responsible for atrial extrasystoles. In keeping with this interpretation is that atenolol did not abolish arrhythmias. A number of clinical and experimental findings[16,17] suggest that ventricular diastolic compliance is abnormal in hypertensive concentric LVH. It might be speculated that the exaggerated "booster pump" action assumed by the atria to keep ventricular filling normal[24] is somehow related to the atrial premature depolarizations detected in group 2. Although atenolol, verapamil, and nifedipine unloaded the left ventricle to a similar extent, atrial extrasystoles were reduced significantly only in the verapamil-treated patients. This makes a relationship between LV afterload and atrial premature depolarizations unlikely and suggests an influence of the drug on the ventricular diastolic properties or on the cardiac pacemaker activity.

In group 3 the predominance of ventricular premature depolarizations was associated with the highest level of end-systolic LV afterload. Differences in the responses to the two calcium antagonists involved both the ventricular unloading and the antiarrhythmic effect. Reduction in end-systolic wall stress after verapamil was not statistically significant, whereas the efficacy of nifedipine on ventricular wall stress was prominent. The number of ventricular extrasystoles in 24 hours from an average of 223 was reduced to an average of 13 in the nifedipine-treated patients, and augmented from 177 to 206 in the 24 hours in those who received verapamil. Couplets and salvos of ventricular tachycardia were still seen in three cases of the latter and one case of the former population. The divergent response of ventricular extrasystoles to the two calcium antagonists is not really explained in terms of antiarrhythmic properties, since nifedipine seems to be devoid of such properties.[25] On the basis of the relationship that seems to exist between ventricular afterload and arrhythmias, the excessive contractile effort of the left ventricle might be interpreted as one of the elicitors of ventricular extrasystoles, and the antiarrhythmic response to nifedipine might be ascribed to a potent unloading effect. The less pronounced efficacy on afterload of verapamil compared with nifedipine can possibly be referred to a lower vasodilating and impedance-reducing potency and to the intrinsic depressant effect of the compound on the myocardium. This latter effect is counterbalanced by the vasodilating response when the function of the heart in the baseline is well preserved, but becomes apparent when the function is impaired.[26]

Under an applicative viewpoint, these findings can imply that the cardiac rhythm in hypertension may present a clinical problem, mostly in the presence of hypertrophy associated with LV cavity enlargement and that a favorable influence on ventricular ectopic activity is an additional reason for considering effective LV unloading compounds as best suited for treating hypertension in the presence of cardiac dilation. This reinforces the concept that treatment of hypertension should be based on individual considerations and that an accurate evaluation of the heart can provide guidelines for more appropriate treatment.

References

1. HARRISON DC, FITZGERALD JW, WINKLE RA: Contribution of ambulatory electrocardiographic monitoring to antiarrhythmic management. Am J Cardiol 1978; 41: 996–1004.

2. LOWN B: Sudden cardiac death: the major challenge confronting contemporary cardiology. Am J Cardiol 1979; 43: 313–328.

3. PAPADEMETRION V, FLETCHER R, KHATRI IM, FREIS ED: Diuretic induced hypokalemia in uncomplicated systemic hypertension: effect of plasma potassium correction on cardiac arrhythmias. Am J Cardiol 1983; 52: 1017–1022.

4. MESSERLI FH, VENTURA HO, ELIZARDI DJ, DUNN FG, FROHLICH ED: Hypertension and sudden death: increased ventricular ectopic activity in left ventricular hypertrophy. Am J Med 1984; 77: 18–22.

5. MESSERLI FH, GLADE LB, VENTURA HO, et al: Diurnal variations of cardiac rhythm, arterial pressure, and urinary catecholamines in borderline and established essential hypertension. Am Heart J 1982; 104: 109–114.

6. LOWN B, LEVINE HD: Atrial arrhythmias, digitalis and potassium. New York: Lansberger, 1958.

7. FISCH C, SURAWICZ B: Digitalis. New York: Grune & Stratton, 1969.

8. DAVIDSON S, SURAWICZ B, KY L: Ectopic beats and atrioventricular conduction disturbances in patients with hypopotassemia. Arch Intern Med 1967; 120: 280–285.

9. GIFFORD RW JR: Combined drug therapy in hypertension. In: Hahnemann Symposium on hypertensive disease (1958). Hypertension. Pennsylvania: W.B. Saunders 1959; 361.

10. Veterans Administration Cooperative Study Group on Antihypertensive Agents: effects of treatment on morbidity in hypertension; further analysis of side effects. Circulation 1972; 45: 991–1004.

11. FREIS ED: Hemodynamics of hypertension. Physiol Res 1960; 40: 27–54.

12. COHN JN, LIMAS CJ, GUIHA NH: Hypertension and the heart. Arch Intern Med 1974; 133: 969–979.

13. KARLINER JS, WILLIAMS G, GORWIT W, CRAWFORD MH, O'ROURKE RA: Left ven-

tricular performance in patients with left ventricular hypertrophy caused by systemic arterial hypertension. Br Heart J 1977; 39: 1239–1245.

14. GUAZZI M, FIORENTINI C, OLIVARI MT, POLESE A: Cardiac load and function in hypertension. Ultrasonic and hemodynamic study. Am J Cardiol 1979; 44: 1007–1012.

15. HANRATH P, MATHEY DG, SIEGERT R, BLEIFELD W: Left ventricular relaxation and filling pattern in different forms of left ventricular hypertrophy: an echocardiographic study. Am J Cardiol 1980; 45: 15–23.

16. DRESLINSKI GR, FROHLICH ED, DUNN FG, MESSERLI FH, SUAREZ DH, REISIN E: Echocardiographic diastolic ventricular abnormality in hypertensive heart disease: atrial emptying index. Am J Cardiol 1981; 47: 1087–1090.

17. OLIVARI MT, FIORENTINI C, POLESE A, GUAZZI MD: Pulmonary hemodynamics and right ventricular function in hypertension. Circulation 1978; 57: 1185–1190.

18. FIORENTINI C, POLESE A, OLIVARI MT, GUAZZI MD: Cardiac performance in hypertension re-evaluated through a combined haemodynamic ultrasonic method. Br Heart J 1980; 43: 344–350.

19. ABI-SAMRA, FOUAD FM, NAKASHIMA Y, TARAZI RC: Determinants of left ventricular hypertrophy and function in hypertension. Am J Cardiol 1982; 49: 951.

20. LOALDI A, PEPI M, AGOSTONI PG, FIORENTINI C, GRAZI S, DELLA BELLA P, GUAZZI MD: Cardiac rhythm in hypertension assessed through 24-hour ambulatory electrocardiographic monitoring. Effects of load manipulation with atenolol, verapamil and nifedipine. Br Heart J 1983; 50: 118–126.

21. DEVEREUX RB, REICHECK N: Repolarization abnormalities of left ventricular hypertrophy. Clinical echocardiographic and hemodynamic correlates. J Electrocardiol 1982; 15: 47–54.

22. GUAZZI MD: Use of calcium channel blocking agents in the treatment of systemic arterial hypertension. In: Stone PH, Antman EM, eds. Calcium channel blocking agents in the treatment of cardiovascular disorders. New York: Futura Publishing, 1983.

23. REICHECK N, WILSON J, SUTTON MSJ, PLAPPERT TA, GOLDBERG S, HIRSHFELD JW: Noninvasive determination of left ventricular end-systolic stress: validation of the method and initial application. Circulation 1982; 65: 99–108.

24. TARAZI RC, MILLER A, FROHLICH ED, DUSTAN HP: Electrocardiographic changes reflecting left atrial abnormality in hypertension. Circulation 1966; 34: 818–822.

25. ANTMAN E, STONE PH, MULLER JE, BRAUNWALD E: Calcium channel blocking agents in the treatment of cardiovascular disorders. Part I: basic and clinical electrophysiologic effects. Ann Intern Med 1980; 93: 875–885.

26. CHEW CVC, HECHT HS, COLLETT JT, McALLISTER RG, SINGH BN: Influence of severity of ventricular dysfunction on hemodynamic responses to intravenously administered verapamil in ischemic heart disease. Am J Cardiol 1981; 47: 917–922.

25

Myocardial Hypertrophy and Cardiac Failure: A Complex Interrelationship

BARRY M. MASSIE, M.D.

The interrelationship between myocardial hypertrophy and myocardial dysfunction is complex. It has long been appreciated that many pathologic processes affecting the heart, such as chronic hypertension, valvular disease, and the cardiomyopathies, produce both cardiac hypertrophy and myocardial failure. In each of these conditions, myocardial hypertrophy may be an important compensation for impaired contractility or excessive loading conditions, but at the same time it may itself become a pathologic process.[1,2]

Figure 1 illustrates the interdependence of myocardial hypertrophy and failure. Often, they result from the same disease process or experimental stimulus. This may be the case in aortic stenosis or systemic hypertension, both of which produce abnormal systolic pressure loads on the left ventricle, and in aortic or mitral regurgitation, which imposes excess volume loading on the same chamber. Despite their different underlying pathophysiologies, each of these processes increases left ventricular (LV) systolic or diastolic circumferential wall stress, which, as defined by the Laplace equation shown, is a function of the product of intracavitary pressure (P) times the chamber radius (R) divided by myocardial wall thickness (h).

$$\text{Stress} = \frac{PR}{2h}$$

Similarly, wall stress of the residual healthy myocardium increases when segmental dysfunction results in chamber dilation and increased diastolic volumes and pressures. Finally, in the failing heart, wall stress is increased as a result of LV dilation. In all of these settings, the increase in wall stress is particularly disadvantageous when myocardial contractility or contractile reserve is impaired, since this excessive loading will further depress cardiac performance.

Increased wall stress is also an important stimulus to left ventricular hypertrophy (LVH), which, by increasing wall thickness, may reduce systolic or diastolic stress, or both, toward normal levels.[3] This unloads the left ventricle and improves cardiac performance.[2] On the other hand, if, as some evidence suggests, hypertrophied myocardium is functionally abnormal, the persistence or progression of hypertrophy may eventually result in worsening cardiac performance.[1]

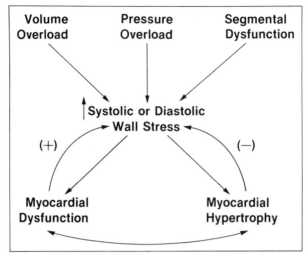

Figure 1. *The complex interrelationship between myocardial dysfunction and myocardial hypertrophy is shown schematically. See text for explanation.*

Much of the work that has provided our present understanding of the hypertrophy process and its interrelationship with myocardial function is experimental. Although this article will consider some of this information, it will focus on the clinically important issues, including the role of hypertrophy as a compensatory mechanism in pressure and volume overload states and myocardial failure, hypertrophy as a pathologic process, and the effect of hypertrophy regression on myocardial function.

Evolution of Cardiac Hypertrophy

The stimulus to hypertrophy in most experimental models and clinical states is an increase in wall stress, generated in diastolic fiber tension in volume overload states with chamber dilation or by an increase in systolic pressure.[3] Some data indicate that factors other than hemodynamic alterations may also lead to hypertrophy.[4] Laks and coworkers[5] have produced LVH with long-term subhypertensive infusions of norepinephrine. This and other inferential evidence support a role for the sympathetic nervous system in the pathogenesis of hypertrophy.

The mechanisms by which the stimulus for hypertrophy is translated into sarcomerogenesis remain speculative. Meerson and Breger[6] hypothesized that the increased energy requirements resulting from the supranormal workload deplete high energy phosphate stores and that this in turn stimulates nuclear and mitochondrial protein synthesis. Others have postulated a role for cyclic adenosine monophosphate and for changes or intercompartmental shifts in calcium ion concentration. [7] Although further substantiation for these hypotheses is required, the biochemical sequence of events leading to hypertrophy is better documented. In the stressed heart, messenger RNA synthesis increases within minutes. In a period of 1 to 3 hours, ribosomal RNA concentration increases. New contractile protein synthesis can be demonstrated within a few hours, and mitochondrial protein and DNA synthesis soon follow. [1]

Since most evidence indicates that myocardial cell division ceases in adult mammalian species, cardiac hypertrophy proceeds predominantly as a result of an increase in the volume of existing myocytes. [3] Newly formed sarcomeres may be added in series or in parallel. Data from human subjects suggest that in the volume-overload heart, with cardiac dilation and a normal or increased chamber diameter to wall thickness ratio (so called eccentric hypertrophy), sarcomerogenesis occurs in series. In contrast, pressure overloaded states produce concentric hypertrophy, characterized by a lower than normal chamber volume to wall thickness ratio as a result of the parallel addition of sarcomeres. [2,8] In either case, as hypertrophy proceeds there is an accompanying deposition of fibrous tissue and hyperplasia of stromal elements, including capillaries, although not always in proportion to the degree of myocyte enlargement. [9,10]

Hypertrophy as a Compensatory Process

Experimental Models: Ontologically, it is attractive to consider myocardial hypertrophy as a compensatory process. [2,3,8] Ample experimental and clinical evidence suggests that this is usually the case. It is most obvious in the hypertrophy that occurs with normal growth or in response to athletic training. It is also seen in the adaptation to increased metabolic demands, such as thyrotoxicosis. In many volume- or pressure-overloaded animal models, hypertrophy serves to normalize or at least minimize the impairment of cardiac pump performance. This has been elegantly demonstrated with long-term aortic constriction in dogs. [11] Immediately after constriction and for the next several days, indices of contractility are decreased and chamber dilation is present. After several weeks, hypertrophy occurs and pump function indices return toward baseline. Calculated wall stress also decreases to preconstriction levels as the chamber radius to wall thickness ratio normalizes. Similarly, in the spontaneously hypertensive rat, global indices of pump function, such as peak stroke volume during fluid loading and maximum developed pressure during aortic occlusion, are normal during the early phases of the disease. During this time period, despite markedly increased systemic arterial pressure, peak systolic stress is maintained within normal limits as a result of progressive hypertrophy. [12] Significant LV dysfunction occurs only at a later stage when hypertrophy does not keep pace with the workload.

Hypertrophy in Human Pressure and Volume Overload States: It has long been recognized that hypertrophy serves a compensatory function

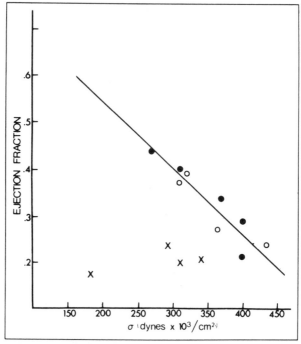

Figure 2. *Ejection fraction is plotted against mean circumferential wall stress. The patients, shown by closed or open circles, improved postoperatively and when measured had an increase in ejection fraction. The patients indicated by X's experienced pump failure perioperatively or showed no postoperative improvement. It was suggested that the preoperative ventricular dysfunction in the first group was due to afterload mismatch with inadequate hypertrophy, whereas in the second group, a primary disorder of myocardial contractility was also present. (Reproduced with permission from Carabello et al.[14])*

in human subjects as well, although several recently published studies have reemphasized this point.[2,3] Grossman and associates[13,14] have investigated the role of LVH in patients with aortic valve disease. They found that before the onset of clinically apparent LV dysfunction, LV wall stress is maintained within the normal range despite markedly increased intracavitary pressures. This is accomplished by concentric hypertrophy with resultant low chamber radius to wall thickness ratios (Fig. 1). When wall stress increases, producing excessive afterload, ejection phase indices of cardiac performance, such as ejection fraction, decrease (Fig. 2). In these patients, hypertrophy has not kept pace with the pressure overload. Carabello et al[14] have also identified another group of subjects in whom systolic performance is inappropriately depressed relative to wall stress (Fig. 2). They speculate that there is associated myocardial dysfunction in these patients and have shown that their prognosis after valve replacement is poor.

In the volume overload setting of aortic insufficiency, hypertrophy appears to play a similar compensatory role.[13] Despite an increase in chamber diameter, systolic wall stress remains normal by virtue of increased wall thickness in compensated patients. However, in an important subset of chronic volume overloaded patients, systolic dysfunction develops, and many of these manifest an abnormally high chamber radius to wall thickness ratio, suggesting inadequate hypertrophy.[15]

Hypertrophy in Congestive Cardiomyopathy: Hypertrophy is also consistently present in the chronic congestive cardiomyopathies, whether they are primary or result from ischemic heart disease.[16,17] As in the previously discussed pressure and volume overload states, hypertrophy appears to play a compensatory role. Thus, Hamby and associates[18] observed that LV wall thickness to volume and mass to volume ratios were higher in compensated than in decompensated subjects with primary myocardial disease. Field and his coworkers[16] performed quantitative angiography on 36 patients with primary cardiomyopathy. They found that in patients with LV mass to volume ratios above 0.9 g/ml the clinical course was more prolonged and subsequent survival better. Furthermore, this measurement provided additional prognostic information even when the patients were subdivided by ejection fraction.

More recently, Benjamin and associates[17] performed a postmortem study to evaluate further the role of hypertrophy in congestive cardiomyopathy. They found that patients who had survived longer had a significantly greater LV mass and mean wall thickness. Although this could reflect progressive hypertrophy over time rather than a protective role for hypertrophy, they also noted that survival was better in patients with a greater wall thickness to chamber diameter ratio and that this measurement had a greater predictive value than either chamber size or LV mass alone. These findings again support the hypothesis that hypertrophy, by preventing excessive wall stress, is an important adaptation to LV dysfunction.

Pathologic Aspects of Cardiac Hypertrophy

Most of the preceding discussion has centered on the compensatory role of hypertrophy in disease states characterized by excessive loading conditions or depressed contractility. However, a considerable body of predominantly experimental and pathologic data indicates that significant abnormalities exist in hypertrophied myocardium.[1,6] Although this information has been extensively reviewed elsewhere, since it remains controversial it will be considered here in brief.

Much of the controversy results from the fact that many findings are not reproducible in different experimental models and that similar data are difficult to obtain in human subjects.[1,2] Various investigators have documented biochemical and histologic abnormalities in hypertrophy and have found associated disorders of contractility, myocardial blood flow, and myocardial metabolism. These abnormalities are generally more prevalent in models in which the stimulus to hypertrophy is abrupt and severe, when it involves a pressure overload, and when small animals are utilized.[1]

Many studies have demonstrated decreased indices of contractility in isolated cardiac muscle from hearts subjected to pressure overload of either the right or left ventricle.[12,19,20] Similar findings have been noted with intact hearts in hypertensive rats.[12] Contractile dysfunction has also been seen in volume-overload models.[21] However, other investigators have found that in some long-term preparations contractility returns to normal as hypertrophy progresses.[11] Hence, the question of whether hypertrophied myocardium functions normally remains unsettled.

A number of workers have shown that depressed contractility in hypertrophied myocardium is associated with decreased myosin adenosine triphosphatase activity and changes in the relative distribution of its isoenzymes.[1] Other biochemical defects in hypertrophied muscle have been described, the best documented of which is a decrease in norepinephrine content.[22] This has been detected in hypertrophied myocardium before the onset of heart failure and becomes more severe with the appearance of overt contractile dysfunction.

Considerable circumstantial evidence suggests that hypertrophied myocardium may have an inadequate energy supply.[6] On the cellular level, workers have noted a decrease in the number of mitochondria and in the activity of mitochondrial enzymes relative to the myofibrillar content.[23] However, whether or not there is any primary metabolic abnormality in myocardial hypertrophy remains controversial.

The increase in cell diameter that particularly characterizes concentric hypertrophy necessarily reduces the cell surface to cell volume ratio.[3] This may impair the transfer of substrates and metabolites in and out of the cell. Histologic studies indicate that capillary density is reduced in experimental pressure overload hypertrophy.[10] This could also impair local perfusion. Mechanical factors, such as an increase in intramyocardial tension in the subendocardium, could also interfere with coronary blood flow and myocardial perfusion. Several groups have in fact documented a reduction in myocardial perfusion and coronary reserve in human subjects with hypertrophy.[16]

Ischemia, for whatever reason, could very well explain the presence of cell necrosis and fibrosis that are usually found in both experimental and clinical hypertrophy.[24,25] This increase in collagen content of hypertrophied myocardium is the likely explanation for the increase in muscle stiffness and reduced diastolic compliance noted in most hypertrophic states.[21] This impairment in diastolic performance may be the earliest detectable change in human hypertrophy and may have important pathophysiologic consequences, as will be discussed.

Left Ventricular Hypertrophy in Hypertension

Evolution of Hypertensive Heart Disease: Chronic hypertension is the most frequent cause of LVH.[26] It has been shown in animal models and, with the availability of echo, in human subjects that hypertrophy occurs early in the clinical course of hypertension.[27,28] Surprisingly, the correlation between the level of blood pressure and the degree of hypertrophy is not close.[4] Since hypertension is a major etiologic factor in many patients with congestive heart failure,[29] the question of whether hypertrophy plays a compensatory or pathologic role is of obvious importance. The evolution of hypertrophy and heart failure has been particularly well studied in spontaneously hypertensive rats.[12,27] In this model, hypertrophy may appear even before the onset of significant hypertension. Between 3 and 9 months of age, hypertension is established and although hypertrophy proceeds, contractility indices are normal or even increased. Subsequently, although the blood pressure shows no further increase, hypertrophy continues to progress. In this phase, contractile function declines and histologic evidence of necrosis and fibrosis appears.

The progression of cardiac involvement in hypertensive human subjects (Table I)[30] appears to parallel that in the spontaneously hypertensive rat. Hypertrophy may precede the appearance of "fixed" hypertension. Early in the course of hypertension, many patients exhibit a hyperkinetic picture characterized by increased blood volume and cardiac output together with supranormal indices of contractility. During the phase of chronic, stable hypertension, hypertrophy proceeds and ventricular performance generally remains normal.[31–33]

In this phase, subtle abnormalities in systolic function can sometimes be detected with stress, such as handgrip or exercise.[31] Interestingly, recent studies have indicated that even in the presence of normal systolic function many patients will manifest abnormalities of diastolic performance, such as a decrease in early diastolic filling rates.[33–35] These, then, are probably the earliest indications of hypertensive heart disease. They may reflect increased chamber stiffness due to the hypertrophy per se or they may reflect decreased compliance due to fibrosis.

Ultimately, overt cardiac dysfunction and clinical congestive heart failure will develop in some patients. However, there is enormous variation in individual responses to hypertension. Some patients will manifest little if any change in LV mass, whereas in others hypertrophy will develop but they will exhibit varying degrees of functional abnormality. Unfortunately, little is known of the factors that produce these variations in the progression of hypertensive cardiac involvement.

As noted previously, Strauer[15] has argued that hypertrophy, by maintaining relatively low systolic wall stress in the presence of increased systolic pressures, reduces afterload and prevents decompensation. However, this simply beneficial role of hypertrophy is belied by its poor prognosis. In the Framingham Study, electrocardiographic evidence of LVH was associated

TABLE I   **Evolution of Hypertensive Heart Disease**

	Early Hypertension	Hypertension	Congestive Heart Failure
Blood pressure	↑	↑	↑ or ←→
Cardiac output	↑ or ←→	←→	←→ or ↓
Left ventricular mass	←→ or ↑	↑	↑
Left ventricular volume	←→ or ↓	←→	↑
Contractility	↑	←→ or ↓	↓
Ejection fraction	←→ or ↑	←→	↓

with an eight fold increase in cardiovascular mortality.[26] Of note is that mortality was twice as high at any blood pressure level when electrocardiographic hypertrophy was present. Thus, it seems that even though an inadequate hypertrophic response to hypertension may lead to LV failure, the pressure of hypertrophy per se is a marker for high risk patients.

Regression of Left Ventricular Hypertrophy: Regression of LVH has been demonstrated in animal hypertension models[36–40] and, more recently, with medical therapy in human subjects.[41,42] In the context of the preceding discussion of the possibly pathologic nature of myocardial hypertrophy, this finding takes on added significance. In both renal hypertensive and spontaneously hypertensive rats, established LVH regresses with antihypertensive therapy.[36–40] As the hypertrophy reverses, previously impaired indices of systolic function return toward normal and the biochemical abnormalities discussed earlier disappear.[37,40,43]

Regression of LVH during antihypertensive therapy is more difficult to demonstrate in human subjects because of the necessity for using more indirect techniques of evaluation. With the availability of echo, several studies have now demonstrated hypertrophy regression, sometimes in surprisingly short periods of follow-up.[41,42] Thus far, regression of hypertrophy has been noted with methyldopa, beta blockers, and thiazide diuretics, and there are not enough data to suggest any advantage to one class of drugs.

Two obvious questions arise in the context of the earlier discussion of the compensatory and pathologic roles played by hypertrophy. The first is whether reversal of hypertrophy may be deleterious if hypertension recurs. A sudden increase in systolic pressure without the protective adaptation of a gradual increase in myocardial mass could result in markedly increased wall stress and might precipitate acute heart failure. Experimental data support this potential risk,[37] but its clinical ramifications remain to be explored. The second point of interest is whether the functional derangements associated with hypertrophy will be reversed. As mentioned previously, animal studies suggest that systolic abnormalities do diminish. The available data in human subjects document little change in systolic function, but the baseline measurements are generally within normal limits. The experimental results suggest that diastolic dysfunction, which presumably reflects increased collagen deposition, may not reverse.[21,40,43] Serial measurements of diastolic function are not yet available in human subjects.

Implications for Antihypertensive Therapy: In conclusion, we must briefly consider the therapeutic implications of the foregoing discussion. The first goal of antihypertensive therapy remains adequate blood pressure control, and the step-care approach provides a rational framework for achieving this. If hypertensive heart disease follows the progression outlined in Table I, it would make sense to employ beta blockers as well as diuretics as initial agents in patients with mild hypertension, normal LV function, and no evidence of LVH. The early use of a beta blocker, or conceivably another sympatholytic agent, might be particularly justified in the mild hypertensive patient with hyperfunction of the left ventricle, with or without hypertrophy. In patients with more significant cardiac involvement, evidenced from definite hypertrophy or LV dysfunction, or both, it might make sense to employ a diuretic plus a sympatholytic agent. Once LV dysfunction has progressed to the point of clinical heart failure, the use of vasodilating drugs that might unload the ventricle to a greater extent for a given degree of blood pressure control may be particularly appropriate.[44]

At this point, it is probably most prudent to consider the regression of hypertrophy, whether it results from valve replacement in aortic stenosis or regurgitation, or from antihypertensive therapy, to be a marker for the successful, long-term reduction of the load on the myocardium. If further studies indicate a dissociation between the level of blood pressure control and the degree of hypertrophy regression in human subjects, we will have to consider whether hypertrophy reversal should be a primary goal of therapy. At present, there is insufficient experience to determine whether a reduction in LV mass is associated with lower incidences of heart failure or mortality than those achieved by adequate blood pressure control alone, but these questions are likely to be addressed in future experimental and clinical studies.

Acknowledgment

This study was supported in part by the National Heart, Lung, and Blood Institute Grant HL28146.

References

1. WIKMAN-COFFELT J, PARMLEY WW, MASON DT: The cardiac hypertrophy process: analysis of factors determining pathologic versus physiological development. Circ Res 1979; 45: 697–707.
2. GROSSMAN W: Cardiac hypertrophy: useful adaptation or pathologic process. Am J Med 1980; 69: 576–584.
3. LINZBACH AJ: Heart failure from the point of view of quantitative anatomy. Am J Cardiol 1960; 5: 370–382.
4. FROHLICH ED, TARAZI RC: Is arterial pressure the sole factor responsible for hypertensive cardiac hypertrophy? Am J Cardiol 1979; 44: 959–963.

5. LAKS MM, MORADY F, SWAN HJC: Myocardial hypertrophy produced by chronic subhypertensive doses of norepinephrine in the dog. Chest 1976; 64: 75.

6. MEERSON FZ, BREGER AM: The common mechanism of the heart's adaptation and deadaptation: hypertrophy and atrophy of the heart muscle. Basic Res Cardiol 1977; 72: 228–234.

7. RASMUSSEN H, GOODMAN DBP: Relationship between calcium and cyclic nucleotides in cell activation. Physiol Rev 1977; 57: 421–509.

8. FORD LE: Heart size. Circ Res 1976; 39: 297–303.

9. BUCCINO RA, HARRIS E, SPANN JF, SONNENBLICK EH: Response of myocardial connective tissue to development of experimental hypertrophy. Am J Physiol 1969; 216: 425–428.

10. GERDES AM, CALLAS G, KASTEN FH: Differences in regional capillary distribution and myocyte sizes in normal and hypertrophic rat hearts. Am J Anat 1979; 156: 523–532.

11. SASAYAMA S, ROSS J, FRANKLIN D, BLOOR CM, BISHOP S, DILLEY RB: Adaptations of the left ventricle to chronic pressure overload. Circ Res 1976; 38: 172–178.

12. BURGER SB, STRAUER BE: Left ventricular hypertrophy in chronic pressure load due to spontaneous essential hypertension. In: Strauer BE, ed. The heart in hypertension. Berlin: Springer-Verlag, 1981; 13–35.

13. GROSSMAN W, JONES D, McLAURIN LP: Wall stress and patterns of hypertrophy in the human left ventricle. J Clin Invest 1975; 56: 56–64.

14. CARABELLO BA, GREEN LH, GROSSMAN W, COHN LH, KOSTER JK, COLLINS JJ: Hemodynamic determinants of prognosis of aortic valve replacement in critical aortic stenosis and advanced congestive heart failure. Circulation 1980; 62: 42–48.

15. STRAUER BE: Myocardial oxygen consumption in chronic heart disease: role of wall stress, hypertrophy and coronary reserve. Am J Cardiol 1979; 44: 730–740.

16. FIELD BJ, BAXLEY WA, RUSSELL RO, ET AL: Left ventricular function and hypertrophy in cardiomyopathy with depressed ejection fraction. Circulation 1973; 47: 1022–1031.

17. BENJAMIN IJ, SCHUSTER EH, BULKLEY BH: Cardiac hypertrophy in idiopathic dilated congestive cardiomyopathy: a clinicopathologic study. Circulation 1981; 64: 442–447.

18. HAMBY RI, CATANGAY P, APIADO O, KHAN AH: Primary myocardial disease. Clinical, hemodynamic, and angiocardiographic correlates in 50 patients. Am J Cardiol 1970; 25: 625–634.

19. SPANN JF, BUCCINO RA, SONNENBLICK WH, BRAUNWALD E: Contractile state of cardiac muscle obtained from cats with experimentally produced ventricular hypertrophy and heart failure. Circ Res 1967; 21: 341–354.

20. CAPASSO JM, STROBECK JE, SONNENBLICK EH: Myocardial mechanical alterations during gradual onset longterm hypertension in rats. Am J Physiol 1981; 241: H435–H441.

21. PINSKY WW, LEWIS RM, HARTLEY CJ, ENTMANN ML: Permanent changes of ventricular contractility and compliance in chronic volume overload. Am J Physiol 1979; 237: H575–H583.

22. RUTENBERG HL, SPANN JF: Alterations of cardiac sympathetic neurotransmitter activity in congestive heart failure. Am J Cardiol 1973; 32: 472–479.

23. RABINOWITZ M, ZAK R: Mitochondria and cardiac hypertrophy. Circ Res 1975; 36: 367–376.

24. REVIS NW, CAMERON AJV: Association of myocardial cell necrosis with experimental cardiac hypertrophy. J Pathol 1979; 128: 193–202.

25. CAREY RA, NATARJAN G, BOVE AA, SANTAMORE WP, SPANN JF: Elevated collagen content in volume overload induced cardiac hypertrophy. J Mol Cell Cardiol 1980; 12: 929–936.

26. KANNELL WB, GORDON T, OFFUTT D: Left ventricular hypertrophy by electrocardiogram. Prevalence, incidence, and mortality in the Framingham Study. Ann Intern Med 1969; 71: 80–101.

27. YAMORI Y, MORI C, NISHIO T, ET AL: Cardiac hypertrophy in early hypertension. Am J Cardiol 1979; 44: 964–969.

28. SCHEIKEN RM, CLARKE WR, LAUER RM: Left ventricular hypertrophy in children with blood pressure in the upper quintile of the distribution. The Muscatine Study. Hypertension 1981; 3: 669.

29. KANNEL WB, CASTELLI WP, McNAMARA PM, McKEE PH, FEINLEIB M: Role of blood pressure in the development of congestive heart failure. N Engl J Med 1972; 227: 782.

30. COHN JN, LIMAS CJ, GUIHA NH: Hypertension and the heart. Arch Intern Med 1974; 133: 969–979.

31. DUNN FG, CHANDRARATNA P, DECARVALHO JGR, BASTA LL, FROHLICH ED: Pathophysiologic assessment of hypertensive heart disease with echocardiography. Am J Cardiol 1977; 39: 789–795.

32. GUAZZI M, FIORENTINI C, OLIVARI MT, POLESE A: Cardiac load and function in hypertension. Ultrasound and hemodynamic study. Am J Cardiol 1979; 44: 1007–1012.

33. DRESLINSKI GR, FROHLICH ED, DUNN FG, MESSERLI FH, SUAREZ DH, REISIN E: Echocardiographic diastolic ventricular abnormality in hypertensive heart disease: atrial emptying index. Am J Cardiol 1981; 47: 1087–1090.

34. FOUAD FM, TARAZI RC, GALLAGHER JH, MACINTYRE WJ, COOK SA: Abnormal left ventricular relaxation in hypertensive patients. Clin Sci 1980; 59: 411s–414s.

35. INOUYE IK, MASSIE BM, LOGE D, ET AL: Abnormal left ventricular filling: an early finding in mild to moderate systemic hypertension. Am J Cardiol 1984; 53: 120–126.

36. SEN S, TARAZI RC, BAMPUS FM: Cardiac hypertrophy and antihypertensive therapy. Cardiovasc Res 1977; 11: 427–433.

37. FERRARIO CM, SPECH MM, TARAZI RC, DOI Y: Cardiac pumping ability in rats with experimental renal and genetic hypertension. Am J Cardiol 1979; 4: 979–985.

38. SEN S, TARAZI RC, BUMPUS FM: Reversal of cardiac hypertrophy in renal hypertensive rats: medical versus surgical therapy. Am J Physiol 1981; 240: H408–H412.

39. PFEFFER JM, PFEFFER MA, FLETCHER P, FISHBEIN MC, BRAUNWALD E: Favorable effects of therapy on cardiac performance in spontaneously hypertensive rats. Am J Physiol 1982; 242: H776–H784.

40. CAPASSO JM, STROBECK JE, MALHOTRA A, SCHEUER J, SONNENBLICK EH: Contractile behavior of rat myocardium after reversal of hypertensive hypertrophy. Am

J Physiol 1982; 242: H882–H889.

41. FOUAD FM, NAKASHIMA Y, TARAZI RL, SALCEDO ED: Reversal of left ventricular hypertrophy with methyldopa. Am J Cardiol 1982; 49: 795.

42. SCHLANT RC, FEINER JM, HEYMSFIELD SB, ET AL: Echocardiographic studies of left ventricular anatomy and function in essential hypertension. Cardiovasc Med 1977; 2: 477–491.

43. SEN S, TARAZI RC, BUMPUS FM: Biochemical changes associated with development and reversal of cardiac hypertrophy in spontaneously hypertensive rats. Cardiovasc Res 1976; 10: 254–261.

44. MASSIE BM, CHAN S: Antihypertensive therapy with prazosin in patients with left ventricular dysfunction. Chest 1981; 80: 692–697.

26

Is Normotensive Aging of the Cardiovascular System a Muted Form of Hypertensive Cardiovascular Disease?

EDWARD G. LAKATTA, M.D.

It has been the consensus of medical clinicians that blood pressure elevation to specified levels above what is construed as normal be designated as "hypertension." It is well established that hypertension causes cardiac hypertrophy, which is accompanied by a reduction in left ventricular (LV) diastolic compliance and early filling rate and in elderly patients is associated with altered properties of the arterial wall, an increase in systemic vascular resistance, and a decline in resting cardiac output (CO). With aging, changes in the arterial wall occur that are similar to those caused by hypertension and are associated with an increase in stiffness[1,2] manifested as an increase in pulse wave velocity.[3–6] It is not entirely clear whether such alterations within the vascular media should be considered to be a manifestation of a "normal" biologic aging process, or whether these, like atherosclerosis, should also be considered pathologic states. Although this alteration in the vasculature media does not directly impact on organ flow, as does advanced atherosclerosis, it seems to be the cause of an increased vascular stiffness and systolic blood pressure within the clinically normal range, even in otherwise healthy subjects who have rigorously been screened for cardiovascular disease.[7] Because of this and the observation that the baroreceptor reflex is attenuated both in patients with hypertension and with advancing adult age in normotensive subjects,[8] aging might be construed as a "muted" form of hypertension;[9] or conversely, hypertension might be viewed as accelerated aging.[10] If either of these hypotheses are correct, similar but less pronounced changes might be demonstrable in the heart with aging in normotensive subjects as those observed in patients with clinical hypertension. What evidence suggests that this may be the case?

In animal models chronic experimental cardiac hypertrophy at a young age produced by creating a ventricular pressure overload results in a prolonged action potential and contraction duration, a reduction in myofibrillar adenosine triphosphatase (ATPase), and diminished rate of protein synthesis (see Gerstenblith et al[4] and Lakatta and Yin[10] for review). Similar findings accompany the cardiac hypertrophy of aging in the normotensive rat model and experimental cardiac hypertrophy has been likened to "premature" aging.[11] More recent studies, however, have demonstrated that cardiac hypertrophy and these other age-related myocardial changes can be dissociated,[12–15] indicating that aging and experimental cardiac hypertrophy due to enhanced ventricular afterloading, although affecting similar changes in the heart, apparently do so via different mechanisms.

Does the modest progressive increment in systolic blood pressure that occurs with aging in man constitute an increase in workload on the heart sufficient to cause an age-related increase in cardiac mass? Stroke work, or stroke volume times blood pressure, is indeed increased with age in normotensive subjects[7,16] and is associated with a moderate but definite increase in LV wall thickness[17–19] and estimated mass.[17,20] In addition, a modest but significant correlation between the level of blood pressure and LV wall thickness among normal individuals can be demonstrated.[21] However, factors other than increased blood pressure, such as an increased level of circulating catecholamines in elderly subjects either at rest or during the routine activities of daily living (vide infra), may contribute to the ventricular hypertrophy.

The early diastolic filling rate at rest, as judged from the maximum E-F slope of the echo[17,18] and from time activity curves of gated blood pool scans[22] decreases with age and the magnitude of this decrease is similar to that observed in persons with hypertension,[23,24] even though the left ventricular hypertrophy (LVH) is greater in elderly patients with hypertension than in elderly normal subjects.[24–28]

Since aging in normotensive subjects is associated with cardiac hypertrophy, a diminution in early diastolic filling rate, and an increase in vascular stiffness and blood pressure, the heart and vasculature of elderly subjects do indeed take on the appearance of "muted" hypertension.[29] Does this analogy hold when other aspects of cardiac function are compared in hypertensive and normotensive subjects studied across a broad age range?

In elderly patients with hypertension (more than 65 years of age) a recent study indicates that CO, heart rate, stroke volume (SV), and renal blood flow were significantly lower and peripheral vascular resistance higher than in younger (less than 42 years of age) patients.[25] Similar findings for CO, SV, and peripheral resistance have also been reported previously in elderly hypertensive subjects.[30,31] A prevalent view among cardiologists, physiologists, and gerontologists is that cardiac index (CI) at rest in healthy elderly subjects exhibits a progressive decline over the adult age range (Fig. 1A). However, recent studies in volunteer subjects who were more rigorously screened for occult coronary artery disease (CAD) and who were more homogeneous with regard to lifestyle variables than in previous studies do not support the notion that an obligatory decline in CI occurs with aging (Fig. 1B). Table I compares other hemodynamic variables in the populations whose CI is illustrated in Figure 1. Note in particular that in population B, the end-diastolic volume was not age related. Thus, at rest, the slowed rate of early ventricular filling noted in comparably screened subjects does not compromise the end-diastolic filling volume, which suggests that atrial contrac-

TABLE I   Effect of Adult Age on Resting Cardiac Function

Parameter	Population A: Institutionalized, Unscreened for Occult CAD (2nd–9th Decade)*	Population B: Active in Community Life Screened for Occult CAD with Cardiovascular Stress (3rd–8th Decade)†
Heart rate	Slight decrease	Slight decrease
Stroke volume	Decrease	Slight increase
End-diastolic volume	Not measured	No effect
Cardiac output	Decrease	No effect
Cardiac index	Decrease	No effect
Peripheral vascular resistance	Increase	No effect
Peak systolic blood pressure	Increase	Increase
Diastolic pressure	No effect	No effect
Stroke work	Increase	Increase
End-systolic volume	Not measured	No effect
Ejection fraction	Not measured	No effect
Maximum filling rate	Not measured	Decrease
Maximum ejection rate	Not measured	No effect

*Data from Brandfonbrener et al.[15]
†Data from Gerstenblith et al[21] and Rodeheffer et al.[6]

tion may make a greater contribution to ventricular filling in elderly than in younger subjects. Note also that indices of pump function, that is ejection fraction and velocity of ejection, are not age related at rest in population B. Thus, the cardiac hypertrophy measured in another subset of this population[18] may be considered an adapative mechanism to reduce toward normal the increased ventricular stress due to enhanced blood pressure, permitting normal ventricular ejection even in the presence of enhanced afterload. Similarly, in moderately hypertensive subjects, ejection fraction is normal at rest.[23]

The population studied in Figure 1B and Table I (population B) also exhibited age-related adaptations to maintain CO during exercise. In previous hemodynamic studies of the effect of age on cardiovascular function during exercise, SV, heart rate and CO declined with advancing age.[32–34] With progressive exercise, in the healthy elderly subjects in the population B in Table I the heart rate failed to increase to the extent that it did in younger subjects, and ventricular dilation, both end-diastolic and end-systolic, occurred. The increase in LV wall thickness with age is a particularly important adaptation to exercise stress, since it would tend to normalize the increase in wall stress due to this cardiac dilation during exercise. Stroke volume did not decline in these subjects, however, but rather increased, and this permitted CO to increase to the same extent in elderly as younger subjects, despite the diminished increment in heart rate. This hemodynamic profile is depicted in Figure 2 in which the slope of the age regression for selected hemodynamic variables is plotted as a function of exercise workload. Although CO is maintained and SV is enhanced, end-systolic volume increases with age during exercise (Figure 3A), whereas at rest heart size at end-systole was not age related. The

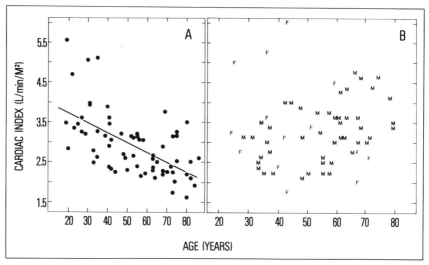

Figure 1. **A:** *The relationship between age and cardiac index, determined by the direct Fick method in 67 "basal" males without apparent circulatory disorders. The line indicates a significant linear regression for the points. (Reprinted with permission from Branfonbrener et al[16]* **B:** *The effect of age on cardiac output at rest determined by radionuclide angiography in BLSA subjects. M = males; F = females. (Reprinted with permission from Rodeheffer et al.[7])*

ejection fraction, although not age related at rest, also declines with age in this population during vigorous exercise (Fig. 3B). However, in contrast to a previous observation,[35] a decrease in ejection fraction from the resting level did not occur in these elderly subjects. Similar observations have recently been made in moderately hypertensive subjects.[23]

On the other hand, there is abundant evidence that demonstrates that the target response to catecholamines diminishes with advancing age in animals,[10] and other studies suggest that this is the case in man.[41,43–46] Infusion of catecholamines produces a diminished heart rate response in elderly versus younger adult normotensive subjects[41,43–46] and animals.[47] This age-related decrease in isoproterenol-induced increment heart rate is exaggerated in hypertensive patients.[41,48] In normotensive men studies[49] indicate that stimulation of cyclic adenosine monophosphate (cAMP) in lymphocytes by isoproterenol decreases with age. (However, young adults were compared to patients in a geriatric unit or residents of an old peoples' home.) Although early studies suggested that the number of beta receptors on circulating lymphocytes decreased with age[50] repeat studies with technologic refinement to measure specific binding indicated that no such age change occurs.[51]

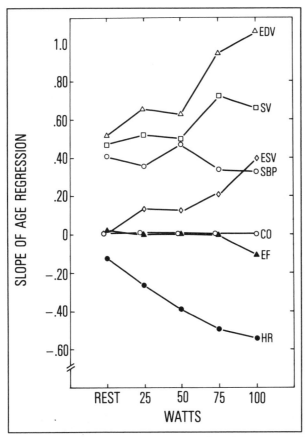

Figure 2. *The slope of the regression functions on age of end-diastolic volume (EDV), end-systolic volume (ESV), stroke volume (SV), systolic blood pressure (SBP), cardiac output (CO), ejection fraction (EF), and heart rate (HR) at incremental workloads from rest to 100 W. At each workload, each parameter was regressed on age and the slope coefficients of the regression function are depicted. For each parameter, an increase or decrease in the slope coefficient with increasing workloads indicates a respective increasing or decreasing age effect. (Reprinted with permission from Rodeheffer et al.[7])*

the absence of catecholamines or exogenous stimulants, declines with age in healthy subjects. Although this cannot be measured precisely in man, there is no support for this notion in animal models.[10]

A growing literature in both man and animal models when considered collectively does indicate that beta-adrenergic modulation of cardiovascular performance declines with age.[36] Indeed, the hemodynamic profile of the

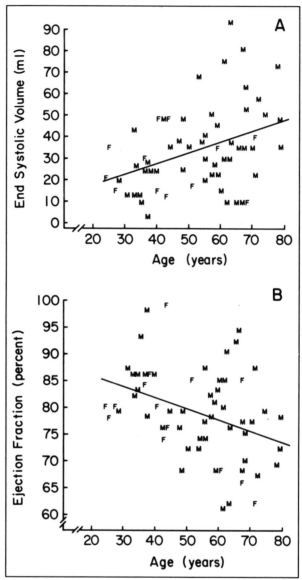

Figure 3. *The effect of age on end-systolic volume (A) and ejection fraction (B) measured via gated blood pool scans during maximum upright bicycle exercise. The population is the same as in Figures 1B, and 2. End-systolic volume (ml) = 6.5 + 0.5 (age), r = .41, p < 0.001. Ejection fraction = 89.9 − 0.21 (age), r = .37, p < 0.003. At rest neither end-systolic volume nor ejection fraction were age related (r = 0.05, p = 0.7 and r = 0.19, p = 0.14, respectively). (Reprinted with permission from Rodeheffer et al.[7])*

elderly subjects indicated by Figure 2, that is, a diminished heart rate, increased end-diastolic volume, and enhanced SV with increased end-systolic volume, resembles that observed during exercise in the presence of beta-adrenergic blockade.[37,38] The apparent age-related reduction in SV and heart rate with age observed in other populations during exercise[32–34] may also be in part attributed to a diminished catecholamine modulation of myocardial contractility and heart rate. In fact, because the age difference observed in cardiovascular performance during exercise was diminished when the subjects exercised in the presence of propranolol, it has been suggested that either failure to elaborate catecholamines or a failure of target organ response to catecholamines in the elderly subjects might explain the result obtained.[32] The former explanation can now be dismissed. Plasma catecholamine levels at rest, although either not age-related or increased in normotensive men, depend on the population studied and the definition of "basal" levels,[39,40] and are not decreased during exercise. Rather they are enhanced with age in a subset of the population. (Fig. 1B, 2, and 3). Plasma catecholamine levels have also been noted to increase with age in response to changes from the basal state in other normotensive populations as well.[39,41] Similarly, in hypertensive subjects basal levels of norepinephrine have been either reported not to be age related or to be increased with age,[41,42] whereas during exercise a substantial age-related increase has been observed.[41]

On the other hand, there is abundant evidence that demonstrates that the target response to catecholamines diminishes with advancing age in animals,[10] and other studies suggest that this is the case in man.[41,43–46] Infusion of catecholamines produces a diminished heart rate response in elderly versus younger adult normotensive subjects[41,43–46] and animals.[47] This age-related decrease in isoproterenol-induced increment heart rate is exaggerated in hypertensive patients.[41,48] In normotensive men studies[49] indicate that stimulation of cyclic adenosine monophosphate (cAMP) in lymphocytes by isoproterenol decreases with age. (However, young adults were compared to patients in a geriatric unit or residents of an old peoples' home.) Although early studies suggested that the number of beta receptors on circulating lymphocytes decreased with age[50] repeat studies with technologic refinement to measure specific binding indicated that no such age change occurs.[51]

Aortic vasodilation in response to beta agonists decreases with age in animal models.[52,53] It is important here to note that characteristic input impedance in the beagle dog during exercise is also apparently dependent on beta-adrenergic stimulation: in the presence of propranolol the characteristic aortic impedance increased in both young and senescent chronically instrumented beagle dogs during exercise, whereas before propranolol, it increased only in the senescent animals.[54] This may be another manifestation of a modification of exercise hemodynamics with aging due to a diminished target response to catecholamines.

The direct action of beta-adrenergic agonists on myocardial contractility has also been demonstrated to diminish with advanced age.[36,55] Both the contractile response to isoproterenol and dibutyryl cAMP are diminished, whereas the response to elevated Ca^{2+} is preserved.[36,56] In this rat model neither the numbers nor affinity of beta receptors, as measured by agonist or antagonist binding, are altered with adult age.[50,54,55] That neither basal cAMP levels nor elevated levels during the response to isoproterenol were age-related[56] and that dibutyryl cAMP, which produced equal activation of cAMP-dependent protein kinase activation, also produced a diminished increment in contractility suggest that with adult aging alterations distal to cAMP formation and protein kinase activation account for the diminished effectiveness of catecholamines to augment myocardial contractility. The affinity for agonist binding to the beta-receptor, however, is decreased when maturational and senescent rats are compared,[57] and the coupling of the receptor to the catalytic unit adenlyate cyclase effected by guanine nucleotides appears to change during maturation.[55]

Summary

The increase in systolic arterial pressure within the normal range, the increase in stroke work, the concomitant cardiac hypertrophy, and the reduced ventricular early diastolic filling rate at rest support the notions that aging is "muted hypertension"[42] or that clinical hypertension is "accelerated aging."[9,27] However, the recent demonstration that CO and SV at rest or during exercise is not necessarily reduced in rigorously screened elderly normotensive subjects (Figs. 1B, 2, and Table I) as it is in hypertensive subjects[27,30,31] seems not to support these hypotheses. Rather, these recent data suggest that variables that modify cardiovascular function other than aging per se, such as lifestyle (nutrition or smoking), physical conditioning status, and occult coronary disease present in less rigorously screened populations (Fig. 1A), have accounted for the diminished cardiac output and stroke volume observed in the elderly subjects in earlier studies.[16,32–34] The prominent age-related change in the hemodynamic profile in response to exercise, that is, a diminished heart rate and enhanced end-systolic volume, resembles that observed when the beta-adrenergic system is pharmacologically inhibited. In some populations, such as that in Figure 2, however, adaptive mechanisms, that is, greater end-diastolic volume and greater SV (Starling mechanism), compensate for these deficiencies and prevent a significant age-related decline of CO during exercise. Thus, although certain characteristic age-related changes can be defined in the cardiovascular system, such as an increase in systolic blood pressure and modest cardiac hypertrophy, these changes per se, at least before about 80 years of age, do not necessarily reduce CO, the raison-d'être of the cardiovascular system, either at rest or during exercise.

Finally, it is emphasized that all of the studies discussed, both those in normotensive and hypertensive subjects, were cross-sectional in design; that is, different younger and older adult men, animals, or animal tissues were compared. Such studies define only the members of a population who are alive at the time of the study and are screened for study by various "filters."

Longitudinal studies, those that measure the variables discussed serially in a given subject, are required to substantiate conclusions regarding the nature of an "aging process" in the cardiovascular system.

References

1. BADER H: Dependence of wall stress in the human thoracic aorta on age and pressure. Circ Res 1967; 30: 354–361.

2. LEAROYD BM, TAYLOR MG: Alterations with age in the visco-elastic properties of human arterial walls. Circ Res 1966; 18: 278–292.

3. AVOLIO AP, CHEN S-G, WANG R-P, ZHANG C-L, LI M-F, O'ROURKE MF: Effects of aging on changing arterial compliance and left ventricular load in a northern Chinese urban community. Circulation 1983; 68: 50–58.

4. GERSTENBLITH G, LAKATTA EG, WEISFELDT ML: Age changes in myocardial function and exercise response. Prog Cardiovasc Res 1976; 19: 1–21.

5. LANDOWNE M: The relation between intra-arterial pressure and impact pulse wave velocity with regard to age and arteriosclerosis. J Gerontol 1958: 13: 153–161.

6. LINZBACH AJ, AKUAMOA-BOATENG E: Die Alternsveranderunger des menschlichen Herzens. I. Das Herzgewicht im Alter. Klin Wochenschr 1973; 51: 156–163.

7. RODEHEFFER RJ, GERSTENBLITH G, BECKER LC, FLEG JL, WEISFELDT ML, LAKATTA EG: Exercise cardiac output is maintained with advancing age in healthy human subjects: cardiac dilatation and increased stroke volume compensate for diminished heart rate. Circulation 1984; 69: 203–213.

8. GRIBBIN B, PICKERING TG, SLEIGHT P, PETO R: Effect of age and high blood pressure on baroreflex sensitivity in man. Circ Res 1971; 29: 424–431.

9. PICKERING GW: High Blood Pressure. London: JA Churchill, 1955; 154–183.

10. LAKATTA EG, YIN FCP: Myocardial aging: functional alterations and related cellular mechanisms. Am J Physiol 1982; 242: H927–H941.

11. MEERSON FZ, JAVICH MP, LERMAN MI: Decrease in the rate of RNA and protein synthesis and degradation in the myocardium under long-term compensatory hyperfunction and on aging. J Mol Cell Cardiol 1978; 10: 145–159.

12. KORECKY B: The effects of load, internal environment, and age on cardiac mechanics. J Mol Cell Cardiol 1979; 11 (suppl 1): 33.

13. LAKATTA EG: Dissociation of hypertrophy and altered function in senescent rat myocardium. In: Jacob R, Gulch RW, Kissling G, eds. Cardiac adaptation to hemodynamic overload, training and stress. Darmstadt: Steinkopff Verlag, 1983; 53–58.

14. SPURGEON HA, STEINBACH MF, LAKATTA EG: Chronic exercise prevents characteristic age-related changes in rat cardiac contraction. Am J Physiol 1983; 244: H513–H518.

15. WEI JY, SPURGEON HA, LAKATTA EG: Excitation-contraction in rat myocardium. Alterations with adult aging. Am J Physiol 1984; 15: H784–H791.

16. BRANDFONBRENER M, LANDOWNE M, SHOCK NW: Changes in cardiac output with age. Circulation 1955; 12: 447–566.

17. GARDIN JM, HENRY WL, SAVAGE DD, WARE JH, BURN C, BORER JS: Echocardiographic measurements in normal subjects: evaluation of an adult population without clinically apparent heart disease. J Clin Ultrasound 1979; 7: 439–447.

18. GERSTENBLITH G, FREDERIKSEN J, YIN FCP, FORTUIN NJ, LAKATTA EG, WEISFELDT ML: Echocardiographic assessment of a normal adult aging population. Circulation 1977; 56: 273–278.

19. SJOGREN AL: Left ventricular wall thickness determined by ultrasound in 100 subjects without heart disease. Chest 1971; 60: 341–346.

20. LAKATTA EG: Alterations in the cardiovascular system that occur in advanced age. Fed Proc 1979; 38: 163–167.

21. FLEG JL, LAKATTA EG: Comparison of the effect of aging on echocardiographic measurements in men and women. In preparation.

22. GERSTENBLITH G, FLEG JL, BECKER LC, et al: Maximum left ventricular filling rate in healthy individuals measured by gated blood pool scans: effect of age. Circulation 1983; 68: III-101.

23. INOUYE I, MASSIE B, LOGE D, et al: Abnormal left ventricular filling: an early finding in mild to moderate systemic hypertension. Am J Cardiol 1984; 53: 120–126.

24. DEVEREUX RB, SAVAGE DD, DRAYER JIM, LARAGH JH: Left ventricular hypertrophy and function in high, normal, and low-renin forms of essential hypertension. Hypertension 1982; 4: 524–531.

25. DRAYER JIM, WEBER MA, DEYOUNG JL: BP as a determinant of cardiac left ventricular muscle mass. Arch Intern Med 1983; 143: 90–92.

26. MESSERLI FH, SUNDGAARD-RIISE K, VENTURA HO, DUNN FG, GLADE LB, FROHLICH ED: Essential hypertension in the elderly: haemodynamics, intravascular volume, plasma renin activity, and circulating catecholamine levels. Lancet 1983; 2: 983–986.

27. SAVAGE DD, DRAYER JIM, HENRY WL, et al: Echocardiographic assessment of cardiac anatomy and function in hypertensive subjects. Circulation 1979; 59: 623–632.

28. SHKHVATSABAYA IK, USUBALIYEV NN, YURENEV AP, PANFILOV VV: The interrelations of cardiac and vascular wall hypertrophy in arterial hypertension. Cardiovasc Rev Rep 1981; 2: 1145–1149.

29. WOLINSKY H: Long-term effects of hypertension on the rat aortic wall and their relation to concurrent aging changes. Morphological and chemical studies. Circ Res 1972; 30: 301–309.

30. TERASAWA F, KURAMOTO K, YING LH, SUZUKI T, KURAMOCHI M: The study of the hemodynamics in old hypertensive subjects. Acta Gerontol Jpn 1972; 56: 47–55.

31. TSUCHIYA M, KAWASAKI S, MASUYA K, et al: Cardiovascular function in hypertension: the effect of aging on the hemodynamics. Jpn J Geriatr 1973; 10: 135–142.

32. CONWAY J, WHEELER R, SANNERSTEDT R: Sympathetic nervous activity during exercise in relation to age. Cardiovasc Res 1971; 5: 577–581.

33. GRANATH A, JONSSON B, STRANDELL T: Circulation in healthy old men, studied by right heart catheterization at rest and during exercise in supine and sitting position. Acta Med Scand 1964; 176: 425–446.

34. JULIUS S, ANTOON A, WHITLOCK LS, CONWAY J: Influence of age on the hemody-

namic response to exercise. Circulation 1967; 36: 222–230.

35. PORT E, COBB FR, COLEMAN RE, JONES RH: Effect of age on the response of the (LV) ejection fraction to exercise. N Engl J Med 1980; 303: 1133–1137.

36. LAKATTA EG: Age-related alterations in the cardiovascular response to adrenergic mediated stress. Fed Proc 1980; 39: 3173–3177.

37. EPSTEIN SE, ROBISON BF, KAHLER RL, BRAUNWALD E: Effects of beta-adrenergic blockade on the cardiac response to maximal and submaximal exercise in man. J Clin Invest 1965; 44: 1745–1753.

38. REYBROUCH T, AMERY A, BILLIET L: Hemodynamic response to graded exercise after chronic beta-adrenergic blockade. J Appl Physiol 1977; 42: 133–138.

39. ROWE JW, TROEN BR: Sympathetic nervous system and aging in man. Endocr Rev 1980; 1: 167–179.

40. TZANKOFF ST, FLEG JL, NORRIS AH, LAKATTA EG: Age-related increase in serum catecholamine levels during exercise in healthy adult men. Physiologist 1980; 23: 50.

41. BERTEL O, BUHLER FR, KIOWSKI W, LUTOLD BE: Decreased beta-adrenoreceptor responsiveness as related to age, blood pressure, and plasma catecholamines in patients with essential hypertension. Hypertension 1980; 2: 130–138.

42. MESSERLI FH, FROHLICH ED, SUAREZ DH, et al: Borderline hypertension: relationship between age, hemodynamics and circulating catecholamines. Circulation 1981; 64: 760–764.

43. KURAMOTO K, MATSUSHITA S, MIFUNE J, SAKAI M, MURAKAMI M: Electrocardiographic and hemodynamic evaluation of isoproterenol test in elderly ischemic heart disease. Jpn Circ J 1978; 42: 955–960.

44. LONDON DM, SAFAR ME, WEISS YA, MILLIEZ PL: Isoproterenol sensitivity and total body clearance of propranolol in hypertensive patients. J Clin Pharmacol 1976; 16: 174–182.

45. VESTAL RE, WOOD AJJ, SHAND DG: Reduced -adrenoceptor sensitivity in the elderly. Clin Pharmacol Ther 1979; 26: 181–186.

46. YIN FCP, SPURGEON HA, RAIZES GS, GREENE HL, WEISFELDT ML, SHOCK NW: Age-associated decrease in chronotropic response to isoproterenol. Circulation 1976; 54 (suppl 2): II-167.

47. YIN FCP, SPURGEON HA, GREENE HL, LAKATTA EG, WEISFELDT ML: Age-associated decrease in heart rate response to isoproterenol in dogs. Mech Ageing Dev 1979; 10: 15–17.

48. IBSEN H, JULIUS S: Pharmacologic tools for assessment of adrenergic nerve activity in human hypertension. Fed Proc 1984; 43: 67–71.

49. DILLON N, CHUNG S, KELLY J, O'MALLEY K: Age and beta adrenoceptor-mediated function. Clin Pharmacol Ther 1980; 27: 769–772.

50. SCHOCKEN DD, ROTH GS: Reduced beta-adrenergic receptor concentration in aging man. Nature 1977; 267: 856–858.

51. ABRASS IB, SCARPACE PJ: Human lymphocyte beta-adrenergic receptors are unaltered with age. J Gerontol 1981; 36: 298–301.

52. FLEISCH JH: Age-related decrease in beta adrenoceptor activity of the cardiovascular system. Trends Pharmacol Sci 1981; 2: 337–339.

53. FLEISCH JH, MALING HM, BRODIE BB: Beta-receptor activity in aorta. Circ Res 1970; 26: 151–162.

54. YIN FCP, WEISFELDT ML, MILNOR WR: Role of aortic input impedance in the decreased cardiovascular response to exercise with aging in dogs. J Clin Invest 1981; 68: 28–38.

55. ABRASS IB, DAVIS JL, SCARPACE PJ: Isoproterenol responsiveness and myocardial β-adrenergic receptors in young and old rats. J Gerontol 1982; 37: 156–160.

56. GUARNIERI T, FILBURN CR, ZITNIK G, ROTH GS, LAKATTA EG: Contractile and biochemical correlates of β-adrenergic stimulation of the aged heart. Am J Physiol 1980; 239: H501–H508.

57. NARAYANAN N, DERBY J-A: Alterations in the properties of β-adrenergic receptors of myocardial membranes in aging: impairments in agonist-receptor interactions and quanine nucleotide regulation accompany diminished catecholamine-responsiveness of adenylate cyclase. Mech Ageing Dev 1982; 19: 127–139.

PART VI
ANTIHYPERTENSIVE
THERAPY
AND THE HEART

27

Hemodynamics of Antihypertensive Therapy

PER LUND-JOHANSEN, M.D.

It is well documented that the cardinal hemodynamic disturbance in nearly all patients considered to need drug treatment for hypertension is an increased total peripheral resistance (TPR).[1-3] Increased arteriolar resistance is present in most vascular beds, such as in the kidneys, in the splanchnic organs, in the skin, and, in advanced hypertension, also in the skeletal muscles.[2,4] In mild to moderate hypertension the cardiac output (CO) during rest is usually normal or only slightly reduced due to a subnormal stroke volume (SV), but during muscular exercise greater reductions in CO and SV are usually found even in young subjects.[1]

When essential hypertension is left untreated over many years, CO and SV decrease, whereas TPR increases, at rest as well as during muscular exercise.[1] The changes in blood pressure may vary, but in most patients with mild and moderate established hypertension (not borderline hypertension) blood pressure will show an increase over 1 to 2 decades. In a 10-year follow-up of 23 untreated patients with mild hypertension, CO decreased by 20% and TPR increased by 30%.[1] The changes seen at the 10-year follow-up had progressed further at the 17-year follow-up.

This review will discuss how we alter central hemodynamics by chronic drug treatment in the typical patients with mild to moderate (diastolic pressure, 100 to 120 mmHg) essential hypertension. The review will be limited to diuretics, alpha and beta blockers, calcium antagonists, converting enzyme inhibitors, and serotonin inhibitors. Over the years, we have studied the hemodynamic responses in about 300 patients. Before treatment, practically all the subjects demonstrated an increased TPR at rest (more than 2800 dyn. s. cm^{-5}. m^2) and also increased values during exercise.

Diuretics

In 1960 Conway and Lauwers[5] showed in their classic study that although blood pressure reduction during the first days of thiazide treatment was associated with a decrease in CO and no change in TPR, prolonged use over several months induced a gradual normalization in central hemodynamics, a decrease in TPR and a gradual increase in CO. Ten years later, we showed that the reduction in exercise blood pressure during chronic thiazide treatment was maintained by the same mechanisms: a decrease in TPR without reduction in CO.[6] The heart rate response to exercise was unchanged. Van Brummelen et al[7] have shown that the decrease in TPR index is greatest in the "responders." In 1980 we demonstrated that a similar hemodynamic response was obtained by another diuretic agent, tienilic acid.[8]

In summary, then, the thiazide diuretics and tienilic acid might be said to induce at least a partial correction of the hemodynamic disturbances: only partial because the subnormal SV and CO during exercise is not corrected.[5–8]

Beta Blockers

It is well known that the acute effect of the first clinically important beta blocker propranolol is an immediate decrease in heart rate and CO without any reduction in blood pressure because of an increase in TPR.[9,10] In another classic study on the hemodynamic effects of antihypertensive agents, Tarazi and Dustan[9] demonstrated that in the "responders" TPR declined during the following months toward pretreatment level and blood pressure decreased.[10] In recent years it has been shown that this decrease in TPR and blood pressure is seen during the first hours after the first oral dose of other beta blockers, such as atenolol[11] and ICI 141-292.[12] From a pharmacologic point of view, one would expect that different types of beta blockers (cardioselective, noncardioselective, with or without intrinsic sympathomimetic activity [ISA]) would induce different chronic hemodynamic responses.[13,14]

Indeed, there are well-documented differences in the hemodynamic responses to the various types of beta blockers during rest. However, during muscular exercise the hemodynamic responses are largely the same, especially during chronic treatment.[15,16]

We studied seven different beta blockers in 89 patients with mild to moderate essential hypertension, all previously untreated. The typical response to chronic treatment with beta blockers without ISA was a blood pressure reduction of about 15% to 20%, a decrease in heart rate and CO of about 20% to 25% during rest. During exercise, there was some compensatory increase in SV and the reduction in CO was somewhat less, but still 15% to 20%. The TPR usually did not decrease below pretreatment levels[16] (Fig. 1).

During rest beta blockers with strong ISA, such as pindolol, usually maintain blood pressure reduction with less decrease in heart rate and CO than beta blockers without ISA. The TPR stays at pretreatment levels or is slightly reduced. During exercise, when sympathetic tone is increased, the reduction in heart rate is significant (-30 to -35 beats/min), but the reduction is usually less than on beta blockers without ISA. The SV increases (compared with pretreatment level), and TPR during exercise decreases slightly below pretreatment level.[16]

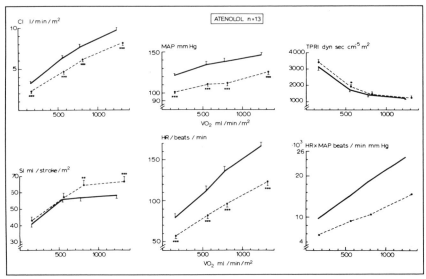

Figure 1. *Hemodynamic changes induced by 1 year of therapy with atenolol in 13 men with essential hypertension. VO$_2$ = oxygen consumption; CI = cardiac index; MAP = mean arterial pressure; TPRI = total peripheral resistance index; SI = stroke index; HR = heart rate. Statistical significance of differences between the first and the last study: *=p < 0.05, **=p < 0.01, ***=p < 0.001. ——— = before therapy, – – – – – = on therapy, partly compensating for the reduction in heart rate. (Reprinted with permission from Lund-Johansen.[16])*

Most investigators have agreed on these hemodynamic changes,[14–16] but some patients responding to beta-blocker therapy even with an increase in CO and a marked decrease in TPR have been described.[17,18] Pretreatment CO is then usually very low, perhaps due to coronary artery disease. However, in patients with mild to moderate essential hypertension, this reaction pattern is rare according to our experience[16] (Fig. 2).

Most studies have shown that chronic beta-blocker treatment causes little change in total oxygen consumption at rest as well as during exercise.[16] Since the cardiac index (CI) is reduced, usually 20% to 25%, this means that the arteriovenous oxygen difference is increased accordingly. The significance of this is not known. Although many patients react initially to beta-blocker therapy with muscular fatigue and cold hands and feet, these complaints often disappear during chronic treatment. Admittedly, cold extremities, most likely due to reduced peripheral blood flow,[16] are an important problem in cold climates. Thus, from a hemodynamic point of view, patients on chronic beta-blocker therapy have had their normokinetic hypertensive circulatory system replaced by a normotensive but hypokinetic system. It is,

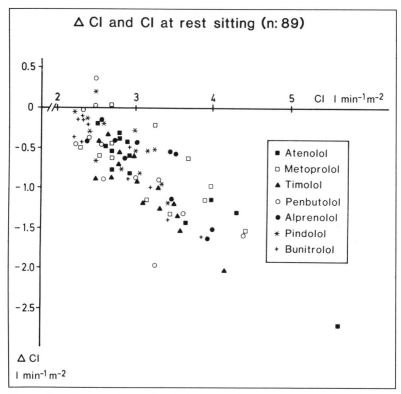

Figure 2. *Changes in cardiac index related to pretreatment cardiac index while sitting in 89 men with mild to moderate essential hypertension treated with different beta blockers. (Reprinted with permission from Lund-Johansen.[16])*

of course, important that the blood pressure-heart rate product be markedly reduced on beta-blocker therapy, especially during muscular exercise when a 40% reduction or more might be seen. This reaction is, of course, most adequate in patients with a compromised coronary circulation.

Alpha Blockers

Entirely different hemodynamic changes are induced by alpha blockers (prazosin and trimazosin). As expected from the pharmacologic effect of alpha blockade, these drugs reduce blood pressure entirely due to reduction in TPR acutely as well as chronically.[19–21] The heart rate and CO remain unchanged during rest. During exercise, post-treatment CO is increased, mainly due to an increase in SV and a slight increase in heart rate. In conclusion, prazosin might be said to restore normal circulation in many patients with mild to moderate essential hypertension. No reduction in renal or peripheral blood flow is seen. [20,21]

A similar reaction pattern is seen on trimazosin. [22–24] In our experience the decrease in blood pressure was less consistent and less pronounced on trimazosin than on prazosin (trimazosin dose, 150 to 600 mg/day, prazosin dose, 3 mg/day). [24] There was a decrease in TPR of about 12% at rest and during exercise. Due to an increase in CO, the decrease in blood pressure was only approximately 7%.

Combination of Alpha and Beta Blockers

When alpha and beta blockade is properly balanced, a marked reduction in blood pressure is often achieved, the blood pressure reduction being partly due to a decrease in TPR and partly due to a decrease in CO. [25] An increase in SV is seen and the decrease in CO during exercise is less than when beta blockers are used alone.

Labetalol, a relatively new drug in the United States but in use in Europe for several years, possesses alpha- and beta-blocker properties in a single molecule. This drug induces blood pressure reduction immediately after intravenous administration, as do alpha blockers, but in contrast to pure beta blockers, [26–29] the blood pressure decrease is partly due to reduction in TPR (via alpha blockade of the arteriolar receptors) and partly due to a decrease in heart rate and CO (due to beta blockade of the heart). [26,27] Labetalol is therefore useful for therapy of hypertensive crisis when immediate but controlled reduction in blood pressure is necessary. [29] During long-term use, there is a progressive reduction in TPR and an increase in SV and CO. [28,30–33] Particularly during exercise, CO is much less reduced than by pure beta blockers. [28,30,33] Together with substantial decrease in blood pressure and in heart rate-blood pressure product, this might be an advantage. (For results of the 6-year follow-up see later. [33])

Calcium Antagonists

In recent years the calcium antagonists have been introduced in therapy of hypertension. Most information is available on verapamil and nifedipine. [34–38] These two drugs reduce blood pressure through reduction in TPR, but the heart rate responses differ. When given acutely, nifedipine (capsule preparation) induces a rapid decrease in TPR. The heart rate increases and partly counteracts the decrease in blood pressure, [37] whereas heart rate is unchanged or decreases with verapamil. [35] However, during chronic therapy, nifedipine, [38] when given in long-acting form, reduces blood pressure 17% during rest without any significant changes in heart rate, SV, or CO (Fig. 3). Verapamil chronically induces similar reduction in TPR, but also about 10% decrease in heart rate. However, this was compensated for by an increase in SV, and CO was unchanged. [36] Thus, the calcium antag-

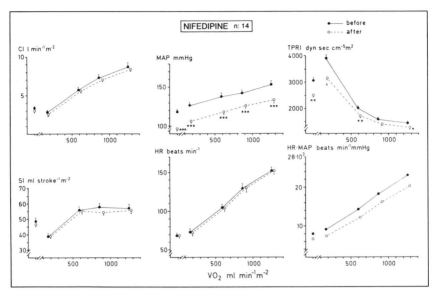

Figure 3. *Hemodynamic changes during chronic treatment with long-acting nifedi-pine in 14 men with essential hypertension. Note the reduction in TPR index, and no significant changes in CI, stroke index, and heart rate. (Reprinted with permission from Lund-Johansen and Omvik.[38])*

onists, like the diuretics, reduce blood pressure by partial correction of the hemodynamic disturbances; the reduction is only partial because the subnormal CO during exercise is not corrected. Their place in treatment of uncomplicated, mild to moderate hypertension is not yet settled.

Converting Enzyme Inhibitors

The converting enzyme inhibitors have been used in therapy of primary as well as secondary hypertension. The reduction in angiotensin II should theoretically induce a decrease in TPR, and a decrease in TPR has indeed been shown in patients with moderate as well as in patients with severe hypertension.[39–44]

In a group of 12 patients with severe therapy-resistant hypertension, captopril plus a diuretic reduced blood pressure while sitting from 205/119 to 174/102 mmHg (15%), entirely due to a decrease in TPR (17%). During mild exercise, a decrease in TPR was seen, but the CI also was decreased (7% at 50 W and 15% at 100 W).[41]

In patients with less severe hypertension treated with enalapril alone or in combination with a thiazide, blood pressure while sitting was reduced from

187/108 to 150/87 mmHg (20%) entirely due to a decrease in TPR.[44] In these patients the changes seen during rest and exercise were similar. In the enalapril-treated patients, no side effects were seen. Similar results have been found in other studies, and a reduction in left ventricular hypertrophy (LVH) has also been demonstrated.[43]

Serotonin Antagonists

Thirty years ago Page[45] suggested that serotonin (5-HT) might play a role in the sustained increase in TPR in chronic hypertension by amplification of the angiotensin and norepinephrine system. Blockade of 5-HT has therefore attracted great interest as another approach to hypertensive treatment, but the blood pressure-lowering effect of ketanserin seems to be rather modest.[46-48]

We studied 13 patients with primary hypertension. The blood pressure while sitting was reduced from 167/101 to 153/91 mmHg (14/10 mmHg). The dose of ketanserin ranged from 40 to 160 mg/day, mean of 84 mg/day. This rather modest reduction in blood pressure was not associated with any really clear-cut hemodynamic changes. There was no significant reduction in TPR, whereas the CO decreased by approximately 8% at rest and by 3% during exercise. Most of the changes were not statistically significant. There was an increase in dose-induced side effects. Thus, the hemodynamic changes caused by chronic ketanserin treatment were small and less characteristic than the changes seen with most other antihypertensive agents.

Hemodynamic Responses to Prolonged Drug Treatment

Since at least some of the hemodynamic abnormalities in established hypertension are thought to be due to structural changes in the heart and in the resistance vessels,[1,4] it could be hoped that permanent blood pressure reduction over several years could induce regression of these changes and also a further normalization of central hemodynamics. We have studied groups of patients treated with different beta blockers (alprenolol, atenolol, or metoprolol) and labetalol, who have had a third hemodynamic study after 3 to 6 years of therapy.[33,49] In patients on atenolol, the results were somewhat disappointing because there was no tendency to increase CO and SV or to decrease TPR from year 1 to year 5. On the other hand, no obvious deterioration had taken place,[49] and the reduction of the workload on the heart was maintained. All these patients had mild hypertension.

In a 6-year follow-up on 15 patients with moderate hypertension treated with labetalol, the responses were somewhat different from those seen on beta-blocker therapy. The blood pressure was controlled over these 6 years and did not change significantly. However, between the first and the sixth

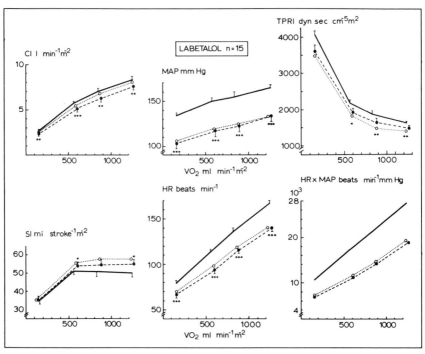

Figure 4. *Hemodynamic changes induced after 6 years of therapy with labetalol in 15 men studied before therapy ———, after 1 year – – – – –, and after 6 years ·········· Mean values and SEM. Small stars show differences between the first and the second study, large stars, between the first and the third studies. Note the gradual decrease in TPR index and a slight increase in SI and CI during the 5 years between the second and the third study.*

year, TPR had decreased at rest as well as during exercise, whereas the stroke index and CI had increased[33] to pretreatment values or higher (Fig. 4).

Comments

This review has shown that most of the commonly used antihypertensive agents may control blood pressure at rest and during exercise, but often only by partially correcting the basic hemodynamic disturbances. Particularly, the beta blockers will usually maintain a subnormal CO at rest and during exercise, and, of course, also a subnormal heart rate. The arteriovenous oxygen difference is increased at rest as well as during exercise. Greater degree of normalization of central hemodynamics is achieved by diuretics, calcium antagonists, and converting enzyme inhibitors, but complete normalization of CO is usually not achieved. In our experience the greatest normalization of central hemodynamics was achieved by the alpha blocker prazosin.

During prolonged treatment for 5 to 6 years, the beta blockers prevented further decrease in SV and further increase in TPR and thus seemed to arrest the changes that could have been expected in untreated subjects.[1] Prolonged therapy with combination of alpha and beta blockade (by use of labetalol) induced a gradual decrease in TPR and a slight increase in CO at rest as well as during exercise. Thus, combination of alpha and beta blockade might induce more adequate responses than beta blockers alone.[33,49]

In this short review only the typical response in patients with mild to moderate essential hypertension has been reported. Most of these patients generally seemed to tolerate the chronic reduction in CO, induced by the beta blockers, surprisingly well, generally with little restriction to their physical activity. In athletes, however, reduction in maximal physical performance is seen.[50]

In special subgroups of patients the use of a wrong antihypertensive agent may induce inappropriate responses, such as a decrease in CI in patients with hypertension and peripheral vascular disorders. In patients with very severe therapy-resistant hypertension, converting enzyme inhibitors are sometimes particularly useful, at least partly normalizing central hemodynamics through reduction in TPR.

Finally it should be emphasized that, although the responses to antihypertensive agents vary greatly from a hemodynamic point of view, other effects of the antihypertensive agents such as 24-hour blood pressure control, tolerability, biochemical side effects, and lipid profile, might, of course, have greater significance for the clinical outcome.

However, at least when dealing with relatively young patients with mild to moderate essential hypertension, where many years (perhaps lifelong) therapy might be necessary, restoration of a normal circulatory system would seem to be the most logical way of treating this condition.

References

1. LUND-JOHANSEN P: State of the art review. Hemodynamics in essential hypertension. Clin Sci 1980; 59: 343.
2. BIRKENHÄGER WH, DE LEEUW PW, SCHALEKAMP MADH: Control mechanisms in essential hypertension. Amsterdam: Elsevier Biomedical Press, 1982.
3. BÜHLER FR: Pathophysiology of primary hypertension: role of adrenoceptors in the transformation from an early high cardiac output into a later high arteriolar resistance phase. In: Amery A, ed. Hypertensive cardiovascular disease: pathophysiology and treatment. The Hague: Martinus Nijhoff 1982; 164.
4. FOLKOW B: Physiological aspects of primary hypertension. Physiol Rev 1982; 62: 347–504.
5. CONWAY J, LAUWERS P: Hemodynamic and hypotensive effects of long-term therapy with chlorothiazide. Circulation 1960; 21: 21–27.
6. LUND-JOHANSEN P: Hemodynamic changes in long-term diuretic therapy of essential hypertension. Acta Med Scand 1970; 187: 509.

7. VAN BRUMMELEN P, MAN IN 'T VELD AJ, SCHALEKAMP MADH: Hemodynamic changes during long-term thiazide treatment of essential hypertension in responders and non-responders. Clin Pharmacol Ther 1980; 27: 328–336.

8. LUND-JOHANSEN P: Hemodynamic and metabolic long-term effects of tienilic acid in essential hypertension. Acta Med Scand [suppl] 1980; 646: 106–114.

9. TARAZI RC, DUSTAN HP: Beta-adrenergic blockade in hypertension. Am J Cardiol 1972; 29: 633–640.

10. TARAZI RC, FOUAD FM, BRAVO EL: Total peripheral resistance and beta-adrenergic blockade. In: Laragh JH, Buhler FR, Seldin DW, eds. Frontiers in hypertension research. Berlin: Springer-Verlag, 1981; 454.

11. SIMON G, FRANCIOSA JA, GIMENEZ HJ, COHN JN: Short-term systemic hemodynamic adaptation to beta-adrenergic inhibition with atenolol in hypertensive patients. Hypertension 1981; 3: 262–268.

12. LUND-JOHANSEN P, OMVIK P, HAUGLAND H: Initial haemodynamic effects of ICI 141 292, a cardioselective beta-blocker with ISA at rest and during exercise in patients with essential hypertension. Acta Med Scand, in press.

13. CLARK BJ: Beta-adrenoceptor-blocking agents: are pharmacologic differences relevant? Am Heart J 1982; 104: 334–346.

14. MAN IN 'T VELD AJ, SCHALEKAMP MADH: How intrinsic sympathomimetic activity modulates the hemodynamic responses to beta-adrenoceptor antagonists. A clue to the nature of their antihypertensive mechanism. Br J Clin Pharmacol (suppl) 1982; 13: 245s–257s.

15. SVENDSEN TL, CARLSEN JE, HARTLING O, McNAIR A, TRAP-JENSEN J: A comparison of the acute haemodynamic effects of propranolol and pindolol at rest and during supine exercise in man. Clin Sci (suppl) 1980; 59: 465s–468s.

16. LUND-JOHANSEN P: Central hemodynamic effects of beta-blockers in hypertension. A comparison between atenolol, metoprolol, timolol, penbutolol, alprenolol, pindolol and bunitrolol. Eur Heart J (suppl) 1983; 4: 1–12.

17. ATTERHØG JH, DUNER H, PERNOW B: Hemodynamic effects of pindolol in hypertensive patients. Acta Med Scand [suppl] 1977; 606: 55–62.

18. GUAZZI M, POLESE A, FIORENTINI C, OLIVARI MT, MAGRINI F: Cardiac performance and beta-adrenergic blockade in arterial hypertension. Am J Med Sci 1977; 273: 63–69.

19. SMITH IS, FERNANDES M, KIM KE, SCHWARTZ C, ONESTI G: A three-phase clinical evaluation of prazosin. Postgrad Med 1975; Spec No: 53–60.

20. LUND-JOHANSEN P: Haemodynamic changes at rest and during exercise in long-term prazosin therapy of essential hypertension. In: Cotton DWK, ed. Prazosin—evaluation of a new antihypertensive agent. Amsterdam: Excerpta Medica, 1974; 43.

21. DE LEEUW PW, WESTER A, STIENSTRA R, FALKE HE, BIRKENHAGER WH: Hemodynamic and endocrinological studies with prazosin in essential hypertension. In: Lund-Johansen P, Mason DT, eds. Recent advances in hypertension and congestive heart failure—prazosin. Amsterdam: Excerpta Medica, 1978; 11.

22. POOL PE, SEAGREN SC, SALEL AF: Clinical hemodynamic profile of trimazosin in hypertension. Am Heart J 1983; 106: 1237–1242.

23. CHRYSANT, SG: Autonomic, systemic, and renal hemodynamic actions of trimazosin in hypertensive patients. Am Heart J 1983; 106: 1243–1250.

24. OMVIK P, LUND-JOHANSEN P: Hemodynamic effects at rest and during exercise of long-term treatment with trimazosin in essential hypertension. 1985; in press.

25. LUND-JOHANSEN P: Haemodynamic long-term effects of prazosin plus tolamolol in essential hypertension. Br J Clin Pharmacol 1977; 4: 141–145.

26. LUND-JOHANSEN P: Haemodynamic effects of labetalol—a review. Drugs 1984; 28 (suppl 2): 35–50.

27. KOCH G: Haemodynamic effects of combined alpha- and beta-adrenoceptor blockade after intravenous labetalol in hypertensive patients at rest and during exercise. Br J Clin Pharmacol 1976; 3 (suppl): 725–728.

28. KOCH G: Haemodynamic adaptation at rest and during exercise to long-term antihypertensive treatment with combined alpha- and beta-adrenoceptor blockade by labetalol. Br Heart J 1979; 41: 192–198.

29. OMVIK P, LUND-JOHANSEN P: Acute hemodynamic effects of labetalol in severe hypertension. J Cardiovasc Pharmacol 1982; 4: 915–920.

30. LUND-JOHANSEN P, BAKKE OM: Haemodynamic effects and plasma concentration of labetalol during long-term treatment of essential hypertension. Br J Clin Pharmacol 1979; 7: 169–174.

31. FAGARD R, LIJNEN P, AMERY A: Response of the systemic and pulmonary circulation to labetalol at rest and during exercise. Br J Clin Pharmacol 1982; 13 (suppl 1): 13s–17s.

32. COHN JN, MEHTA J, FRANCIS GS: A review of the haemodynamic effects of labetalol in man. Br J Clin Pharmacol 1982; 13 (suppl 1): 198–268.

33. LUND-JOHANSEN P: Short- and long-term (six year) haemodynamic effects of labetalol in essential hypertension. Am J Med 1983; 75 (suppl): 24–31.

34. DOYLE AE, ANAVEKAR SN, OLIVER LE: A clinical trial of verapamil in treatment of hypertension. In: Zanchetti A, Krikler DM, eds. Calcium antagonism in cardiovascular therapy: experience with verapamil. Amsterdam: Excerpta Medica, 1981; 252.

35. DE LEEUW PW, SMOUT AJPM, WILLEMSE PJ, BIRKENHÄGER WH: Effects of verapamil in hypertensive patients. In: Zanchetti A, Krikler DM, eds. Calcium antagonism in cardiovascular therapy: experience with verapamil. Amsterdam: Excerpta Medica, 1981, 233.

36. LUND-JOHANSEN P: Hemodynamic long-term effects of verapamil in essential hypertension at rest and during exercise. Acta Med Scand [suppl] 1983; 681: 109–115.

37. OLIVARI MT, BARTORELLI C, POLESE A, FIORENTINI C, MORUZZI P, GUAZZI MD: Treatment of hypertension with nifedipine, a calcium antagonistic agent. Circulation 1979; 59: 1056–1062.

38. LUND-JOHANSEN P, OMVIK P: Haemodynamic effects of nifedipine in essential hypertension at rest and during exercise. J Hypertens 1983; 1: 159–163.

39. TARAZI RC, BRAVO EL, FOUAD FM, OMVIK P, CODY RJ JR: Hemodynamic and volume changes associated with captopril. J Hypertens 1980; 2: 576–585.

40. FAGARD R, BULPITT C, LIJNEN P, AMERY A: Response of the systemic and pulmonary circulation to converting-enzyme inhibition (captopril) at rest and during exercise in hypertensive patients. Circulation 1982; 65: 33–39.

41. OMVIK P, LUND-JOHANSEN P: Combined captopril and hydrochlorothiazide therapy in severe hypertension: long-term haemodynamic changes at rest and dur-

ing exercise. J Hypertens 1984; 2: 73–80.

42. DE LEEUW PW, HOOGMA RPLM, VAN SOEST GAW, VAN ES PN, BIRKENHAGER W: Physiological effects of short-term treatment with enalapril in hypertensive patients. J Hypertens 1983; (suppl 1): 87–91.

43. DUNN FG, et al: Enalapril improves systemic and renal hemodynamics and allows regression of left ventricular mass in essential hypertension. Am J Cardiol 1984; 53: 105–108.

44. LUND-JOHANSEN P, OMVIK P: Haemodynamic long-term effects of enalapril in essential hypertension at rest and during exercise. J Hypertens 1984; 2 (suppl 2): 49–56.

45. PAGE IH: Serotonin (5-hydroxy-tryptamin) Physiol Rev 1954; 34: 563–588.

46. FAGARD R, FIOCCHI R, LIJNEN P, et al: Haemodynamic and humoral responses to chronic ketanserin treatment in essential hypertension. Br Heart J 1984; 51: 149–156.

47. WENTING GJ, SCHALEKAMP MADH: Serotonin (5-HT) and blood pressure, treatment of hypertension with a highly selective 5-HT receptor antagonist. Eur J Clin Invest 1982; 12 (suppl II): 46.

48. OMVIK P, LUND-JOHANSEN P: Long-term effects on central haemodynamics and body fluid volumes of ketanserin in essential hypertension studies at rest and during dynamic exercise. J Hypertens 1983; 1: 405–412.

49. LUND-JOHANSEN P: Hemodynamic consequences of long-term beta-blocker therapy: a 5-year follow-up study of atenolol. J Cardiovasc Pharmacol 1979; 1: 487–495.

50. BENGTSSON C: Impairment of physical performance after treatment with beta blockers and alpha blockers. Br Med J 1984; 288: 671–672.

28

Regression of Left Ventricular Hypertrophy by Medical Treatment: Present Status and Possible Implications

ROBERT C. TARAZI, M.D.

The recent surge of clinical interest in reversibility of cardiac hypertrophy stemmed initially from the conveyance of two apparently unrelated advances, the development of effective antihypertensive drugs and the application of ultrasonography to quantitative studies of left ventricular (LV) mass and function. This interest was certainly not new, but earlier studies had been hampered by the animal models used, by the difficulties in quantitating left ventricular hypertrophy (LVH), and by the seemingly small effect of inotropic drugs.[1,2] Moreover, the first reports describing unequivocal reversal of hypertrophy by medical therapy also raised important questions of both theoretic and practical importance.[1,3] The regression of hypertrophy was found to involve, in many cases, more factors than a simple reduction of the load that had initially caused the increase in myocardial mass.[3-5] Alterations in myocardial composition were also documented with regression of hypertrophy that raised questions regarding its functional implications.[3]

This review will address some specific questions regarding (1) the relation of blood pressure to ventricular hypertrophy and the role of neurohumoral factors in favoring or hindering the regression of hypertrophy, and (2) the impact of that regression on ventricular function and coronary blood flow. The answer to the latter question, which is not yet completely answered, would be of particular importance in the choice of antihypertensive therapy; the final answer may well determine whether or not regression of cardiovascular hypertrophy should be an additional goal of antihypertensive therapy alongside blood pressure control. Cardiac hypertrophy in hypertension cannot be considered in isolation of structural changes in both the large windkessel arteries and the small resistance vessels. Changes in either vascular segment will deeply influence the evolution of hypertension.

Role of Blood Pressure Control and Antihypertensive Therapy

Many approaches have been used to induce regression of hypertrophy[6] (Table I). Interference with protein synthesis is a highly experimental ap-

TABLE I   **Regression of Myocardial Hypertrophy**

1. Control or cure of primary cause
   Medical treatment
   Surgical cure
2. Inhibition of protein synthesis
3. Use of cardiotonic agents
4. Control of secondary or modulating factors

proach and has been used more in the prevention than in the treatment of cardiac hypertrophy.[7] Inotropic agents, such as digitalis, have not proved very successful in general.[1,2,8] The basic reason for many of the questions raised in this review lies in the discrepancies repeatedly documented in both man and animals between control of arterial pressure and regression of hypertrophy;[1,3,4,9–11] similar discrepancies have also been described in the results of successful aortic valve replacement.[12,13] The lack of a close correlation between the degree of pressure overload and that of consequent hypertrophy[4,14,15] implies either that overload was not accurately quantified or that other factors modulate the hypertrophic response to variations in cardiac load.

With regard to the first possibility, there is little doubt that arterial pressure levels alone do not adequately reflect the cardiac pressure load.[16] The latter are certainly more closely related to the systolic pressure than to the diastolic or mean arterial pressure. Left ventricular load is best assessed from calculations of LV wall stress[16,17] or of aortic impedance.[18] The latter is difficult to obtain in man, and little has been reported regarding its relationship to LV mass. The utilization of different indices of LV wall stress has not materially improved the correlation with LV mass,[15] possibly because of the dual relationship involved; hypertrophy resulting from the increased stress can help to normalize it.[16,17] Returning to blood pressure levels, there is some evidence that a better correlation with LV mass can be obtained from longer term blood pressure monitoring (2 to 24 hours) than from casual measurements.[19,20] The practical implications of these observations are many, including particularly that systolic blood pressure levels be included in the strategy of antihypertensive therapy[16,21] and that home blood pressure determinations[22,23] or preferably long-term automatic recordings[16,21] be used in evaluating patients whose LVH persists despite treatment.

However, even after accounting for the imprecisions of the common pressure load indices, important discrepancies still remain between change in pressure load and variations in LV mass. These were first described in spontaneously hypertensive rats[3,24] (Table II). In contrast, the cardiac response of renovascular hypertensive rats showed a very close correlation between blood pressure level and cardiac weight both in untreated rats and in rats treated by unilateral nephrectomy, coverting enzyme inhibitors or a calcium entry blocker.[25–27] This contrast underlines the inhomogeneity of cardiac responses in different types of hypertension.[28,29] Moreover, in addition to differences in response to different forms of therapy and to differences be-

TABLE II   Antihypertensive Therapy and Cardiac
Hypertrophy in Spontaneously
Hypertensive Rats (SHR)

Group	Blood Pressure (mmHg)	Ventricular Weight (mg/g)
Normal	120	2:6
SHR	188	3:4
Methyldopa	149	2:7
Hydralazine	123	3:4
Minoxidil	130	3:8

Results of antihypertensive therapy indicate that reversal of cardiac hypertrophy is not dependent on blood pressure control alone. Data reproduced with permission from Sen et al.[24]

tween different models of hypertension, a striking difference is also emerging in the response of subjects receiving the same therapy. This was noted not only in clinical studies,[10] but also in some experimental models.[6] In addition, myocardial alterations have been described following experimentally induced narrowing of large vessels in the ventricle on which no pressure load was imposed; thus, increased LV collagen was found after banding of the pulmonary artery to produce right ventricular hypertrophy.[30]

Factors Modulating Reversal of Cardiac Hypertrophy

The factors that can modulate the response of cardiac hypertrophy to medical therapy have been recently reviewed.[6,28] Of particular importance among them is the role of adrenergic influences discussed by Sen.[31] Adrenergic stimuli, however, are not the only neurohumoral factors that could modulate the cardiac hypertrophic response to altered loads. Angiotensin II might be involved either through its potentiation of sympathetic effects or by an independent stimulating effect on myocardial protein synthesis.[32] Converting enzyme inhibition had led to reduction in LV mass in some patients with essential hypertension;[33] it was also found to reverse cardiac hypertrophy in both spontaneous and renovascular hypertensive rats without significant alterations in myocardial catecholamines.[34] The reported data as yet are much too sparse to draw final conclusions in this regard for either the renin-angiotensin system or other hormones reported to influence muscle hypertrophy.[35]

A large body of evidence has been developed in the past few years confirming suggestions proposed by Raab in the 1950s[36] regarding the importance of catecholamines in hypertensive heart disease, in both the development[29,37] and regression[6,29] of LVH. Yamori et al[37] reported that the increase in cardiac weight produced by continuous norepinephrine infusions in rats was not prevented when the pressor effects were blunted by concomitant alpha-adrenergic blockade. Conversely, the increase in cardiac mass induced by norepinephrine was significantly less when beta blockers were given concurrently, although the latter did not prevent the increase in blood pressure.

It is important to note in this context that the relationship between catecholamines and cardiac hypertrophy is bimodal and not restricted to the influence of the first on the latter.[38] Cardiac hypertrophy can, in turn, lead to altered myocardial catecholamines[30,39] and diminished inotropic response to adrenergic stimuli.[40]

Functional Sequelae of Regression of Hypertrophy

These have been mostly studied in hypertensive conditions. The results must be carefully assessed in order to differentiate the effect of a reduction in LV mass on ventricular function from the impact of the concomitant reduction in arterial pressure. The need for precise answers in this area has been made more urgent by the demonstration that increases in LV mass can occur in early childhood or adolescent hypertension[41] and that LV mass can be altered differently by different antihypertensive drugs.[6,42] If regression of hypertrophy is beneficial per se, this could influence both the indications and planning of antihypertensive therapy.

Effects on ventricular function: Cardiac hypertrophy in hyperthyroid animals regresses after correction of the metabolic disorder, but contractility remains depressed.[42] On the other hand, Cooper et al[43] reported normalization of myocardial contractility after obtaining relief of a right ventricular pressure overload; similar results were attained by Capasso et al[44] following reversal of LVH via surgical cure of renovascular hypertension in rats.

Overall ventricular performance in man, assessed by LV percent shortening at rest, was not altered with reduction in LV mass.[10,45] Studies in animals revealed a more complex picture. Cardiac performance was evaluated in rats in terms of the maximum cardiac output achieved by rapid blood transfusion (peak output).[46] Reversal of hypertrophy by methyldopa treatment in spontaneously hypertensive rats led to higher peak output levels for the same LV end-diastolic pressure; although the ventricles were reduced in mass, this did not apparently impair their ability to sustain increased volume loads compared with hypertrophied controls.[46] These results were recently confirmed in renovascular hypertensive rats also treated with methyldopa.[47] However, this improvement in pumping ability was probably related to blood pressure control, as shown by repeating the same study while arterial pressure was increased by an infusion of phenylephrine.[46] The increase in blood pressure led to a greater reduction of peak output in hearts with reversed hypertrophy than in either untreated spontaneously hypertensive rats or untreated normotensive controls (Fig. 1).

On the other hand, studies of the maximum LV force developed by nonejecting beats revealed a different picture. In the hypertrophied left ventricle of renovascular hypertensive rats, much higher systolic pressures de-

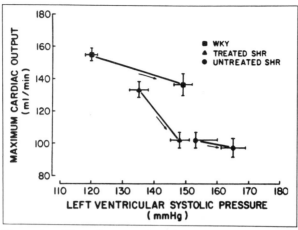

Figure 1. *Effect of pressure load stress on the peak pumping ability of Wistar-Kyoto (WKY) controls, treated spontaneously hypertensive rats (SHR), and untreated hypertensive controls.* **Arrows** *denote direction of the change in performance following infusion of phenylephrine hydrochloride.* **Ordinate,** *peak cardiac output;* **abscissa,** *LV systolic pressure at plateau of the function curve. (Reprinted with permission from Ferrario et al.[46])*

veloped than in normotensive controls, albeit at the expense of higher end-diastolic pressure.[6] Following treatment with a converting enzyme inhibitor, ventricular weight was reduced to normal and so were the left ventricular end-diastolic pressure and the maximum LV developed pressure during transient aortic occlusion. The correlation between ventricular weight and developed pressure remained similar to that found before reversal, suggesting that this aspect of ventricular performance was not adversely affected by regression of hypertrophy.[6,48]

On balance, it would appear as if regression of hypertrophy did not significantly influence the heart's overall performance. However, in my opinion, the results available are still sketchy, and more studies are needed to evaluate both the systolic and diastolic functions of the heart and to differentiate carefully the effects of pressure reduction and the lingering action of antihypertensive agents from possible changes due to regression of hypertrophy.

Inotropic responsiveness to adrenergic stimulation. In many studies in both spontaneously hypertensive rats and renovascular hypertensive rats (2-kidney 1-clip, Goldblatt), a reduced inotropic responsiveness of the hypertrophied hearts to isoproterenol has been described.[48–51] This reduction was significantly correlated with LV weight in renovascular hypertensive rats.[48] The results were confirmed by studies in vitro (Langendorff isolated hearts) and related in part to a reduction in density of beta-adrenergic receptors.[40,52] In contrast, hypertrophied hearts from the same model of hypertension maintained a normal response to such other inotropic agents as calcium and the cardiac glycoside scillaren.[40]

It is conceivable that the reduced response to beta-adrenergic stimulation might play a role in the progression of hypertensive heart disease,[48] since adrenergic mechanisms play an important role in helping the heart meet with increased stress.[53] Regression of LVH induced by either nephrectomy of the clipped kidney or by the administration of captopril restored responsiveness of isoproterenol to or near normal.[52]

Coronary circulation and regression of left ventricular hypertrophy. The effects of antihypertensive therapy and associated regression of LVH on coronary blood flow depends on a number of factors. These include the degree of alterations in coronary flow due to the hypertrophy itself[54,55] and the anatomic changes due to hypertension in the small coronary vessels,[56] as well as the pharmacologic properties of the drug utilized.[27] Few studies have been reported on all these aspects simultaneously.

Most investigators would agree that, expressed per unit weight of myocardial mass, coronary blood flow at rest remains, by and large, normal in hypertrophied ventricles.[54,55] However, the ability of the coronary vessels to dilate in response to either pharmacologic agents, transient occlusion, or increased myocardial demands (coronary vascular reserve) has been questioned. Marcus et al[54] reported that pressure-induced hypertrophy was associated with a reduction in coronary vascular reserve. This reduction was documented in some experimental and clinical studies,[57] but not in all.[55,58] The general tendency was toward some reduction, but statistical significance was not achieved in many studies. Several factors can account for the wide spectrum of reported results, including differences in techniques as well as in type and degree of hypertrophy.

Of particular importance with regard to the consequences of the reversal of hypertrophy is the influence on the coronary circulation of the ratio of the driving head of pressure to the ventricular mass[55] (Fig. 2). In our experience, coronary vascular reserve remained mostly within normal limits in those conditions in which the pressure load on the heart, the degree of LVH, and the driving head of pressure for the coronary circulation were closely related. When, however, the level of systemic (and, therefore, of coronary) arterial pressure and the degree of LVH were dissociated, significant alterations occurred in coronary vascular reserve. A reduction in arterial pressure without a change in LV mass was associated with a reduction in coronary vascular reserve.[26]

If the results are confirmed in man, they will have important clinical implications; coronary flow reserve after antihypertensive therapy would remain normal if the decrease in blood pressure is associated with a parallel regression of hypertrophy. Conversely, coronary flow reserve could be altered if the treatment normalized blood pressure, but not LV mass, such as might occur with some vasodilators (hydralazine, minoxidil).[3,9] In aortic stenosis or regurgitation, the coronary flow reserve would also be reduced since coronary perfusion pressure is normal or low while LV mass is augmented.

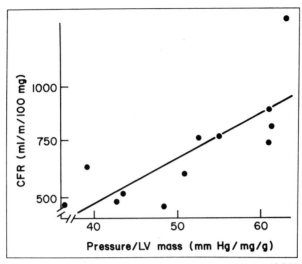

Figure 2. *Correlation between coronary flow reserve (CFR) and the ratio of coronary pressure to LV mass; the lower the ratio, the greater the reduction in coronary flow during maximal vasodilation. (Reprinted with permission from Yamori et al.[55])*

Vascular Hypertrophy

Of particular importance in a discussion of the regression of cardiac hypertrophy is the possible relationship between the structural responses of the heart and of the vessels to hypertension. Folkow[59] was the first to point out the dynamic role played in the evolution of hypertension by alterations in the structure and geometry of resistance vessels; he stressed that they should not be considered as late irreversible changes but rather as important active forces that can influence even the early evolution of the disease. The same could be said of the heart.[60] It would be most important to define whether the response of cardiac hypertrophy to treatment mirrors or differs from that of the peripheral or central arteries.

The studies by Yamori and collaborators[61] of arterial responses to antihypertensive therapy suggested a close relationship among alterations, reversal in cardiac mass, and reduction of protein synthesis in the mesenteric arteries of spontaneously hypertensive rats. From their observation on the importance of neural influences in modulating the regression of vascular hypertrophy, they came to the same conclusions as we did in our studies of reversal of cardiac hypertrophy. Wolinsky[62] reported that in rats the increased aortic medial wall thickness, as well as total dry weight associated with renovascular hypertension, regressed partially toward normal with reversal of hypertension. The restoration of aortic wall thickness to normal was more complete in female than in male rats and was less complete the longer the duration of hypertension.[63] The work of Columbo and coworkers[64] also revealed some differences between cardiac and aortic wall responses to antihypertensive treatment. More detailed studies are obviously needed.

This discussion has both theoretical and practical implications; the importance of identifying factors that modulate cardiac and vascular smooth muscle hypertrophy hardly needs stressing. As more is learned, one is tempted to speculate that antihypertensive therapy may eventually be guided by more than its effects on blood pressure alone.

Acknowledgment

This study was supported in part by grants 6835 and 15837 from the National Heart, Lung and Blood Institute and from the American Heart Association, Northeast Ohio Affiliate, Cleveland, Ohio.

I gratefully acknowledge my indebtedness to my many colleagues who collaborated and participated so much in the studies reported here, particularly Dr. Subha Sen for the experimental data, Dr. Fetnat M. Fouad for the studies in patients, and Dr. M. Hani Ayobe for the beta-receptor studies. Miss Kathy Akiya was of great help in the preparation of the manuscript.

References

1. TARAZI RC: Reversal of cardiac hypertrophy; possibility and clinical implications. In: Roberton JIS, Caldwell ADS, eds. Left ventricular hypertrophy in hypertension. London: Academic Press and the Royal Society of Medicine, 1979; 55–65.

2. WILLIAM JF JR, BRAUNWALD E: Studies on digitalis: effects of digitoxin on the development of cardiac hypertrophy in the rat subjected to aortic constriction. Am J Cardiol 1965; 16: 534–539.

3. SEN S, TARAZI RC, KHAIRALLAH PA, BUMPUS FM: Cardiac hypertrophy in spontaneously hypertensive rats. Circ Res 1974; 35: 775–781.

4. FROHLICH ED, TARAZI RC: Is arterial pressure the sole factor responsible for hypertensive cardiac hypertrophy? Am J Cardiol 1979; 44: 959–963.

5. TARAZI RC, SEN S: Catecholamines and cardiac hypertrophy. In: Mezey KC, Caldwell ADS, eds. Catecholamines and the heart. London: Academic Press and Royal Society of Medicine, 1979; 48–57.

6. TARAZI RC, SEN S, FOUAD FM, WICKER P: Regression of myocardial hypertrophy: conditions and sequelae of reversal in hypertensive heart disease. In: Alpert NR, ed. Perspective in cardiovascular research, myocardial hypertrophy and failure. New York: Raven Press, 1983; 637–652.

7. BARTOLOME J, HUGUENARD J, SLOTKIN TA: Role of orinthine decarboxylase in cardiac growth and hypertrophy. Science 1980; 210: 793–794.

8. TARAZI RC, MASSON GMC: Prophylatic digitalis in hypertension. N Engl J Med 1972; 287: 1355.

9. KAZDA S, GARTHOFF B, THOMAS G: Antihypertensive effect of calcium antagonists in rats differs from that of vasodilators. Clin Sci 1982; 63: 363s–365s.

10. FOUAD FM, NAKASHIMA Y, TARAZI RC, SALCEDO EE: Reversal of left ventricular hypertrophy with methyldopa. Am J Cardiol 1982; 49: 795–801.

11. CUTILLETTA AF, DOWELL RT, RUDNIK M, ARCILLA RA, ZAK R: Regression of myocardial hypertrophy. I. Experimental model, changes in heart weight, nucleic acids and collagen. J Mol Cell Cardiol 1975; 7: 761–780.

12. KENNEDY JW, TWISS RD, BLACKMAN JR, MENEDINO KA: Hemodynamic studies one year after homograft aortic valve replacement. Circulation 1968; 37, 38 (suppl): II110–II118.

13. BAXLEY WA, DODGE HT: Relationship of left ventricular performance and hypertrophy in humans. In: Alpert NR, ed. Cardiac hypertrophy. New York: Academic Press, 1971; 425–431.

14. SAVAGE DD, DRAYER JIM, HENRY WL, et al: Echocardiographic assessment of cardiac anatomy and function in hypertensive subjects. Circulation 1979; 59: 623–632.

15. ABI-SAMRA F, FOUAD FM, TARAZI RC: Determinants of left ventricular hypertrophy and function in hypertensive patients: an echocardiographic study. Am J Med 1983; 75 (suppl 3A): 26–33.

16. TARAZI RC, LEVY MN: Cardiac responses to increased afterload. Hypertension 1982; 4 (suppl II): II-8–II-18.

17. GROSSMAN W, JONES D, MCLAURIN LP: Wall stress and patterns of hypertrophy in human left ventricle. J Clin Invest 1975; 56: 56–64.

18. MILNOR WR: Arterial impedance as ventricular afterload. Circ Res 1975; 36: 565–569.

19. DEVEREUX RB, PICKERING TG, HARSHFIELD GA, et al: Relation of hypertensive left ventricular hypertrophy to 24-hour blood pressure (abstr). Circulation 1981; 64 (suppl IV): IV–321.

20. DRAYER JIM, WEBER MA, DEYOUNG JL: BP as a determinant of cardiac left ventricular mass. Arch Intern Med 1983; 143: 90–92.

21. TARAZI RC, FERRARIO CM, DUSTAN HP: The heart in hypertension. In: Genest J, Koiw E, Kuchel O, eds. Hypertension, physiopathology and treatment. New York: McGraw-Hill, 1977; 738–754.

22. IBRAHIM MM, TARAZI RC, DUSTAN HP, GIFFORD RW JR: Electrocardiogram in evaluation of resistance to antihypertensive therapy. Arch Intern Med 1977; 137: 1125–1129.

23. JULIUS S, ELLIS CN, PASCUAL AV, et al: Home blood pressure determination. JAMA 1974; 229: 663–666.

24. SEN S, TARAZI RC, BUMPUS FM: Cardiac hypertrophy and antihypertensive therapy. Cardiovasc Res 1977; 11: 427–433.

25. SEN S, TARAZI RC, BUMPUS FM: Reversal of cardiac hypertrophy in renal hypertensive rats: medical versus surgical therapy. Am J Physiol 1981; 240: H409–H412.

26. WICKER P, TARAZI RC, KOBAYASHI K: Coronary blood flow during the develop-

ment and regression of left ventricular hypertrophy in renovascular hypertensive rats. Am J Cardiol 1983; 51: 1744–1749.

27. KOBAYASHI K, TARAZI RC: Effect of long-term nitrendipine therapy on coronary blood flow and left ventricular hypertrophy in renovascular hypertension. Hypertension 1983; 5 (suppl II): II-45–II-51.

28. TARAZI RC, SEN S, FOUAD FM: Regression of myocardial hypertrophy. In: Braunwald E, Mock MB, Watson J, eds. Congestive heart failure: current research and clinical applications. New York: Grune & Stratton, 1982; 151–163.

29. SEN S, TARAZI RC: Myocardial catecholamines in hypertensive ventricular hypertrophy. In: Tarazi RC, Dunbar JB, eds. Perspectives in cardiovascular research. Vol 8. Cardiac hypertrophy in hypertension. New York: Raven Press, 1983; 309–318.

30. SPANN JF JR, SONNENBLICK EH, HARRIS ED JR, BUCCION RA: Connective tissue of the hypertrophied heart. In: Alpert NR, ed. Cardiac hypertrophy. New York: Academic Press, 1971; 141–145.

31. SEN S: Regression of cardiac hypertrophy: experimental animal model. Am J Med 1983; 75 (suppl 3A): 87–93.

32. KHAIRALLAH PA, KANABUS J: Angiotensin and myocardial protein synthesis. In: Tarazi RC, Dunbar JB, eds. Perspectives in cardiovascular research. Vol 8, Cardiac hypertrophy in hypertension. New York: Raven Press, 1983; 337–347.

33. NAKASHIMA Y, FOUAD FM, TARAZI RC, BRAVO EL: Left ventricular function with reversal of left ventricular hypertrophy in hypertensive patients (abstr.). J Am Coll Cardiol 1983; 1: 598.

34. SEN S, TARAZI RC, BUMPUS FM: Effect of converting enzyme inhibitor (SQ 14225) on myocardial hypertrophy in spontaneously hypertensive rats. Hypertension 1980; 2: 169–176.

35. WHITEHORN WV: Effects of hypophyseal hormones on cardiac growth and function. In: Alpert NR, ed. Cardiac hypertrophy. New York: Academic Press, 1971; 27–37.

36. RABB W: Hormonal and neurogenic cardiovascular disorders. Baltimore: Williams & Wilkins, 1953.

37. YAMORI Y, TARAZI RC, OOSHIMA A: Effect of β-receptor blocking agents on cardiovascular structural changes in spontaneous and nonadrenaline-induced hypertension in rats. Clin Sci 1981; 59: 457s–460s.

38. TARAZI RC, SEN S, SARAGOCA M, KHAIRALLAH PA: The multifactorial role of catecholamines in hypertensive cardiac hypertrophy. Eur Heart J 1982; 3: 103–110.

39. FISCHER JE, HORST W, KOPIN IJ: Norepinephrine metabolism in hypertrophied rat hearts. Nature 1965; 207: 951–953.

40. AYOBE MH, TARAZI RC: Beta-receptors and contractile reserve in left ventricular hypertrophy. Hypertension 1983; 5 (suppl II): I-192–I-197.

41. CULPEPPER WS, SODT PC, MESSERLI FH, RUSCHHAUPT DG, ARCILLA RA: Cardiac status in juvenile borderline hypertension. Ann Intern Med 1983; 98: 1–7.

42. DEVEREUX RB, SAVAGE DD, SACHS I, LARAGH JH: Effects of blood pressure control on left ventricular hypertrophy and function in hypertension (abstr). Circulation 1980; 62 (suppl II): II—36.

43. COOPER G, SATAVA RM, HARRISON CE, COLEMAN HN: Normal myocardial func-

tion and energetics after reversing pressure-overload hypertrophy. Am J Physiol 1974; 226: 1158–1165.

44. CAPASSO JM, STROBECK JE, MALHOLTRA A, SCHEUER J, SONNENBLICK ED: Contractile behavior of rat myocardium after reversal of hypertensive hypertrophy. Am J Physiol 1982; 242: H882–H889.

45. SCHLANT RC, FELNER JM, BLUMENSTEIN BA, et al: Echocardiographic documentation of regression of left ventricular hypertrophy in patients treated for essential hypertension. Eur Heart J 1982; 3 (suppl A): 171–175.

46. FERRARIO CM, SPECH MM, TARAZI RC, DOI Y: Cardiac pumping ability in rats with experimental renal and genetic hypertension. Am J Cardiol 1979; 44: 979–985.

47. KUWAJIMA I, KARDON MB, PEGRAM BL, SESOKO S, FROHLICH ED: Regression of left ventricular hypertrophy in 2-kidney, 1-clip Goldblatt hypertension. Hypertension 1982; 4 (suppl II): II-113–II-118.

48. SARAGOCA MA, TARAZI RC: Left ventricular hypertrophy in rats with renovascular hypertension. Alterations in cardiac function and adrenergic responses. Hypertension 1981; 3 (suppl II): II-171–II-176.

49. PFEFFER MA, PFEFFER JM, FROHLICH ED: Pumping ability of the hypertrophying left ventricle of the spontaneously hypertensive rat. Circ Res 1976; 38: 423–429.

50. KUNOS G, ROBERTSON B, KAN WH, PREIKSAITIS H, MUCCI L: Adrenergic reactivity of the myocardium in hypertension. Life Sci 1978; 22: 847–854.

51. SARAGOCA MA, TARAZI RC: Impaired cardiac contractile response to isoproterenol in the spontaneously hypertensive rats. Hypertension 1981; 3: 380–385.

52. AYOBE MH, TARAZI RC, KHAIRALLAH PA: Alterations of beta-adrenergic receptors with development and reversal of cardiac hypertrophy (abstr). J Mol Cell Cardiol 1982; 14: 23.

53. BRAUNWALD E, ROSS J, SONNENBLICK EH: Mechanisms of contraction of the normal and failing heart. Boston: Little Brown, 1967; 157–163.

54. MARCUS ML, MUELLER TM, GASCHO JA, KERBER RE: Effects of cardiac hypertrophy secondary to hypertension on the coronary circulation. Am J Cardiol 1979; 44: 1023–1028.

55. WICKER P, TARAZI RC: Coronary blood flow in left ventricular hypertrophy: a review of experimental data. Eur Heart J 1982; 3: 111–118.

56. YAMORI Y, MORI C, NISHIO T, et al: Cardiac hypertrophy in early hypertension. Am J Cardiol 1979; 44: 964–969.

57. STRAUER BE: Ventricular function and coronary hemodynamics in hypertensive heart disease. Am J Cardiol 1979; 44: 999–1006.

58. BACHE RJ, VROBEL TR, RING WS, EMERY RW, ANDERSON RW: Regional myocardial blood flow during exercise in dogs with chronic left ventricular hypertrophy. Circ Res 1979; 48: 76–87.

59. FOLKOW B: Cardiovascular structural adaptation: its role in the initiation and maintenance of primary hypertension. Clin Sci Mol Med 1979; 55: 3S–22S.

60. TARAZI RC: The role of the heart in hypertension. Clin Sci 1982; 63: 347S–358S.

61. YAMORI Y, NAKADA T, LOVENBERG W: Effect of antihypertensive therapy on lysine incorporation into vascular protein in the spontaneously hypertensive rat. Eur J Pharmacol 1976; 38: 349–355.

62. WOLINSKY H: Effects of hypertension and its reversal on the thoracic aorta of male and female rats. Circ Res 1971; 28: 622–636.

63. WOLINSKY H, MENARD J: Influence of the duration of hypertension on the reversibility of vascular changes in the female rat aorta: role of connective tissue. In: Milliez P, Safar M, eds. Recent advances in hypertension. France: Boehringer Ingelheim, 1975; 151–159.

64. COLUMBO M, PADDOCK J, MAGRAJ S, HOLLANDER W: Effects of hydralazine and propranolol on hypertensive cardiovascular disease in the SHR (abstr). Circulation 1979; 60 (part II): II-10.

29

Regression of Left Ventricular Hypertrophy: General Aspects

JAN I. M. DRAYER, M.D.
MICHAEL A. WEBER, M.D.
JULIUS M. GARDIN, M.D.

Cardiac left ventricular hypertrophy (LVH) is known to be a significant risk factor of cardiovascular complications in patients with hypertension. The presence of signs of left ventricular hypertrophy on the electrocardiogram (ECG) represents a residual three fold increased risk of clinically overt coronary heart disease after adjustment for the effect of coexisting hypertension.[1]

Both ECG and echo signs of cardiac hypertrophy often are seen in patients with borderline, mild, moderate, or severe hypertension.[2–5] It is evident that the incidence of cardiac hypertrophy in hypertensive patients has been underestimated using the ECG in the diagnosis of LVH. Echo techniques have been shown to be much more specific than the ECG in the detection of LVH in patients with hypertension. We have shown previously that the incidence of ECG-hypertrophy in treated and untreated patients with hypertension was less than one tenth of the true incidence of hypertrophy as measured by echo. Data obtained in the general population confirm the greater sensitivity of echo in the detection of LVH.[6] We have shown that the degree of cardiac hypertrophy was not significantly different between treated and untreated patients.[5] Others also have reported that the incidence of LVH is not related to the presence of antihypertensive therapy.[7] In fact, the correlation between blood pressure levels and the degree of cardiac hypertrophy was fairly poor in both treated and untreated hypertensive patients. Postmortem studies also have revealed a lack of association between left ventricular (LV) weight and any measurement of blood pressure.[8]

Others have confirmed that blood pressure levels are not the sole contributors to the process of cardiac hypertrophy. Cardiac hypertrophy has been observed in hypertensive patients even before the development of high blood pressure levels.[9] In addition, LVH is found in many adolescent patients with very mild or borderline hypertension.[3,4,10,11] The importance of factors other than blood pressure has further been emphasized by the observation that certain antihypertensive agents may not lower blood pressure but at the same time may cause regression of hypertrophy.[12] Other antihypertensive agents have been shown to lower blood pressure effectively, but treatment with these drugs did not necessarily lead to regression of cardiac muscle mass.[13–15] Thus, the relationship between drug-induced changes in blood pressure and concomitant changes in cardiac muscle mass, as measured using echo, is not strong. Similar observations have been made when the ECG was used in the detection of cardiac hypertrophy.[16,17] Although the correlation coefficient between changes in blood pressure and changes in cardiac muscle mass does not reach statistical significance in individual studies, combined data from several studies show a significant relationship between these parameters.[18]

The effects of antihypertensive drugs on cardiac muscle mass is most clearly observed in patients who exhibited frank hypertrophy on the ECG or on echo before the start of antihypertensive therapy. Indeed, in a number of studies in patients with hypertension, a significantly positive relationship has been reported between the degree of cardiac hypertrophy before treatment and the changes in cardiac muscle mass observed during therapy.[3,19] However, decreases in LV muscle mass also have been observed in hypertensive patients with a pretreatment muscle mass, which was in the range found in normotensive control subjects. These findings support the fact that, even in patients who develop only mild changes in cardiac muscle mass during the evolution of the hypertension, therapy may result in some decrease in muscle mass.

Recently, we presented echo data obtained in 51 male hypertensive patients during their course of antihypertensive therapy.[20] Antihypertensive therapy resulted in a decrease in cardiac muscle mass in 29 patients (59%). As in other studies, the changes in cardiac muscle mass were not related to changes in blood pressure. The decrease in blood pressure observed in patients who experienced a decrease in muscle mass was not different from the decrease in blood pressure seen in patients who did not show a decrease in muscle mass during therapy (Table I). Pretreatment blood pressures also were similar between the two groups. However, patients with regression of muscle mass had a significantly greater muscle mass before the start of the

TABLE I   Clinical Data on 29 Patients with a Decrease and 22 Patients with no Change or Increase in Cardiac Muscle Mass During Antihypertensive Therapy

	Responders (Decrease in Muscle Mass)	p	Nonresponders (Increase in Muscle Mass)
Control systolic blood pressure (mmHg)	153 ± 16	NS	147 ± 15
Control diastolic blood pressure (mmHg)	102 ± 8	NS	99 ± 6
Control left ventricular muscle mass (g)	267 ± 46	p < 0.01	213 ± 54
Change in systolic blood pressure (mmHg)	−16 ± 18	NS	−13 ± 15
Change in diastolic blood pressure (mmHg)	−10 ± 7	NS	−12 ± 7

study. Control muscle mass was greater than that predicted on the basis of data obtained in normotensive control subjects of the same sex and body weight: 267 ± 46 g (SD) versus 233 ± 54 g. Muscle mass was greater than this standard of normalcy in 19 of the 29 patients, but in the remaining 10 patients cardiac muscle mass was within or even below normal. In addition, many of the responders had a cardiac muscle mass that was within range of normalcy accepted by echo laboratories.

Thus, the presence of a relatively normal control muscle mass in patients who did not show a decrease in muscle mass during antihypertensive therapy cannot be regarded as the main reason for this absence of response during effective antihypertensive therapy. In fact, in our study, muscle mass tended to increase during therapy in this subgroup. The increase in muscle mass probably was related to the significant increase in LV dimension observed in these patients (+4 ± 5 mm, p < 0.05). In addition, these patients showed signs of mild volume retention; venous hematocrit decreased in this subgroup to a greater extent than in patients in whom muscle mass and LV dimension decreased. Indeed, concomitant diuretic therapy was less often prescribed in the former (7 of 22 patients) than in the latter group (18 of 29 patients). Thus, the presence of diuretic therapy in patients treated with a centrally acting sympatholytic drug or a vasodilator may promote regression of LVH. This observation contrasts with the relative lack of regression of muscle mass observed in patients treated with a diuretic only.[13–15] The presence of nondiuretic antihypertensive agents probably is related to the disparity of the response of muscle mass during these forms of antihypertensive therapy.

It has been postulated that the decreases in muscle mass found during antihypertensive therapy are directly related to drug-induced decreases in end systolic wall stress. In our study, we did not find a significant relationship between changes in wall stress and changes in cardiac muscle mass (r = 0.02, NS). However, changes in wall stress were related to changes in systolic blood pressure (r = 0.36, p < 0.05). In addition, changes in wall stress were related to changes in cardiac function, such as fractional shortening (r = 0.63, p < 0.01). The consequence of this relationship is that cardiac function deteriorates in patients in whom wall stress increases significantly during antihypertensive therapy. It must be emphasized that a deterioration of cardiac function has not been observed during antihypertensive therapy of patients with mild to moderate hypertension. However, deterioration of cardiac function is likely to occur in patients with an inappropriately low LV muscle mass or in patients with marked LV dilation.[21]

Abnormalities in cardiac function have been observed in hypertensive patients with and without LVH. Characteristics of diastolic LV filling have been shown to be abnormal in many hypertensive patients. This abnormality is not dependent on blood pressure levels and can be found in patients with a normal LV mass and in whom systolic function is preserved.[22–24] Obviously, an abnormal cardiac function is more often found in hypertensive patients with LVH. This decrease in LV function may be related to the reduction in beta-adrenergic receptor responsiveness, impaired coronary vasodilatory responses, increases in connective tissue, and decreases in capillary density found in the hypertrophied heart. In addition, the presence of overt or subclinical coronary artery disease will contribute to the ultimate determination of LV function. It must be emphasized that it is extremely unlikely that a 5% to 15% reduction in cardiac muscle mass will lead to significant deterioration of cardiac function. Unloading of the heart by means of antihypertensive therapy will lead to decreases in muscle mass, and the concomitant changes in blood pressure will cause wall stress not to change, and, hence, cardiac function will be preserved.

However, if a decrease in blood pressure occurs without a decrease in muscle mass, a low stress form of hypertrophy will be present, cardiac function will be normal, and cardiac oxygen consumption may be decreased. In contrast, if a decrease in muscle mass occurs in the absence of a decrease in blood pressure, then a high stress form of hypertrophy is present with a decrease in cardiac function and an increase in oxygen consumption.[21] This might be an important consideration, especially in cases in which cardiac function already is compromised because of coexisting coronary artery disease, as in many elderly patients with hypertension or with additional valvular heart disease. In this analysis, it is not important whether changes in blood pressure itself or other factors have caused the changes in cardiac muscle mass in the hypertensive patient.

It may be concluded that factors other than blood pressure are important in the development and regression of cardiac muscle mass. The most important factor probably is the sympathetic nervous system.[25] Increases in sympathetic activity often are found in young patients with mild or borderline hypertension. In these patients sympathetic nervous system activity and to a lesser extent the blood pressure level per se may be responsible for the increased muscle mass. Animal experiments have clearly demonstrated that catecholamines and specifically norepinephrine play a major role in the growth of cardiac muscle.[26,27] Simpson[28] has shown that stimulation of post synaptic alpha-1 receptors by norepinephrine results in growth of cultured cardiac muscle cells. Stimulation or blockade of postsynaptic beta receptors did not alter this growth process. These findings help to explain why treatment with centrally acting sympatholytic agents, such as alpha-methyldopa, causes regression of cardiac muscle mass even in the absence of blood pressure control.[12,29,10] We have observed regression of cardiac muscle mass during long-term therapy with a diuretic and alpha-methyldopa. In these patients, regression of cardiac muscle mass was most pronounced at the level of the interventricular septum.[30] The presence of the sympatholytic agent was believed to be more important in causing regression of muscle mass than the drug-induced decreases in blood pressure. Similarly, the effect of other classes of antihypertensive agents on cardiac muscle cells are, at least in part, mediated through the effects of these drugs on the sympathetic nervous system rather than through drug-induced changes in blood pressure. Thus, the absence of regression of cardiac muscle mass during diuretic or vasodilatory therapy may be related to the stimulatory effect of these agents on catecholamines.[13-15] The role of beta-adrenergic antagonists in this respect is less clear.

Regression of cardiac muscle mass has been observed during treatment with atenolol,[19] metoprolol,[31] nadolol,[32] and timolol,[33] but regression was not observed during therapy with pindolol.[34] We have given acebutolol to 7 hypertensive patients whose blood pressure was not controlled with a diuretic. Addition of the beta-blocker did not lead to regression of muscle mass. In these patients cardiac muscle mass was 233 ± 13 g before and 246 ± 17 g during therapy with acebutolol. Both pindolol and acebutolol are beta-adrenergic blocking agents that exhibit intrinsic sympathomimetic activity. This may lead to increased catecholamine-induced receptor stimulation of muscle cells, and it may prevent regression of muscle mass. Indeed, others have shown that although treatment with acebutolol may cause regression of cardiac muscle mass, the regression was directly related to drug-induced changes in heart rate.[35] The presence of marked intrinsic sympathomimetic activity will not lead to decreases in heart rate, and regression of muscle mass was not observed in such patients. However, other effects of beta blockers may lead to regression of muscle mass; the blood pressure-lowering effect of beta blockers, the inhibitory effect of these drugs on norepinephrine release at nerve terminals, the blockade of the activity of the renin-angiotensin system, and the effect of beta blockers on cardiac work and cardiac oxygen consumption may result in decreases in muscle mass. Regression in muscle mass observed in patients treated with metoprolol was closely related to drug-induced changes in total peripheral resistance.[31]

Treatment with inhibitors of the renin-angiotensin system, such as the converting enzyme inhibitor enalopril, has been shown to cause significant decreases in blood pressure and in cardiac muscle mass.[36,37] In contrast, drugs that do not always lead to regression of muscle mass, such as diuretics and vasodilators, have been shown to increase the activity of the renin system.[14]

Finally, whole blood viscosity also has to be taken into account in the evaluation of treatment-induced changes in cardiac muscle mass. We have shown that blood viscosity is increased in many hypertensive patients, and that whole blood viscosity is directly related to the degree of cardiac hypertrophy found in these patients.[38] The fact that diuretics may increase and sympatholytic agents decrease blood viscosity may well have contributed to the opposite effect that these drugs have on cardiac muscle mass.

Calcium channel blockers are now being used in the treatment of hypertensive patients. These drugs lower blood pressure through their vasodilatory effect. This effect might be related to selective inhibition of the vasoconstriction induced by stimulation of $alpha_2$ adrenergic receptors by (nor)epinephrine. These receptors do not block $alpha_2$ receptors, but they prevent the stimulation of contractile proteins.[39] In contrast, verapamil has been shown to inhibit stimulation of $alpha_1$ more clearly than stimulation of $alpha_2$ receptors.[40] One would expect that the effects of calcium channel blockers on blood pressure and on alpha receptors would permit muscle mass to regress during therapy. Preliminary results of treatment with calcium channel blocker nitrendipine does not support this thesis, since long-term treatment did not lead to regression of muscle mass. Left ventricular muscle mass was 233 ± 51 before and 236 ± 52 $(n = 18)$ after therapy.[41] Increases in heart rate and in renin activity and possibly mild volume retention observed during therapy with various calcium channel blockers may explain this discrepancy.

Summary

Recent studies that included echo examination of hypertensive patients before and during effective antihypertensive therapy have provided a first glance at the complex relationship between blood pressure, the sympathetic nervous system, the renin system, blood viscosity, and the many other factors involved in the control of growth of cardiac muscle cells. A preliminary conclusion is that the actions of antihypertensive agents on these parameters should be examined to allow insight into the actions of these agents on cardiac muscle mass. In addition, the use of techniques that allow a better definition of the antihypertensive effect of these drugs, such as ambulatory blood pressure monitoring techniques, might help to improve the determination of the relationship between blood pressure and the degree of cardiac hypertrophy.[42] Finally, it seems likely that computerized analyses of two-dimensional echo techniques will enhance the sensitivity of this tool in the assessment of drug-induced changes in muscle mass.

References

1. KANNEL WB, GORDON T, CASTELLI WP, MARGOLIS JR: Electrocardiographic left ventricular hypertrophy and risk of coronary heart disease. The Framingham Study. Ann Intern Med 1970; 72: 813–822.

2. CULPEPPER WS, SODT PC, MESSERLI FH: Cardiac status in juvenile borderline hypertension. Ann Intern Med 1983; 98: 1–7.

3. JOHNSON GL, KOTCHEN JM, MCKEAN HE, COTTRILL CM, KOTCHEN TA: Blood pressure related echocardiographic changes in adolescents and young adults. Am Heart J 1983; 105: 113–118.

4. NIEDERLE P, WIDIMSKY J, JANDORA R, RESSO J, GROSPIC A: Echocardiographic assessment of the left ventricle in juvenile hypertension. Int J Cardiol 1982; 2: 91–101.

5. SAVAGE DD, DRAYER JIM, HENRY WL, MATHEWS EC JR, WARE JH, GARDIN JM: Echocardiographic assessment of cardiac anatomy and function in hypertensive subjects. Circulation 1979; 59: 623–632.

6. SAVAGE DD, ABBOTT RD, PADGETT S, GARRISON RJ: Epidemiologic aspects of left ventricular hypertrophy in normotensive and hypertensive subjects. In: J Schipperheyn, and ter Keurs H, eds. Left ventricular hypertrophy. The Hague: Martinus Nijhoff, 1983; 2–15.

7. ABI-SAMRA F, FOUAD FM, TARAZI RC: Determinants of left ventricular hypertrophy and function in hypertensive patients. An echocardiographic study. Am J Med 1983; 75 (suppl 3A): 26–33.

8. DEAN JH, GALLAGHER PJ: Cardiac ischemia and cardiac hypertrophy. An autopsy

study. Arch Pathol Lab Med 1980; 104: 175–178.

9. SPARROW D, THOMAS HE, ROSNER B, WEISS ST: The relationship of the baseline ECG to blood pressure change. JAMA 1983; 250: 1285–1288.

10. SCHIEKEN RM, CLARKE WR, PRINEAS R, KLEIN V, LANER RM: Electrocardiographic measures of left ventricular hypertrophy in children across the distribution of blood pressure: the Muscatine Study. Circulation 1982; 66: 428–432.

11. ZAHKA KG, NEILL CA, KIDD L, CUTILLETTA MA, CUTILLETTA AF: Cardiac involvement in adolescent hypertension. Echocardiographic determination of myocardial hypertrophy. Hypertension 1981; 3: 664–668.

12. FOUAD FM, NAKASHIMA Y, TARAZI RC, SALCEDO EE: Reversal of left ventricular hypertrophy in hypertensive patients treated with methyldopa. Am J Cardiol 1982; 49: 795–801.

13. DRAYER JIM, GARDIN JM, WEBER MA, ARONOW WS: Changes in ventricular septal thickness during diuretic therapy. Clin Pharmacol Ther 1982; 32: 283–288.

14. DRAYER JIM, GARDIN JM, WEBER MA, ARONOW WS: Changes in cardiac muscle mass during vasodilation therapy of hypertension. Clin Pharmacol Ther 1983; 33: 727–732.

15. WOLLAM GL, HALL WD, PORTER VD, et al: Time course of regression of left ventricular hypertrophy in treated hypertensive patients. Am J Med 1983; 75: 100–110.

16. DERN PL, PRYOR R, WALKER SH, SEARLS DT: Serial electrocardiographic changes in treated hypertensive patients with reference to voltage criteria, mean QRS vectors, and the QRS-T angle. Circulation 1967; 36: 823–826.

17. LEISHMAN AWD: The electrocardiogram in hypertension. Q Med 1951; 20: 1–11.

18. DRAYER JIM, GARDIN JM, WEBER MA: Echocardiographic left ventricular hypertrophy in hypertension. Chest 1983; 84: 217–221.

19. IBRAHIM MM, MADKOUR MA, MOSSALLAM R: Factors influencing cardiac hypertrophy in hypertensive patients. Clin Sci 1981; 61: 105S–108S.

20. DRAYER JIM, GARDIN JM, WEBER MA: Antihypertensive therapy and changes in echocardiographic left ventricular muscle mass. Clin Pharmacol Ther 1984; 35: 236.

21. STRAUER BE: Ventricular function and coronary hemodynamics in hypertensive heart disease. Am J Cardiol 1979; 44: 999–1006.

22. FOUAD FM, TARAZI RC, GALLAGHER JH, MACINTYRE WJ, COOK SA: Abnormal left ventricular relaxation in hypertensive patients. Clin Sci 1980; 59: 411S–414S.

23. INOUYE I, MASSIE B, LOGE D, et al: Abnormal left ventricular filling: an early finding in mild to moderate systemic hypertension. Am J Cardiol 1984; 53: 120–126.

24. SMITH VE, SCHULMAN P, KARIMEDDNI MV, WHITE WB, MEERAN M, KATZ AM: Left ventricular filling in mild to moderate hypertension. Circulation 1983; 67: 223.

25. FROHLICH ED, TARAZI RC: Is arterial pressure the sole factor responsible for hypertensive cardiac hypertrophy? Am J Cardiol 1979; 44: 959–963.

26. TARAZI RC, SARAGOCA M, KHAIRALLAH P: The multifactorial role of catecholamines in hypertensive cardiac hypertrophy. Eur Heart J 1982; 3: 103–110.

27. OSTMAN-SMITH I: Cardiac sympathetic nerves as the final common pathway in the induction of adaptive cardiac hypertrophy. Clin Sci 1981; 61: 265–272.

28. SIMPSON P: Norepinephrine-stimulated hypertrophy of cultured rat myocardial cells is an alpha-1 adrenergic response. J Clin Invest 1983; 72: 732–738.

29. REICHEK N, FRANKLIN BB, CHANDLER T, MUHAMMAD A, PLAPPERT T, ST. JOHN SUTTON M: Reversal of left ventricular hypertrophy by antihypertensive therapy. Eur Heart J 1982; 3 (suppl A): 165–169.

30. DRAYER JIM, WEBER MA, GARDIN JM, LIPSON JL: The effect on long-term antihypertensive therapy on cardiac anatomy in patients with essential hypertension. Am J Med 1983; 75: 116–120.

31. WIKSTRAND J, TRIMARCO B, BUZZETTI G, et al: Increased cardiac output and lowered peripheral resistance during metoprolol treatment. Acta Med Scand 1983; 672 (suppl): 105–110.

32. ROWLANDS DB, IRELAND MA, GLOVER DR, McLEAY RAB, STALLARD TJ, LITTLER WA: The relationship between ambulatory blood pressure and echocardiographically assessed left ventricular hypertrophy. Clin Sci 1981; 61: 101–103.

33. HILL LS, MONAGHAN M, RICHARDSON PJ: Regression of left ventricular hypertrophy during treatment with antihypertensive agents. Br J Clin Pharmacol 1979; 7: 255–259.

34. PLOTNICK GD, FISHER ML, WOHL B, HAMILTON JH, HAMILTON BP: Improvement in depressed cardiac function in hypertensive patients during pindolol treatment. Am J Med 1984; 76: 25–30.

35. TRIMARCO B, RICCIARDELLI B, DeLUCA N, et al: Effect of acebutolol on left ventricular hemodynamics and anatomy in systemic hypertension. Am J Cardiol 1984; 53: 791–796.

36. FOUAD FM, NAKASHIMA Y, TARAZI RC, SALCEDO EE: Reversal of left ventricular hypertrophy in hypertensive patients treated with methyldopa. Am J Cardiol 1982; 49: 795–801.

37. DUNN FG, OIGMAN W, VENTURA HO, MESSERLI FH, KOBRIN I, FROHLICH ED: Enalopril improves systemic and renal hemodynamics and allows regression of left ventricular mass in essential hypertension. Am J Cardiol 1984; 53: 105–108.

38. DRAYER JIM, DEVEREUX RB, DeYOUNG JL, LETCHER RL, CHIEN S, PICKERING TG: Whole blood viscosity as a determinant of cardiac hypertrophy. Clin Pharmacol Ther 1983; 33: 204.

39. VAN MEEL JC, DeJONGE A, KALKMAN HO, WILFFERT B, TIMMERMANS PB, VAN ZWIETEN PA: Vascular smooth muscle contraction initiated by post synaptic alpha 2 adrenergic activation is induced by an influx of extracellular calcium. Eur J Pharmacol 1981; 69: 205–208.

40. VANHOUTTE PM: Heterogeneity of postjunctional vascular alpha-adrenoceptors and handling of calcium. J Cardiovasc Pharmacol 1982; 4: S91–S96.

41. DRAYER JIM, GARDIN JM, WEBER MA, BREWER DD: Cardiac muscle mass reduction during calcium channel blocker therapy: importance of age. Clin Pharmacol Ther 1984; 35: 236.

42. DRAYER JIM, WEBER MA, DeYOUNG JL: Blood pressure as a determinant of cardiac left ventricular muscle mass. Arch Intern Med 1983; 143: 90–92.

30

Cardiac Function after Reversal of Left Ventricular Hypertrophy

JOSEPH M. CAPASSO, Ph.D.

Concentric hypertrophy is a characteristic fundamental response of the myocardium to chronic systemic hypertension. This adaptive increase in myocardial mass is beneficial in that it allows the heart to maintain normal pump function when confronted with abnormal hemodynamics (that is, pressure overload).[1,2] Although many models of myocardial hypertrophy have been utilized to assess alterations in contractile performance,[3-7] results have been inconsistent due to variations in the severity and duration of the inciting stimulus.[8-10] Moreover, most studies of hypertrophy have involved the acute imposition of a load. This may produce initial pump failure with focal myocardial damage and subsequent recovery with residual scarring and hypertrophy.

Using the isolated left ventricular (LV) papillary muscle to assess myocardial contractile performance, we have chosen to evaluate a more pertinent model of hypertrophy in which the myocardial stress is applied gradually, simulating conditions observed in human hypertensive hypertrophy. The model used is the 2-kidney Goldblatt renovascular hypertensive rat,[11,12] which develops systolic hypertension over 3 to 5 weeks. This gradual-onset model avoids the acute myocardial damage and depression of contractility associated with other more rapid onset models, and the rapid increase in connective tissue content that may result from a severe and acute overload is avoided.[1,13,14]

Despite the similarity to forms of human hypertension and myocardial hypertrophy, little is known in this model of pressure overload of the changes in myocardial contractile performance during the development of a gradual onset hypertensive hypertrophy and during regression of developed hypertrophy.[14-19]

An essential consideration relative to therapy and outcome of the hypertrophic process depends on what is reversible and what is irreversible. Accordingly, we have chosen to examine the mechanical, electrical, and biochemical events associated with the transition to hypertrophy in chronic systemic hypertension and to identify points in the process at which they are irreversible. Of central pathophysiologic importance to the problem of hypertrophy and resultant myocardial failure is the understanding of what factors lead to irreversible depression of myocardial function and ultimate pump failure in the compensatory hypertrophic response to chronic systemic hypertension.

The present investigation reports the course of myocardial functional alterations accompanying chronic systemic hypertension before and after normalization of blood pressure in female Wistar rats.

Methods

Basic Study Design: One hundred and twenty female Wistar rats purchased at 6 weeks of age were housed in our animal facility. At 8 weeks of age, 70 animals underwent surgical constriction of the left renal artery. Animals were made hypertensive by placing a silver clip with a 0.25 mm aperture around the left renal artery. The contralateral kidney was left untouched. Using the tail cuff method,[20] systolic blood pressure was measured under light ether anesthesia before clipping and once weekly thereafter. This method avoids the stress-related increase in blood pressure seen in unanesthetized restrained animals and correlates well with direct measurements of arterial pressure in unanesthetized rats.[21] Rats were considered hypertensive when systolic arterial pressure increased to 150 mmHg within 3 to 5 weeks after clipping and remained at or above this level until the time of study. Hypertension was produced in approximately 75% of all clipped animals 3 to 5 weeks after renal artery constriction. At 10 weeks after the onset of hypertension (13 to 15 weeks after surgery), hypertensive animals were removed from these groups for mechanical, electrophysiologic, and biochemical studies. Age-matched unoperated rats from the same initial groups were used as controls. All hypertensive animals studied displayed significant (40% or greater) left ventricular hypertrophy (LVH).

The mechanical, electrical, and biochemical effects of a reduction in blood pressure were studied in this same group of rats. At 10 weeks after the onset of hypertension, hypertensive animals were randomly selected for unilateral nephrectomy of the ischemic kidney.[22] Normotension resulted in these animals within 24 hours, and blood pressure remained below 150 mmHg until the time of study 10 weeks later. Blood pressure was monitored within 24 hours and then twice weekly for the following 10 weeks. At the end of 10 weeks of normotension (systolic blood pressure 150 mmHg or less), the nephrectomized animals were removed for mechanical, electrophysiologic, and biochemical studies. Age-matched unoperated rats and animals hypertensive for 20 weeks were used for comparison. Ten weeks postnephrectomy, systolic blood pressure was not significantly different from that of control animals. All nephrectomized animals studied displayed regression of functional alterations seen in hypertensive animals (for simplicity, called reversals).

All electrical and biochemical data presented from the five animal groups at 10 and 20 weeks were obtained from the same hearts that were utilized for mechanical recordings.

Instrumentation and Mechanical Recordings: Animals were anesthetized with ether. The hearts were rapidly excised and placed in oxygenated Tyrode's solution. Left ventricular papillary muscles were removed and suspended horizontally in a continuous perfusion muscle bath.[23–28] Care was taken to select muscles of cylindrical uniformity whose cross-sectional area was less than 1.0 mm^2 to ensure adequate oxygenation of central fibers.[29,30] The muscles were continuously perfused with Tyrode's solution of the following composition in mM: Na$^+$, 151.3; Ca^{2+}, 2.4; K$^+$, 4.0; Mg^{2+}, 0.5; Cl$^-$, 147.3; H$_2$PO$_4$, 12.0; and dextrose, 5.5. This solution was maintained at 30°C and bubbled with 95% oxygen and 5% carbon dioxide, which yielded a pH of 7.4. The nontendinous end of the papillary muscle was inserted into a spring-loaded stainless steel clip that was mounted at the end of a micrometer assembly that was used to adjust external muscle length. The tendinous end of the muscle was tied to a light steel wire with a short length of wetted Ethicon 5–0 braided silk. The wire was attached to a 2 cm stainless steel lever that was connected to a servo-controlled galvanometer (Cambridge Technology, Cambridge, MA). Total frictional torque of the lever was calculated at less than 5 mg/cm based on system geometry. The position of the lever was measured by a variable capacitor positioned at the rear of the galvanometer's moving iron core. Force at the tip of the lever was determined by scaling and amplifying the error signal produced in the position servo-section of the control circuitry during the contraction. Control circuitry permitted operation in either afterloaded isotonic or isometric modes.

This system allows servo-control of length, velocity, or force by employing the signals of length and force as negative feedback elements. A step function of length or force can be imposed on a muscle at any time during a contraction and the galvanometer (servo-motor) will complete this step in 500 μs. This allows extension of the force-velocity relation to very light loads, and unloaded velocity of shortening can be measured by electronically reducing preload force to near zero early in the contraction.

Velocity of shortening was determined by electronic differentiation of the muscle length signal (lever position). The rate of force change was determined by differentiation of the force signal.

The actively developed and passive length-tension relationships were obtained after an equilibrium period of 120 minutes during which the muscle contracted isometrically with a resting tension of 1 g. The length-tension curve was generated by reducing muscle length in 0.1 mm steps from the length associated with maximum developed isometric force (L$_{max}$) to approximately 80% of L$_{max}$ while recording resting and developed force. The relationship between force (load) and velocity of muscle shortening for a series of afterloaded contractions was established at L$_{max}$ by progressively increasing the total load on the muscle from preload to the isometric level by varying the current passed through the servo-motor. Isotonic contractions were interposed after ten sequential isometric beats to minimize the effects of prior loading history on contractile activity.

Electrical recordings were obtained during isometric and isotonic contractions with microelectrodes filled with 3 M potassium chloride (KCl). Transmembrane potential was measured as the voltage difference between the intracellular electrode and a sintered silver/silver chloride (Ag/AgCl) ground electrode (immersed in the fluid perfusing the tissue) which served as a reference.[25] The 3 M KCl filled electrode was connected via a 3 M KCl Ag/AgCl bridge to a preamplifier. The microelectrode amplifier (Rockefeller University) has input capacity neutralization to permit accurate measurement of the upstroke velocity of the transmembrane action potential.

The parameters of muscle force and its first derivative, muscle length, velocity, and transmembrane electrical events were displayed as a function of time on a multichannel storage oscilloscope (Tektronix, 5115). At the completion of each experiment, the muscle length at L_{max} was measured and the muscle was then blotted dry and weighed. The cross-sectional area of the muscle was calculated, assuming the geometry of a cylinder with a specific gravity of 1.0. Force and the rate of force change were divided by the cross-sectional area to obtain tension and rate of tension change. Velocity was normalized by division by muscle length at L_{max}. Photographic records were obtained with a Tektronix C5A Polaroid oscilloscopic camera.

Studies of Contractile Proteins: Hearts were stored at $-80°C$ in 50% glycerol containing 50 mM KCl and 10 mM potassium phosphate (KPO_4), pH 7.0, before the extracts were prepared. In all cases the hearts that were examined for calcium activated adenosine triphosphatase (ATPase) activity were the same hearts from which papillary muscles were removed and utilized for mechanical and electrical studies.

The methods for preparing and analyzing cardiac actomyosin from individual hearts have been described previously.[31] The advantage of this preparation is that individual hearts can be analyzed, and, therefore, it is not necessary to pool hearts, which is required for purification of myosin. Actomyosin ATPase has been shown generally to correlate with the calcium ATPase of myosin and actin-activated magnesium ATPase activity of myosin.[32] The ventricles were minced and homogenized in 0.05 M KCl, 0.01 M KPO_4 (pH 7.0) and centrifuged. The pellets were further treated with 0.05 M KCl, 0.01 M KPO_4, and 2 mM ethylene glycol-bis (beta-aminolthyl ether)-N,N'-tetraacetic acid (EGTA), pH 7.0, followed by washing with buffer containing 0.1% Triton X-100. Actomyosin was extracted and isolated from the myofibrils with 10 volumes of 0.6 M KCl, 10 mM imidazole, and 1.0 mM dithiothreotol (DTT), pH 7.0 for 20 hours.

The extract was centrifuged at 10,000 × g for 30 minutes. The supernatant was diluted ten fold with cold deionized water containing 10 mM imidazole and 1.0 mM DTT (pH 7.0). The precipitated actomyosin was redissolved in 1.0 M KCl and 20 mM imidazole (pH 7.0) and the volume adjusted to bring the KCl concentration to 0.6 M. The dilution-precipitation cycle was repeated once more. The final precipitate was dissolved in 0.6 M KCl, 10 mM imidazole, 1.0 mM DTT (pH 7.0) and used as actomyosin. All the homogenization, centrifugation, and extraction procedures were carried out in the cold (4°C).

Measurements of ATPase activity were performed in a final volume of 2.0 ml at pH 7.6 and 30°C. For the Ca^{2+}-dependent ATPase of actomyosin, the reaction mixture consisted of 0.3 M KCl, 0.05 M Tris- Cl, pH 7.6, 0.01 M CaCl$_2$, 0.005 M Na$_2$-ATP and 75 to 100 μg of actomyosin. The reaction was initiated by the addition of the substrate and terminated after 10 minutes by the addition of 1.0 ml of cold 10% trichloroacetic acid. Inorganic phosphate (Pi) was determined by the method of Fiske and Subbarow.[33] Protein concentration was determined by the biuret technique using bovine serum albumin as a standard. Results are expressed as micromoles of Pi liberated per minute per milligram of protein at 30°C.

Data Analysis: Parameters used to characterize animal groups were body weight, dry heart weight, heart weight to body weight ratio, and blood pressure. Parameters used to characterize individual papillary muscles were muscle length, muscle weight, and muscle cross-sectional area.

For isometric contractions, the following parameters were measured: resting tension, peak isometric developed tension, time to peak tension, and time to one-half relaxation. For isotonic contractions, the following parameters were measured: peak isotonic shortening, time to peak shortening, velocity of isotonic shortening, and velocity of isotonic relaxation.

Parameters dependent on muscle length and load were computed at intervals of 1% L$_{max}$ and 5% relative load [(total isotonic load/total isometric load) $\times$ 100], respectively, by linear interpolation of experimental data.

The following action potential parameters were measured: total amplitude and resting membrane potential and duration to 50% and 75% of complete repolarization. The result reported for each action potential parameter is the mean value from three separate impalements along the length of each muscle.

Values obtained from mechanical determinations are presented as mean $\pm$ SE. The statistical significance of differences in mean values for mechanical parameters was assessed by Student's *t*-test.[34] Measured data were analyzed by one-way analysis of variance and the Scheffe multiple comparison test or by two-way analysis of variance.[35] A p value of <0.05 was considered statistically significant.

Results

General Features: General features of the experimental model of renovascular hypertension and its regression are shown in Table I. Results of body weight, heart weight, heart weight to body weight ratio, blood pressure, and bilateral kidney measurements are shown for control and hypertensive animals at 10 weeks after the development of hypertension and after the subsequent reduction of systolic blood pressure (150 mmHg or less) in hypertensive animals for an additional 10 weeks. Heart weights of hypertensive animals were significantly greater than of control animals. Similarly, heart weight to body weight ratios of hypertensive animals were significantly greater than of age-matched controls. Blood pressure values of hypertensive animals showed persistent elevations above controls throughout the 20-week study.

TABLE I   General Features of Control, Hypertensive, and Reversal Animals*

	10 Weeks (n = 8)		20 Weeks (n = 10)		
	Control	Hypertensive	Control	Hypertensive	Reversal
Body weight (g)	267	271	285	280	286
	±5.3	±4.6	±5.7	±6.0	±6.3
p		NS		NS	NS
Heart weight (g)	0.66	0.98	0.68	0.96	0.72
	±0.03	±0.04	±0.02	±0.04	±0.02
p		<0.01		<0.01	<0.01
Heart weight to body weight ratio (mg/g)	2.47	3.62	2.39	3.42	2.51
	±0.08	±0.09	±0.10	±0.10	±0.08
p		<0.01		<0.01	<0.01
Systolic blood pressure (mmHg)	125	186	122	193	120
	±5.0	±5.6	±4.3	±7.1	±6.7
p		<0.01		<0.01	<0.01
Right kidney (g)	0.93	1.25	1.00	1.45	2.13
	±0.01	±0.07	±0.02	±0.05	±0.04†
p		<0.01		<0.01	<0.01
Left kidney (g)	0.95	0.91	0.98	0.81	—
	±0.02	±0.03	±0.04	±0.03	
p		NS		<0.01	

NS = not significant.
*Values are from female animals and are means ± SE.
†Significantly different from control.

Because the left kidney was uniformly involved in the surgical renal artery stenosis, its weight progressively decreased during the course of hypertension, whereas the contralateral kidney increased in weight significantly above the control level (Table I). At 20 weeks after the onset of hypertension, heart weights of reversal animals were virtually identical to control animals. Blood pressure values of hypertensive animals decreased precipitously on removal of the left kidney. Blood pressure decreased to control levels within 24 hours after nephrectomy.

Myocardial Performance: Isometric contractions. Isometric contraction data obtained for all experimental groups are shown in Table II. Also shown are average muscle length, muscle weight, and calculated cross-sectional area. Muscle weight in hypertensive animals was significantly greater than controls, although no difference in muscle length was observed. Therefore, muscle from hypertensive animals displayed a significantly greater cross-sectional area.

Developed tension remained similar in all groups throughout the 20-week study. Time to peak tension (TPT) and time to one-half relaxation (T1/2R) increased in hypertensive muscles, whereas reversal preparations showed values similar to those of controls. Of note was the fact that TPT and T1/2R did not show progressive change between 10 and 20 weeks of hypertension in the hypertensive group.

Significant differences were noted in the peak rate of tension decay among the groups throughout the 20-week period. The time to peak rate of tension

TABLE II   **Isometric Data from Control, Hypertensive, and Reversal Animals***

	10 Weeks (n = 8)		20 Weeks (n = 10)		
	Control	Hypertensive	Control	Hypertensive	Reversal
Muscle length (mm)	6.0	6.1	5.7	6.1	6.2
	±0.3	±0.3	±0.3	±0.3	±0.3
p		NS		NS	NS
Muscle weight (mg)	5.1	6.4	5.5	6.6	6.0
	±0.3	±0.4	±0.4	±0.4	±0.4
p		<0.05		<0.05	NS
Muscle cross-sectional area (mm^2)	0.85	1.05	0.96	1.08	0.97
	±0.06	±0.07	±0.07	±0.07	±0.07
p		<0.05		NS	NS
Resting tension (g/mm^2)	1.94	2.01	2.10	2.05	1.97
	±0.34	±0.40	±0.24	±0.30	±0.31
p		NS		NS	NS
Developed tension (g/mm^2)	6.30	6.70	7.30	7.89	7.21
	±0.56	±0.51	±0.62	±0.67	±0.45
p		NS		NS	NS
Time to peak tension (ms)	119	153	125	155	123
	±1.8	±2.3	±2.1	±2.3	±1.8
p		<0.01		<0.01	<0.01
Time to ½ relaxation (ms)	143	165	146	170	144
	±2.8	±3.0	±2.7	±2.4	±2.1
p		<0.01		<0.01	<0.01
Peak rate of tension rise (g/mm^2/s)	101	96	96	89	97
	±6.3	±5.6	±6.4	±5.7	±5.6
p		NS		NS	NS
Peak rate of tension decay (g/mm^2/s)	56	44	53	41	55
	±2.0	±2.4	±1.8	±2.4	±2.1
p		<0.05		<0.05	<0.05
Time to peak rate of tension rise (ms)	48	68	50	71	48
	±0.3	±0.4	±0.5	±0.7	±0.4
p		<0.01		<0.01	<0.01
Time to peak rate of tension decay (ms)	123	145	126	151	123
	±2.1	±3.1	±2.5	±3.4	±2.3
p		<0.01		<0.01	<0.01

NS = not significant.

*Values are from female animals and are means ± SE. All values are obtained at L$_{max}$.

rise and the time to peak rate of tension decay were significantly prolonged in hypertensive animals when compared with control or reversal preparations. Data from reversal animals were virtually identical to those of controls (Table II).

Passive and active length-tension relationships among the experimental groups show no differences in resting length-tension relationships at 10 or 20 weeks after the onset of hypertension among control, hypertensive, and reversal animals. Analysis of developed tension showed no significant differences among any of the groups studied.

The time course of representative isometric contractions from muscles removed from control, hypertensive, and reversal groups is depicted in Figure 1A. This figure depicts, in addition, the method for measurement of

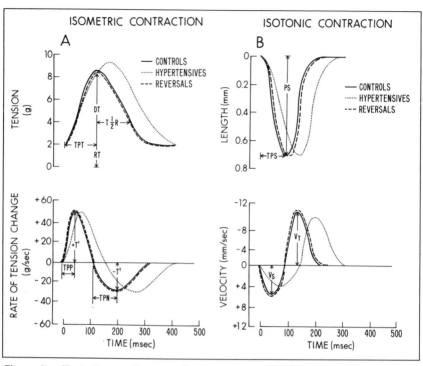

Figure 1. *Illustrative papillary muscle contractions at L_{max} from female animals during the 20-week study (similar results were seen in males). A: Isometric contractions from female control, hypertensive, and reversal preparations. Tension **(upper panel)** and the rate of tension change **(lower panel)** are plotted against time. Mechanical parameters are indicated by arrows pointing to the control trace. RT = resting tension; DT = developed tension; TPT = time to peak tension; T1/2R = time to one-half relaxation (50% DT); +T' = peak rate of tension rise; −T' = peak rate of tension decay; TPP = time to +T'; TPN = time to −T'. B: Isotonic contractions from female control, hypertensive, and reversal preparations. Relative loads [(total isotonic load/total isometric load) × 100] were identical for control, hypertensive, and reversal preparations. Muscle length **(upper panel)** and velocity **(lower panel)** are plotted against time. PS = peak shortening; TPS = time to peak shortening; Vs = peak velocity of shortening; Vr = peak velocity of relengthening.*

various parameters of isometric force development and the rate of force development.

Isotonic contractions. Data from isotonic contractions obtained at an external bath calcium of 2.4 mM are shown in Table III. No significant differences among control, hypertensive, and reversal preparations were observed in the amount of shortening from preload alone at L_{max}. Time to peak shortening (TPS), on the other hand, was significantly prolonged in muscles from hypertensive animals at both study points. Peak velocity of shortening (Vs) at a relative load of 50% was significantly depressed in muscles from

TABLE III   **Isotonic Data from Control, Hypertensive, and Reversal Animals***

	10 Weeks (n = 8)		20 Weeks (n = 10)		
	Control	Hypertensive	Control	Hypertensive	Reversal
Peak shortening muscle length (%)	5.8	5.6	5.9	6.1	6.2
	±0.3	±0.4	±0.3	±0.4	±0.3
p		NS		NS	NS
Time to peak shortening (ms)	121	160	124	162	127
	±3.1	±5.0	±2.3	±5.6	±3.0
p		<0.01		<0.01	<0.01
Peak velocity of shortening	0.77	0.61	0.75	0.59	0.76
(muscle length/s)	±0.02	±0.02	±0.02	±0.02	±0.02
p		<0.01		<0.01	<0.01
Peak velocity of relengthening	0.98	0.95	0.94	0.93	0.95
(muscle length/s)	±0.04	±0.03	±0.03	±0.03	±0.03
p		NS		NS	NS
Time to peak velocity of	67	72	71	75	69
shortening (ms)	±3.0	±2.9	±2.8	±2.5	±2.5
p		NS		NS	NS
Time to peak velocity of	48	58	52	61	50
relengthening (ms)	±2.0	±1.0	±2.1	±2.3	±1.8
p		<0.05		<0.05	<0.05

NS = not significant.
*Values are from female animals and are means ± SE. All values are obtained at an initial muscle length of L_{max} and of a relative load [(total isotonic load/total isometric load) × 100] of 50%.

hypertensive animals at 10 and 20 weeks after the onset of hypertension. Time to peak shortening and Vs values for reversal animals were virtually identical to those of age-matched controls.

Representative isotonic contractions for muscles from all groups, shown in Figure 1B, depict the general character of an isotonic contraction. They also illustrate the method for measuring length and velocity of shortening. Force-velocity curves comparing data of hypertensive and control rats at 10 and 20 weeks after the onset of hypertension were significantly depressed in the hypertensive muscles at all relative loads studied. Force-velocity curves of muscles from reversal animals were similar to controls at all relative loads.

Tables II and III show that the contractile alterations observed in hypertrophied muscles reverse when hypertrophy regresses and that even after 20 weeks of hypertension, tension and peak shortening do not change. Thus, the prolonged course of tension development, relaxation, shortening, and relengthening seen in hypertensive animals 20 weeks after the onset of hypertension is not seen in reversal muscles that have timing parameters similar to control muscles.

Electrical Characteristics: General characteristics of the transmembrane action potential from control, hypertensive, and reversal animals are shown in Table IV. At the 10-week time point, there was no significant difference in the values for resting membrane potential or amplitude. Similarly, there was no significant difference in the values for resting membrane potential and amplitude at 20 weeks. Typical tracing of isometric tension and simultaneously recorded action potentials from control, hypertensive, and

TABLE IV   **Electrical Data from Control, Hypertensive, and Reversal Animals***

	10 Weeks (n = 10)		20 Weeks (n = 10)		
	Control	Hypertensive	Control	Hypertensive	Reversal
Resting membrane potential (mV)	83	83	84	82	79
	±3.0	±3.0	±4.0	±3.0	±3.0
p		NS		NS	NS
Amplitude of transmembrane action potential (mV)	110	115	110	113	109
	±4.0	±5.0	±5.0	±4.0	±4.0
		NS		NS	NS
Action potential duration at 50% repolarization (ms)					
Isometric	23.8	61.6	26.9	70.0	27.5
	±1.1	±2.1	±1.0	±2.0	±1.5
p		<0.01		<0.01	<0.01
Isotonic	21.0	52.9	22.9	60.3	24.4
	±1.0	±2.2	±1.0	±2.2	±1.1
p		<0.01		<0.01	<0.01
Action potential duration at 75% repolarization (ms)					
Isometric	48.9	107.1	58.4	116.6	55.6
	±2.3	±2.1	±1.5	±2.1	±1.8
p		<0.01		<0.01	<0.01
Isotonic	44.9	98.0	50.9	108.3	50.6
	±1.0	±2.1	±1.3	±2.0	±1.7
p		<0.01		<0.01	<0.01

*Values are from male animals and are means ± SE. Resting membrane potential and amplitude of the transmembrane action potential were obtained during isometric contractions at a muscle length of L_{max}. Isotonic data were obtained at an initial muscle length of L_{max} and an afterload that was set at preload.

reversal preparations reveal that the action potential recorded from preparations from animals hypertensive for 20 weeks is substantially longer than that recorded from control muscles. The prolonged action potential of the hypertensive muscle is accompanied by an isometric contraction that is similar in developed tension to that of control preparations. However, a longer time is required to reach this level of peak tension. In contrast, the action potential and isometric contraction recorded from reversal muscles are virtually identical to control traces.

Table II shows that animals hypertensive for 10 weeks have significantly longer action potentials than age-matched controls and that the action potentials recorded during isotonic contractions are significantly shorter than those observed during isometric contraction. The fact that a significant interaction is present between groups and type of contraction indicates that the significant difference is probably between isometric and isotonic contractions of hypertensive muscles.

Table II also shows that the action potential prolongation observed in hypertrophied fibers reverses after regression of hypertrophy. Thus, action potentials of hypertensive muscles are significantly longer than those of both

TABLE V   **ATPase Data from Control, Hypertensive, and Reversal Animals***

	10 Weeks		20 Weeks		
	Control	Hypertensive	Control	Hypertensive	Reversal
ATPase†	0.705	0.523	0.669	0.560	0.668
	±0.006	±0.017	±0.008	±0.023	±0.017
p		<0.01		<0.01 <0.05	
Number hearts	5	4	7	12	9

*Values are obtained from hearts from female rats and are means ± SE.
†ATPase is actomyosin calcium. ATPase activity is expressed as micromole of p/mg/min.

control and reversal muscles during both isometric and isotonic contractions. In contrast, the duration of action potentials of reversal and control muscles is almost identical during both isometric and isotonic contractions.

Contractile Protein Biochemistry: Table V shows actomyosin ATPase activity of preparations from the hearts of control, hypertensive, and reversal animals. Actomyosin ATPase activity was significantly depressed in preparations from hearts of all groups of hypertensive animals. Actomyosin ATPase activity in preparations from the hearts of reversal animals was not significantly depressed compared with the actomyosin ATPase activity in preparations from control animals. The sodium dodecyl sulfate gel electrophoretic bands for myosin from control, hypertensive, and reversal animals did not show any visible differences.

Comment

A good deal of controversy still exists regarding the effects of hypertrophy on myocardial contractile force expressed per unit mass. In previous studies LVH was induced in the rat by banding the ascending aorta and it was found that an increase in the isometric force developed per unit of muscle weight.[36] However, other investigators found no difference in peak isometric-developed tension of LV papillary muscles from rats with moderated LVH (10%) produced by either exercise or aortic coarctation.[37] Furthermore, Spann et al[7] reported a reduction in the peak preloaded shortening velocity, the rate of isometric tension development, and peak isometric tension of right ventricular (RV) papillary muscle obtained from cats with 90% hypertrophy after experimentally produced pulmonary artery stenosis. In the same study, a more severe decrease in contractile indices was observed when congestive heart failure developed. These results were similar to those of Bing[1] utilizing the isolated LV trabeculae carnae muscle of male Wistar rats.

Initial depression of the contractile state of hypertrophied heart muscle may not always persist, since myocardial contractility returned to normal when the acutely induced overload was sustained for longer periods of time. Williams and Potter[38] found that 6 weeks after acute banding of the cat pulmonary artery, which resulted in a 69% increase in RV mass, the active length-tension curve, maximal rate of increase of isometric force, force-velocity relations, and isometric force during paired stimulation of the papillary muscle were reduced. These parameters returned to control levels by 24 weeks after pulmonary artery banding. However, the degree of hypertrophy after 24 weeks had curiously decreased from 69% to 38%. Jouannot and Hatt[19] observed a similar recovery of an initially depressed contractile state.

In studies utilizing pulmonary artery banding, unloaded velocity of shortening and rate of force development were decreased, although force per unit area of muscle was only slightly reduced.[6,7] When congestive heart failure ensued, all of these measurements were further depressed. Force-frequency relations were subtly altered, but increased extracellular calcium returned performance to normal.[6,7] In addition, myofibrillar ATPase was depressed, catecholamines were depleted from the myocardium, and the connective tissue was increased.[6,7,14] The damaging effects that an acute severe systolic overload might produce[6,7] and the reversibility of the process were not explored at this time. However, common to all these studies was the fact that the load was suddenly placed on the myocardium rather than applied gradually, as occurs with essential hypertension.

A precise definition of the course and degree of contractile alterations in the hypertrophied heart is important in the critical evaluation and treatment of clinical conditions associated with pressure overloads. In the present study the gradual application of a pressure overload was accomplished by the creation of left renal artery stenosis. Ten weeks after the development of hypertension, normalization of systolic blood pressure was produced by unilateral nephrectomy of the ischemic kidney, and experiments were conducted to determine the reversibility of contractile abnormalities. In comparison to acute banding[14,39] this model more closely simulates a gradual pressure overload, as occurs with chronic systemic hypertension or valvular stenosis.

In examining the effects of pressure overload on cardiac function in dogs 3 days after bilateral renal artery constriction, Ferrario et al[40] found that the relationship described by stroke volume and end-diastolic pressure was shifted downward and to the right. In the same study, dogs with severe hypertension had significantly greater LV end-diastolic pressure (12 ± 2 mmHg) compared with animals with moderate hypertension (7 ± 3 mmHg). Furthermore, under conditions of fluid loading, hypertensive animals were unable to increase cardiac output to a similar degree as control animals.

Utilizing bilateral renal artery constriction in rats, Ferrone et al[8] found that renovascularly hypertensive, spontaneously hypertensive, and control animals had similar cardiac outputs. Although these investigators studied the effects of hypertension only 14 days after the initiation of the pressure overload, they did find that total peripheral resistance was elevated significantly and to the same degree in either model of hypertension. Using a 2-kidney, 1-clip Goldblatt hypertensive rat, other workers[11] determined from cardiac function curves that chronic renovascular hypertension was associated with a depressed cardiac reserve due either to diminished contractility or reduced ventricular compliance. In addition to significant hypertrophy (44%) in this model, there was a two fold increase in myocardial connective tissue, and both these factors may account for the observed reduction in ventricular compliance. In addition, the rate of increase of blood pressure and the duration of hypertension before study was highly variable (6 to 22 weeks after the onset of hypertension) and may have significantly affected their results.

Examining a model of pressure overload hypertrophy created by surgical constriction of the pulmonary artery in cats, Spann et al[6,7] and Carey et al[41] have shown, using isolated RV papillary muscles, that contractility is depressed, whereas Natarajan et al[42] concluded that this depression may, in part, be due to an increase in the stiffness of hypertrophied muscles. However, this point was addressed recently in a study conducted by Bing et al[13] in which the lathyrogen beta-amino proprionitrile, which inhibits the cross-linking of both collagen and elastin, was fed to rats 14 to 21 days after surgical coarctation of the ascending aorta. This study showed that blocking collagen synthesis in the renovascular hypertensive rat model did not alter the functional alterations as the hearts hypertrophied. These data suggest that the increase in extracellular connective tissue associated with the hypertrophic process is not responsible for alterations in myocardial contractility observed in later stages of myocardial hypertrophy. In addition, others, studying chemically skinned RV muscle bundles from hypertrophied rabbit hearts, found a 34% reduction in Vs and a similar depression in the calcium and actin-activated myosin ATPase activity.[43] However, no depression in force was seen in hypertrophied myocardium.

In the present study as well as in an earlier investigation,[23–25] we have confirmed that hypertrophied myocardium produced by gradual-onset renovascular hypertension in rats also displays significant reductions in muscle speed but muscle force development is well maintained. Previous studies from our laboratory suggest that with gradual application of a pressure overload, little if any acute myocardial damage occurs, because peak force development at 5 weeks of hypertension was elevated above controls and no changes were seen in the force-velocity relationship between hypertensive and control animals. However, with extension of the duration of hypertension to 10 weeks, although force development was maintained above control levels, significant depression of the force velocity relationship was observed along with significant prolongation of the TPT. Sampling animals from the same initial group after 20 and 30 weeks of hypertension revealed a progressive depression of force-velocity characteristics, whereas force development remained above control level. This finding suggests that a dissociation between commonly used measures of contractility, that is, peak force development and velocity of shortening, occurs during gradual-onset myocardial hypertrophy. The dissociation may result from membrane alterations, already found to produce prolongation of action potential duration,[25,44] that can permit maintenance of force development whereas contractile protein alterations, occurring simultaneously, lead to depressions of velocity of shortening and myosin ATPase activity.[24] If this were the case, one would expect longer term studies to show late deterioration of force-development capacity as the contractile proteins defect worsened. Studies of this nature are currently under way and should help explain apparent discrepancies noted on the directional changes of force development and velocity of shortening during the early period (5 to 30 weeks) after the development of stable hypertensive hypertrophy. When force-velocity curves were expressed and analyzed as a function of relative load, the highly significant depression of preloaded velocity of shortening in hypertensive muscles remained. This strongly suggests that these muscles in fact had different zero-load velocity intercepts and therefore exhibited different levels of contractility.

The mechanism of the alterations in force-velocity relations seen in this model of hypertension remains obscure. A major assumption made in the present study is that the localized damage produced by clamping of the muscle ends[45,46] is similar in all groups studied. Although direct studies of sarcomere dynamics would be desirable to solve this potential complexity in the present study, the muscles derived from the left ventricle are generally too large to be studied in this manner. In recent studies[26] internal shortening was analyzed by measuring the separation between two fine markers inserted into the undamaged midregion of the muscle. These types of studies have shown that no noticeable differences exist between control and experimental groups in damage due to clamping the ends of the muscle. Morphologic studies of hypertrophied myocardium from renovascular rats[47] have shown that average sarcomere length determined in both control and hypertensive animals after 8 weeks of hypertension was not changed from the control value. However, the ratio of myofibrillar volume to total cell volume in the hypertrophic muscle was significantly higher than controls at both 8 and 24 weeks of hypertrophy. The increase in myofibrillar volume occurred at the expense of mitochondrial volume, which was decreased in comparison to the control hearts, at each study point. In this study,[47] hearts hypertrophied for 24 weeks showed heterogeneity in their histologic appearance. Some animals showed vessel-wall alterations and diffuse fibrosis, whereas others showed only the characteristic changes of cellular enlargement and no connective tissue changes. It was in the group showing significant extracellular disturbance that mechanical alterations were the most pronounced. These findings suggest that any progressive mechanical alterations seen with pressure overload hypertrophy may occur as a result of an increase in extracellular connective tissue and vessel wall alterations that lead to myocardial ischemia.[47]

These aberrations are invariably accompanied by a significant prolongation in the duration of contraction and a slowing of isotonic and isometric measures of relaxation. The reductions in actomyosin ATPase activity observed in this study correlate and may be responsible for the depressions in muscle Vs but do not explain the unaltered force development capacity or the prolongation of contraction.[48–55]

Our studies have also shown that all of the observed mechanical alterations in this model are reversible after 10 weeks of hypertension if blood pressure is normalized for 10 weeks. Irreversible myocardial dysfunction, therefore, does not result from 10 weeks of hypertension if blood pressure is normalized for 10 weeks. What duration of hypertension or, more importantly, what specific factor is associated with the development of irreversible contractile alterations in chronic systemic hypertension-induced myocardial hypertrophy is the subject of current studies in our laboratory.

Acknowledgment

Supported in parts by NIH Grants # HL 21993-03, # HL 07071-05, and # HL 18824-08. Dr. Joseph M. Capasso is a recipient of a Herman Raucher Investigatorship Award of the New York Heart Association.

References

1. BING OHL, MATSHUSHITA S, FANBURG BL, LEVINE HJ: Mechanical properties of rat cardiac muscle during experimental hypertrophy. Circ Res 1971; 28: 234–245.
2. MEERSON FZ, KAPELKO VI: The contractile function of the myocardium in two types of cardiac adaptation to a chronic load. Cardiology 1972; 57: 183–199.
3. ALPERT NR, HAMRELL B, HALPERN W: Mechanical and biochemical correlates of cardiac hypertrophy. Circ Res 1974; 34: 71–82.
4. COOPER G IV, SATAVA M, HARRISON CE, COLEMAN HN III: Mechanisms for the abnormal energetics of pressure-induced hypertrophy of the cat myocardium. Circ Res 1973; 33: 213–233.
5. SASAYAMA S, ROSS J, FRANKLIN D, BLOOR CM, BISHOP S, DILLEY RB: Adaptations of the left ventricle to chronic pressure overload. Circ Res 1977; 38: 172–178.
6. SPANN JF, CHIDSEY CA, POOL PE, BRAUNWALD E: Mechanism of norepinephrine depletion in experimental heart failure produced by aortic constriction in the guinea pig. Circ Res 1965; 17: 312–321.
7. SPANN JF, COVELL JW, ECKBERG DL, SONNENBLICK EH, ROSS J, BRAUNWALD E: Contractile performance of the hypertrophied and chronically failing cat ventricle. Am J Physiol 1972; 233: 1150–1157.
8. FERRONE RA, WALSH GM, TSUCHIYA M, FROHLICH ED: Comparison of hemodynamics in conscious spontaneous and renal hypertensive rats. Am J Physiol 1979; 236: H403–H408.
9. LUND DD, TWIETMEYER TA, SCHMILD PG, TOMANEK RJ: Independent changes in cardiac muscle fibers and connective tissue in rats with spontaneous hypertension, aortic constriction and hypoxia. Cardiovasc Res 1979; 13: 39–44.
10. WEIGMAN DL, JOSHUA IG, MORFF RJ, HARRIS PD, MILLER FN: Microvascular responses to norepinephrine in renovascular and spontaneously hypertensive rats. Am J Physiol 1979; 236: H545–H548.
11. AVERILL DB, FERRARIO CM, TARAZI RC, SEN S, BAJBUS R: Cardiac performance in rats with renal hypertension. Circ Res 1976; 38: 280–288.
12. WOLINSKY H: Effects of hypertension and its reversal on the thoracic aorta of male and female rats. Circ Res 1971; 28: 622–636.
13. BING OHL, FANBURG BL, BROOKS WW, MATSHUSHITA S: The effect of the lathyrogen b-amino proprionitril (BAPN) on the mechanical properties of experimentally hypertrophied rat cardiac muscle. Circ Res 1978; 43: 632–637.

14. Buccino RH, Harris E, Spann JF, Sonnenblick EH: Response of myocardial connective tissue to development of experimental hypertrophy. Am J Physiol 1969; 216: 425–428.

15. Bishop SP: Structural alterations of the myocardium induced by chronic work overload. In: Bloor CM, ed. Comparative pathophysiology of circulatory disturbances. New York: Plenum Press, 1972; 289–314.

16. Coulson RL, Yazdanfar S, Rubio E, Bove AA, Lemole GM, Spann JF: Recuperative potential of cardiac muscle following relief of pressure overload hypertrophy and right ventricular failure in the cat. Circ Res 1977; 40: 41–49.

17. Hatt PY, Jouannot P, Moraves J, Perennec J, Laplace M: Development and reversal of pressure-induced cardiac hypertrophy. Basic Res Cardiol 1978; 73: 405–421.

18. Hickson RC, Hammons GT, Holloszy JO: Development and regression of exercise-induced cardiac hypertrophy in rats. Am J Physiol 1979; 236: H268–H272.

19. Jouannot P, Hatt PY: Rat myocardial mechanics during pressure-induced hypertrophy development and reversal. Am J Physiol 1975; 299: 355–364.

20. Williams JR Jr, Harrison TR, Grollman A: Simple method for determining systolic blood pressure of unanesthetized rat. J Clin Invest 1939; 18: 373–376.

21. Bunag RD, McCubbin JW, Page IH: Lack of correlation between direct and indirect measurement of arterial pressure in unanesthetized rats. Cardiovasc Res 1971; 5: 24–31.

22. Thurston H, Bing RF, Surales SD: Reversal of two-kidney one clip renovascular hypertension in the rat. Hypertension 1980; 2: 256–265.

23. Capasso JM, Strobeck JE, Sonnenblick EH: Myocardial mechanical alterations during gradual onset long-term hypertension in rats. Am J Physiol 1981; 241: H435–H441.

24. Capasso JM, Strobeck JE, Malhotra A, Scheuer J, Sonnenblick EH: Contractile behavior of rat myocardium after reversal of hypertensive hypertrophy. Am J Physiol 1982; 242: H882–H889.

25. Capasso JM, Aronson RS, Sonnenblick EH: Reversible alterations in excitation-contraction coupling during myocardial hypertrophy in rat papillary muscle. Circ Res 1982; 51: 189–195.

26. Capasso JM, Krueger JW, Sonnenblick EH: Distinctions between internal shortening and contractile element dynamics in isolated heart muscle. Fed Proc 1982; 41: 1014.

27. Capasso JM, Remily RM, Sonnenblick RM: Alterations in mechanical properties of rat papillary muscle during maturation. Am J Physiol 1982; 242: H359–H364.

28. Capasso JM, Sonnenblick EH: Post-natal developmental changes in myocardial contractility in the female Wistar rat. Exp Gerontol 1982d; 17: 195–203.

29. Pool PE, Chandler BM, Sonnenblick EH, Braunwald E: Integrity of energy stores in cat papillary muscle. Effects of temperature and frequency of contraction on high energy phosphate stores. Circ Res 1968; 22: 213–219.

30. Whalen WJ: Oxygen availability in muscle. In: Tanz RJ, Kavaler F, Roberts J, eds. Factors influencing myocardial contractility. New York: Academic Press, 1967; 395–400.

31. Bhan AK, Scheuer J: Effect of physical training on cardiac actomyosin adenosine

triphosphate activity. Am J Physiol 1972; 223: 1486–1490.

32. MALHOTRA A, PENPARGKUL S, FEIN FS, SONNENBLICK EH, SCHEUER J: Effects of streptozocin-induced diabetes in rats on cardiac proteins. Circ Res 1981; 49: 1243–1250.

33. FISKE CH, SUBBAROW Y: The colorimetric determination of phosphorus. J Biol Chem 1925; 66: 375–400.

34. NIE NH, HULL CH, JENKINS JG, STEINBRENNER K, BENT DH: Statistical package for the social sciences. New York: McGraw-Hill, 1970.

35. SNEDECOR GW, COCHRAN WG: Statistical methods. Ames: The Iowa State University Press, 1980; 215–237.

36. KERR AA, WINTERBERGER AR, GIANBATTISTA SM: Tension developed by papillary muscles from hypertrophied rat hearts. Circ Res 1951; 9: 103–105.

37. GRIMM AF, KUBOTA R, WHITEHORN WV: Properties of the myocardium in cardiomegaly. Circ Res 1963; 12: 118–124.

38. WILLIAMS JP, POTTER RD: Normal contractile state of hypertrophied myocardium after pulmonary artery constriction in the cat. J Clin Invest 1974; 54: 1266–1272.

39. BEZNAK M, KORECKY B, THOMAS G: Regression of cardiac hypertrophies of various origins. Can J Physiol Pharmacol 1969; 47: 579–586.

40. FERRARIO CM, KOSOGLOV A, BAJBUS R, MADZAN GR: Ventricular performance after onset of renal hypertension. Clin Sci Mole Med 1976; 51 (suppl): 141–143.

41. CAREY RA, BOVE AA, COULSON RL, SPANN JF: Recovery of myosin ATPase after relief of pressure-overload hypertrophy and failure. Am J Physiol 1978; 234: H711–H717.

42. NATARAJAN N, BOVE AA, COULSON RL, CAREY RA, SPANN JF: Increased passive stiffness of short term pressure-overload hypertrophied myocardium in the cat. Am J Physiol 1979; 237: H676–H680.

43. MAUGHAN D, LOW E, LITTEN R, BRAYDEN J, ALPERT NR: Calcium activated muscle from hypertrophied rabbit hearts. Circ Res 1979; 44: 279–287.

44. ARONSON RS: Characteristics of action potentials of hypertrophied myocardium from rats with renal hypertension. Circ Res 1980; 47: 443–454.

45. DONALD TC, REEVES DNS, REEVES RC, WALKER AA, HEFFNER LL: Effect of damaged ends in papillary muscle preparations. Am J Physiol 1980; 238: H14–H23.

46. KRUEGER JW, POLLACK GH: Myocardial sarcomere dynamics during isometric contraction. J Physiol (Lond) 1975; 251: 627–643.

47. WENDT-GALLITELLI MF, EBRECHT G, JACOB R: Morphological alterations and their functional interpretation in the hypertrophied myocardium of Goldblatt hypertensive rats. J Mol Cell Cardiol 1979; 11: 275–287.

48. ALPERT NR, GALE HH, TAYLOR N: The effect of age on contractile protein ATPase activity and the velocity of shortening. In: Tanz RD, Kavaler F, Roberts J, eds. Factors influencing myocardial contractility. New York: Academic Press, 1967; 127–133.

49. BARANY M: ATPase activity of myosin correlated with speed of muscle shortening. J Gen Physiol 1967; 50: 197–218.

50. BODEM R, SONNENBLICK EH: Mechanical activity of mammalian heart muscle; variable onset, species difference and the effect of caffeine. Am J Physiol 1975; 228: 250–261.

51. BREISCH EA, BOVE AA, PHILLIPS SJ: Myocardial morphometrics in pressure over-

load left ventricular hypertrophy and regression. Cardiovasc Res 1980; 14: 161–168.

52. DELCAYRE C, SWYNGHEDAUW B: A comparative study of heart myosin: ATPase and light subunits from different species. Pfluegers Arch 1975; 355: 39–47.

53. SORDHAL LA, McCOLLUM WB, WOOD WG, SCHWARTZ A: Mitochondria and sarcoplasmic reticulum function in cardiac hypertrophy and failure. Am J Physiol 1973; 224: 497–502.

54. SPECH MM, FERRARIO CM, TARAZI RC: Cardiac pumping ability following reversal of hypertrophy and hypertension in spontaneously hypertensive rats. Hypertension 1980; 2: 75–82.

55. WEBER K, OSBORN M: Reliability of molecular determinations of dodecyl sulfate polyacrylamide gel electrophoresis. J Biol Chem 1969; 224: 4406–4412.

31

Regression of Cardiac Hypertrophy: Experimental Animal Model

SUBHA SEN, Ph.D., D.Sc

Cardiac hypertrophy is generally viewed as a compensatory process as a result of the stress imposed on the heart by various disease processes. The compensatory response maintains cardiac function initially, but after the heart is exposed to prolonged stress, cardiac decompensation ultimately supervenes. The relationship between cardiac hypertrophy and decompensation is quite complex and there is still controversy concerning the efficiency of the hypertrophied heart.[1-3] Deterioration of cardiac function as a pump, resulting from cardiac hypertrophy, may be prevented or reversed by appropriate interventions. Pfeffer et al[4] reported that chronic treatment with guanethidine prevented the deterioration in cardiac pumping performance observed in spontaneously hypertensive rats (SHR) with fixed hypertension and hypertrophy. Wicker et al[5] have shown that in hypertensive heart disease, the return of coronary flow reserve to normal was dependent on normalization of the ratio of left ventricular (LV) mass to systemic arterial pressure.

Reversal of cardiac hypertrophy would therefore appear to be a desirable goal because reversing the structural changes of the disease is a better therapeutic achievement than simply arresting its progress. Myocardial hypertrophy can result from many causes or stimuli. The present review is restricted to myocardial hypertrophy in hypertension and its regression in experimental animal models.

Reversal of Myocardial Hypertrophy

Several methods have been used to achieve reversal or prevention of hypertrophy in hypertension, including surgical removal of the causal factor with antihypertensive therapy and prevention of an increase in protein synthesis in the experimental hypertensive rat model.

Patton et al[6] reported regression of hypertrophy following removal of the clipped kidney in the renovascular hypertensive rat model, which later was confirmed by Hall et al.[7] Recently, we have shown[8] that in the renal hypertensive rat, regression of myocardial hypertrophy can be achieved either by

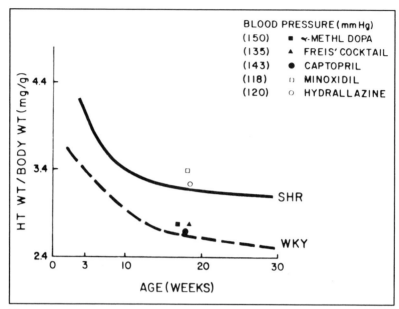

Figure 1. *Effect of antihypertensive drug therapy on heart weight of spontaneously hypertensive rats (SHR) on the background of regression lines of the heart weight to body weight ratio during evolution of hypertrophy and hypertension of SHR and Wistar-Kyoto rats (WKY) (256 rats). Each symbol represents mean heart weight of at least 12 rats.*

removal of the clipped kidney or by therapy with captopril, a converting enzyme inhibitor.

Sen et al[9] have shown that cardiac hypertrophy in SHR can be prevented or reversed by antihypertensive treatment. This has been confirmed by other investigators[10] both in experimental animal models and in humans. One of the most significant results was the marked diversity among various antihypertensive drugs in reversing cardiac hypertrophy, although all reduce arterial pressure to the same degree (Fig. 1). With methyldopa pressure was lowered and cardiac weight was reversed to normal; with hydralazine pressure was controlled but hypertrophy was not reversed;[11] and with minoxidil pressure was lowered but cardiac weight was actually increased.[9] Similar observations have been reported by Yamori et al[12] and Ishise et al.[13] Tomanek et al[10] have shown that regardless of blood pressure control, the use of alpha-methyldopa caused a reversal of hypertrophy in SHR. The varied effects of different antihypertensive drugs on cardiac hypertrophy may conceivably be related to several factors, including effects on catecholamines, hemodynamic changes, cardiac output, heart rate, reflex sympathetic stimulation, and effect on biochemical alteration of cardiac muscles. The striking differences in degree of reversal of hypertrophy between neural blocking agents (20% with methyldopa, 13% with reserpine, and 5% with propranolol) warrant further studies.

Biochemical Changes during Reversal of Myocardial Hypertrophy

In general, to define the biochemical composition, DNA, RNA, and hydroxyproline are measured by most investigators to define alteration in myocardial composition. The DNA concentration serves as an index to differentiate hypertrophy from hyperplasia and RNA serves to assess changes in protein synthesis. The latter changes are also investigated more directly by measuring the rate of incorporation of labeled amino acid to specific proteins. The collagen formation and, by inference, deposition of fibrous tissue are evaluated from changes in ventricular hydroxyproline. Rabinowitz and Zak[14] have shown a direct correlation of change in RNA content with cardiac hypertrophy and its reversal. During development of hypertrophy after aortic banding there was an increase in both RNA concentration and content in the hypertrophied myocardium, which was reversed after surgical removal of the banding. The reversal of hypertrophy under these circumstances probably occurred as a result of inhibition or reduction in protein synthesis. It has been shown repeatedly that the reversal of myocardial hypertrophy is not a result of changes in water content because there is no alteration of the ratio of dry weight to wet weight in all hypertrophied models studied to date. Therefore, the reduction in the heart site is due to reduction in muscle mass. The reduction in muscle mass, again, may be a result of reduction in myosin or collagen content, or both, of the heart as demonstrated by different investigations in different models of myocardial hypertrophy.

Sen and Bumpus[15] have shown an alteration in the rate of collagen synthesis in SHR during the evolution of hypertension. Increase in the rate of synthesis of collagen and a parallel increase in collagen content were observed in young, 4- to 8-week-old SHR as well as in 24-week-old SHR. In young animals, the increase in collagen synthesis occurred in the absence of hypertension, whereas in older animals the collagen increase can be attributed to long-standing hypertension because the increase in the second phase of collagen synthesis is prevented by antihypertensive therapy with alpha-methyldopa and the converting enzyme inhibitor, captopril.[15] Furthermore, Sen[16] has shown that the collagen phenotypic pattern in older SHR differs significantly from that of the Wistar-Kyoto control rats. Again, the alteration of phenotypic pattern can be prevented by therapy with alpha-methyldopa.

Several investigators have reported an early increase in protein synthesis in response to various types of experimental cardiac stress.[17] Nair et al[18] described the sequential changes in DNA, RNA, and DNA-dependent RNA polymerase activity and hydroxyproline content of the heart after banding of the ascending aorta in normal rats. They found an acute increase in DNA, RNA, and hydroxyproline content of the heart within 24 hours of aortic constriction, which reached a maximum level on the second day and was maintained for 2 weeks of the observation period. After removal of the banding, the biochemical pattern returned almost to normal within a short period of time. Grimm et al[19] reported lower myocardial concentration of both DNA and RNA in Wistar rats 5 to 6 months after banding of the abdominal aorta. In contrast with such studies of experimental hypertrophy in SHR, Sen et al[20] have shown that the increase in RNA concentration persists for months. Thus, the rate of variation among biochemical factors appears to differ, depending on the types of stress, whereas RNA concentration was reported to return to normal rapidly after aortic ligation. The increase in RNA with naturally developing hypertension decreased slowly with age despite the persistence of load.

Recently, several investigators reported that myosin, the contractile element of the heart, exists in three different forms of isozymes, V_1, V_2, and V_3, designated according to their electrophoretic mobility, V_1 being the fastest in an electric field and V_3 the slowest. Adenosine triphosphatase (ATPase) activity is highest in V_1 and lowest in V_3. It has been postulated that a heart composed of a higher proportion of V_3 should have less contractile ability. Martin et al[21] have shown a 100% shift in the ratio of V_1 to V_3 in hypertrophied hearts in rabbits after banding of the aorta, compared with nonhypertrophied hearts. Recently, Lompre et al[22] reported a significant shift in the ratio of V_1 to V_3 in 52-week old SHR. Recent data from our laboratory show a significant shift of V_1 to V_3 in 24-week-old SHR.

The importance of alteration in the biochemical composition of the myocardium after reversal of hypertrophy is its implication of functional alteration. It is generally believed that collagen concentration or content may influence the functional capacity of the heart. The thick ventricles secondary to pressure overload contain more collagen than normal, as do the heavy ventricles associated with minoxidil therapy, and regression of hypertrophy and reduction of contractile protein would leave behind an increased concentration of hydroxyproline. This was observed, in fact, in SHR treated with alpha-methyldopa[20] after surgical removal of the clipped kidney in renovascular hypertension[8] and after unbanding the aorta.[23] The lack of regression of collagen after surgical correction or aortic stenosis or after reversal with alpha-methyldopa can be explained by the hypothesis that collagen once formed and extruded into the interstitial space is not accessible to removal, as are the cellular components. This was postulated by Cutiletta et al.[24] However, our studies with the converting enzyme inhibitor captopril do not support this hypothesis.[25] The effects of different antihypertensive drugs on myocardial weight and parallel changes in collagen concentration and content are summarized in Table I. Treatment with alpha-methyldopa and captopril reversed hypertrophy to the same extent in SHR, but the biochemical profile of the myocardium is quite different. Treatment with alpha-methyldopa resulted in an increase in collagen, whereas captopril therapy actually reduced the collagen content of the heart. Therapy with hydralazine, despite normalization of blood pressure, did not alter collagen content or heart weight in SHR. Duration of therapy and age of the animals studied, as well as

TABLE I   Effect of Antihypertensive Drug Therapy on Myocardial Collagen

Therapy SHR	Duration of Treatment (weeks)	Heart Weight/ Body Weight (mg/g)	Collagen	
			Concentration (mg/g)	Content (mg)
No treatment	6	3.5 ± .06	4.0 ± .13	3.70 ± .20
Alpha-methyldopa	6	2.8 ± .05*	4.89 ± .26†	3.80 ± .18
Captopril	6	2.9 ± .04*	4.1 ± .15	3.10 ± .05†
Hydralazine	6	3.4 ± .04	4.1 ± .05	3.8 ± .20

*p < 0.01 compared with untreated controls.
†p < 0.05 compared with untreated controls.

duration of hypertension before therapy is begun, are some of the factors that need further examination to determine the circumstances of reversibility of cardiac collagenous tissue. Specific drug effects may also play an important role, for the type and distribution of collagen fiber appear to be important factors in defining its role in myocardial function.

The relationship of catecholamine to cardiac hypertrophy is a complex, multifaceted interaction, as reviewed by Tarazi et al.[26] Catecholamines can be viewed as inducers of hypertrophy, but, on the other hand, disturbances in cardiac catecholamines can occur secondary to cardiac hypertrophy and show many patterns, depending on the stage and cause of disease, as well as treatment used.

Myocardial Catecholamines in Different Types of Ventricular Hypertrophy

Fischer et al[27] demonstrated that cardiac norepinephrine concentration is reduced with the increase in heart weight secondary to aortic constriction. Subsequently, Spann et al[28] found similar results in hypertrophy secondary to banding of the pulmonary artery. From these and similar results with deoxycorticosterone acetate (DOCA) salt in hypertensive rats, Fanburg[29] concluded that, as a rule, catecholamines are reduced in experimental cardiac hypertrophy. The reduction was attributed to the dilution of the sympathetic nerves due to the increased cardiac mass, since total cardiac norepinephrine was unchanged in moderate hypertrophy.

In contrast to this picture, the relationship between myocardial catecholamine and hypertrophy associated with hypertension is quite different. The amount and concentration of cardiac catecholamines can vary significantly between three different models of hypertension and hypertrophy, as reported by Sen and Tarazi[30] (Table II). In renal hypertensive rats, findings were similar to those resulting from experimental aortic or pulmonary banding. Ventricular catecholamine concentration was reduced, but the total catecholamine content was within normal limits. In SHR, however, the catecholamine concentration was not significantly different from matched controls, resulting in a significantly higher ventricular catecholamine content. In the

TABLE II   **Ventricular Norepinephrine in Hypertensive Rats**

Group	Heart Weight/Body Weight	Norepinephrine (mg/g)
SHR	3.45	580
Renal hypertensive rat	3.3	420*
DOCA salt	3.6	268*
Wistar control	2.8	505

*Statistically significantly different from control.

DOCA salt model, the relationship between catecholamines and hypertrophy was entirely different from the other two models. There was a significant reduction in both ventricular concentration and total content of catecholamines. A similar reduction in norepinephrine content of the heart in the DOCA salt model was reported by deChamplain et al.[31] Thus, the concentration of cardiac catecholamines does not have the same physiologic significance in all types and stages of hypertrophy.

Factors Modulating Myocardial Hypertrophy and Its Regression

Humoral Factors as Inducer: The suggestion that a neurohumoral factor may play an important role in the initiation of hypertrophy was based not only on the discrepancies between blood pressure level and ventricular mass, but also on the observations in experimental conditions that increased sympathetic activity also resulted in an increase in myocardial mass. Laks et al[32] induced hypertrophy by infusion of norepinephrine in dogs and suggested norepinephrine as a myocardial hypertrophic hormone. Ostman-Smith[33] could prevent exercise-induced cardiac hypertrophy in rats by treatment with guanethidine and recently reviewed the evidence for involvement of cardiac sympathetic nerves in the induction of adoptive cardiac hypertrophy. Khairallah et al[34] reported that angiotensin II increases myocardial protein synthesis, and both Gross[35] and Sen et al[11] found a significant positive relationship between plasma renin and heart weight in hypertensive rats. However, it is not clear whether the effect of angiotensin on cardiac hypertrophy can be dissociated from its effect on blood pressure or its potentiation of adrenergic influences. Angiotensin II potentiates sympathetic effects by both a pheripheral and a central action of the autonomic nervous system and stimulates secretion of catecholamines by the adrenal medulla. In order to dissociate these various factors, Sen et al[36] demonstrated that SHR treated for 5 weeks with an angiotensin II antagonist, [Sar^1, Ile^8] angiotensin II, resulted in a significant increase in heart weight associated with an increase in blood pressure. To evaluate further the role of blood pressure in myocardial hypertrophy when the angiotensin antagonists were administered to the normotensive rat, we showed[37] that two of the three analogs used, namely, [Sar^1, Ile^8 and Sar^1, Ala^8] angiotensin II, led to an increase in myocardial protein synthesis and cardiac hypertrophy, whereas the third, [Sar^1, Thr^8]

angiotensin II, left the heart weight unchanged. None of the analogs led to a significant change in blood pressure. The differences in cardiac effect were related to stimulation of catecholamine release by Ile^8 and Ala^8 analogs, since the hypertrophy produced was associated with an increase in concentration of cardiac catecholamine, and that could have been prevented by prior bilateral adrenalectomy. The third analog [Sar^1, Thr^8] did not increase myocardial catecholamine and did not produce hypertrophy. These results appear to minimize a direct role for angiotensin in the induction of hypertrophy.

Catecholamines and Reversal of Cardiac Hypertrophy by Medical Therapy: Our experience with SHR clearly showed that blood pressure control alone was not sufficient to bring about regression of hypertrophy. Both methyldopa and hydralazine lowered blood pressure significantly, but ventricular weight was reduced only in rats treated with methyldopa. Similar results were obtained with other sympatholytic agents, such as reserpine, whereas minoxidil actually increased the ventricular weight despite its excellent blood pressure control. As summarized in Table III, reversal of cardiac hypertrophy was obtained whenever ventricular catecholamine was reduced, and, as demonstrated, the reversal of hypertrophy had no obvious relationship to degree of blood pressure control. When the effect of propranolol was considered in this context, it was evident that propranolol did not control blood pressure, and the myocardial weight was reduced only to a questionable degree. However, when propranolol was given in a varying ratio with hydralazine in SHR,[38] neither propranolol alone (750 mg/liter, which reduced myocardial catecholamine but left blood pressure unchanged) nor hydralazine alone (80 mg/liter, which controlled blood pressure hypertension but increased myocardial catecholamine) altered ventricular weight.[38] Significant reversal of cardiac hypertrophy occurred only when these drugs were used in the ratio (750 mg/liter propranolol and 30 mg/liter hydralazine) that caused a moderate reduction in blood pressure and prevented an increase in catecholamines, demonstrating that in SHR a moderate control of blood pressure is necessary along with reduction of catechol-

TABLE III   **Effect of Antihypertensive Therapy on Ventricular Catecholamines and Cardiac Hypertrophy in SHR**

Treatment	Blood Pressure (mmHg)	Ventricular Weight (mg/g)	Ventricular Catecholamine (mg/g)
None	198	3.5	540
Sympatholytics			
Alpha-methyldopa	140*	3.8*	203*
Reserpine	175*	3.1*	188*
Vasodilators			
Hydralazine	120*	3.5*	718*
Minoxidil	118*	3.8*	—
Beta-Blocker			
Propranolol	188	3.2	451*

*$p < 0.01$ compared with untreated controls. Ventricular weight calculated relative to body weight (mg/g).

amine to achieve a significant reversal of hypertrophy. These observations suggest that adrenergic factors play an important role in modulating structural cardiac response to variations in arterial pressure.

The relationship between catecholamine concentration and reversal of hypertrophy in the renal hypertensive rat is quite different from that observed in SHR.[9] Reversal was achieved surgically by removing the clipped kidney or medically with the use of captopril. When the relationship between catecholamine level and reduction in heart weight was correlated, it was found that reversal was achieved whether catecholamine level was unaltered (captopril-treated) or reduced via nephrectomy. Therefore, it appears that in contrast to conditions in SHR, ventricular hypertrophy associated with renovascular hypertension is influenced predominantly by the blood pressure load.[9]

In mineralocortic hypertension, the relationship between catecholamine level and heart weight was found to be entirely different from that in the foregoing two models.[9] In DOCA hypertension, the reduction in heart weight was associated with reduction in catecholamine, although the catecholamine content of the myocardium was initially lower.

In conclusion, much more needs to be done to define the role of catecholamines in cardiac hypertrophy in order to unravel the part reflecting the causal disease, that which is secondary to simple increase in cardiac output, and that which might play a possible trophic role in the myocardium.

Conclusion

Regression of cardiac hypertrophy has been proved to occur in experimental animals following some types of antihypertensive therapy. However, no direct and necessary correlation can be found between hypertension and cardiac hypertrophy.

Different antihypertensive drugs have varied effects on regression of cardiac hypertrophy despite same degree of hypertensive controls. Therapy with alpha-methyldopa resulted in reversal of hypertrophy with effective blood pressure control, whereas treatment with vasodilators, namely, hydralazine and minoxidil, either did not alter (hydralazine) degree of myocardial hypertrophy or increase it (minoxidil), despite normalization of blood pressure.

The biochemical profile of the myocardium after regression of hypertrophy following antihypertensive therapy is not homogeneous. For example, reversal with alpha-methyldopa is associated with increased collagen content, whereas reversal with captopril did not alter collagen content of the heart.

Adrenergic factors seem to play an important role in the modulation of myocardial structure to variations in arterial pressure.

Results to date suggest that regression of myocardial hypertrophy can be influenced by many factors, namely, degree of adrenergic blockade, site of action of the drug used, and type and stage of evolution of hypertension. Duration of therapy, as well as age when treatment starts, are also important factors. Adrenergic stimuli are certainly not the only neurohumoral factors that may modulate myocardial hypertrophy. Recent data[35] suggest that angiotensin II may be involved either through its potentiation of sympathetic effect or by an independent stimulating effect on myocardial protein synthesis. Furthermore, in each type of hypertrophy in hypertension, a combination of different factors might be responsible, and it may not be correct to assume that the same factors must be involved in the regression of all types of myocardial hypertrophy.

Acknowledgment

Supported in part by NIH Grant HL-6835.
The author gratefully acknowledges Dr. B. C. Pakrashi, Staff Cardiologist, St. Vincent Charity Hospital and Health Center, Cleveland, Ohio, for his valuable suggestions and help in the preparation of this manuscript.

References

1. Ross J, Sobel BE: Regulation of cardiac function. Am Rev Physiol 1972; 34: 47–90.
2. Parmley WW, Tybert JV, Glantz SA: Cardiac dynamics. Am Rev Physiol 1977; 39: 277–299.
3. Tarazi RC, Levy MN: Cardiac responses to increased afterload hypertension. Hypertension 1981; 3: 8–18.
4. Pfeffer J, Pfeffer MA, Fletcher P, et al: Favorable effects of therapy on cardiac performance in spontaneously hypertensive rats. Am J Physiol 1982; 242: H776–H784.
5. Wicker P, Tarazi RC, El-Khair M: Coronary blood flow with reversal of left ventricular hypertrophy (abstr). Clin Res 1981; 29: 250A.
6. Patton HS, Page EW, Ogden E: The results of nephrectomy on experimental renal hypertension. Surg Gynecol Obstet 1943; 76: 494–496.
7. Hall O, Hall CE, Ogden E: Cardiac hypertrophy in experimental hypertension and its regression following reestablishment of normal blood pressure. Am J Physiol 1953; 174: 175–178.
8. Sen S, Tarazi RC, Bumpus FM: Reversal of cardiac hypertrophy in renal hypertensive rats: medical vs surgical therapy. Am J Physiol 1981; 240: H408–H412.
9. Sen S, Tarazi RC, Bumpus FM: Cardiac hypertrophy and antihypertensive therapy. Cardiovas Res 1977; 11: 427–433.
10. Tomanek RJ, Davis JR, Anderson SC: The effect of α-methyldopa on cardiac hypertrophy in SHR. Cardiovasc Res 1979; 13: 172–182.
11. Sen S, Tarazi RC, Bumpus FM: Cardiac hypertrophy in SHR. Circ Res 1974; 35: 775–781.
12. Yamori Y, Morichuzo, Nishio T: Cardiac hypertrophy in early hypertension. Am J Cardiol 1979; 44: 964–969.
13. Ishise S, Pegram BL, Frolich ED: Disparate effects of methyldopa and clonidine on cardiac mass and hemodynamics in rats. Clin Sci 1980; (suppl 6): 50.

14. RABINOWITZ M, ZAK R: Biochemical and cellular changes in cardiac hypertrophy. Ann Rev Med 1972; 23: 245–262.

15. SEN S, BUMPUS FM: Collagen synthesis in development and reversal of cardiac hypertrophy in SHR. Am J Cardiol 1979; 44: 954.

16. SEN S: Alteration in myocardial collagen phenotype in SHR. Mol and Cell Cardiol 1982; 14 (suppl I): 60.

17. MEERSON FZ: Compensatory hyperfunction of the heart and cardiac insufficiency. Circ Res 1962; 10: 250–258.

18. NAIR KG, CUTILLETTA AF, ZAK R, KOIDET, RABINBOWITZ M: Biochemical correlates of cardiac hypertrophy (I). Circ Res 1968; 23: 451–462.

19. GRIMM A, KUBOTA R, WHITEHORN WV: Ventricular nuclei acid and protein levels with myocardial growth and hypertrophy. Circ Res 1966; 19: 552–558.

20. SEN S, TARAZI RC, BUMPUS FM: Biochemical changes associated with development and reversal of cardiac hypertrophy in SHR. Cardiovasc Res 1976; 10: 254–261.

21. MARTIN AF, PAGANI ED, SOLARO RJ: Thyroxine-induced redistribution of isozymes of rabbit ventricular myosin. Circ Res 1982; 50: 117–124.

22. LOMPRE A, SCHWARTZ K, D'ALBIS A, LACOMBE G, THIEM NV, SWYNGHEDAUW B: Myosin isozymes redistribution in chronic heart overload. Nature 1979; 282: 105–107.

23. GROVE D, NAIR KG, ZAK R: Biochemical correlates of cardiac hypertrophy (III). Circ Res 1969; 25: 463–471.

24. CUTILLETTA AF, DOWELL RT, RUDRIK M, ARCHILLA RA, ZAK R: Regression of myocardial hypertrophy (I). J Mol Cell Cardiol 1979; 7: 761–780.

25. SEN S, TARAZI RC, BUMPUS FM: Effect of converting enzyme inhibitor (SQ14,225) on myocardial hypertrophy in SHR. Hypertension 1980; 2: 169–176.

26. TARAZI RC, SEN S: Catecholamines and cardiac hypertrophy. In: Hezey KC, Caldwell ADS, eds. Catecholamines and the heart. London: Academic Press and Royal Society of Medicine, 1979; 47–57.

27. FISCHER JE, HORST WD, KOBIN IJ: Norepinephrine metabolism in hypertrophied rat hearts. Nature 1955; 207: 952–953.

28. SPANN JF JR, BUCCINO RA, SONNENBLICK EH, BRAUNWALD E: Contractile state of cardiac muscle obtained from cats with experimentally produced ventricular hypertrophy and heart failure. Circ Res 1967; 21: 341–354.

29. FANBURG BL: Experimental cardiac hypertrophy. N Engl J Med 1970; 282: 723–732.

30. SEN S, TARAZI RC: Myocardial catecholamines in hypertensive ventricular hypertrophy: In Perspectives in cardiovascular research. Tarazi RC, Dunbar JB (eds.) New York, Raven Press, 1983; 8: 309–318.

31. DECHAMPLAIN J, KRAKOFF L, AXELROD J: Interrelationship of sodium intake, hypertension and norepinephrine storage in the rats. Circ Res 1969; 24, 25 (suppl I): 75–92.

32. LAKS MM, MORADY F, SURANT HSC: Myocardial hypertrophy produced by chronic infusion of subhypertensive dose of norepinephrine in the dog. Chest 1973; 64: 75–80.

33. OSTMAN-SMITH I: Prevention of exercise induced cardiac hypertrophy in rats by chemical sympathectomy. Neuroscience 1976; 1: 497–507.

34. KHAIRALLAH PA, ROBERTSON AL, DAVILLA D: Effect of angiotensin II on DNA, RNA, and protein synthesis. In: Genest J, Koiw E, eds. Hypertension. New York: Springer-Verlag, 1972; 212–220.

35. GROSS F: The renin-angiotensin system and hypertension. Ann Intern Med 1971; 75: 777–787.

36. SEN S, KHAIRALLAH PA, TARAZI RC, BUMPUS FM: Effect of chronic administration of Sar^1, Ile^8-angiotensin II in rats (abstr). Circulation 1975; 51, 52: 98.

37. SEN S, TARAZI RC, BUMPUS FM: Cardiac effects of angiotensin antagonists in normotensive rats. Clin Sci 1979; 56: 439–444.

38. SEN S, TARAZI RC: Regression of cardiac hypertrophy and influence of β-adrenergic system. Am J Physiol 1983; H13: H97–H101.

32

Cardiovascular Adjustment to Antiadrenergic Agents

BARBARA L. PEGRAM, Ph.D.,
EDWARD D. FROHLICH, M.D.

Adaptive cardiac hypertrophy is an increase in heart size that occurs in response to a physiologic or pathologic increase in the workload of the heart. Hemodynamically then, the left ventricular hypertrophy (LVH) that occurs as a consequence of long-standing essential or experimental hypertension is related to an increased (or increasing) total peripheral resistance (TPR). Recent reports have also indicated that the course of LVH is influenced not only by increased afterload but by a number of other factors, which include the severity and duration of the increased afterload, neurohumoral substances, age, race, sex, and obesity, as well as the coexistence of other diseases.[1–4]

During the last 15 to 20 years, an experimental model of hypertension has been developed that resembles in many respects the disease in man with essential hypertension.[5] The spontaneously hypertensive rat (SHR), originally bred by Okamoto and Aoki[6] from the Wistar-Kyoto (WKY) rat, is an inbred strain with a naturally occurring, slowly progressing form of systemic hypertension with associated development of LVH. When compared with the normotensive WKY, the SHR exhibits a progressive increase in arterial pressure that stabilizes at approximately 25 weeks of age. There is also a proportional increase in left ventricular (LV) mass and left ventricle to body weight (LV/BW) ratio that continues to increase even after arterial pressure has stabilized.[7] Similarly, increases in arterial pressure, LV mass and LV/BW ratio can be observed in other forms of experimental hypertension.

The question then arises: what happens to the hemodynamic profile and to LVH when antihypertensive drugs are administered? There is considerable evidence that certain antihypertensive drugs or combinations thereof will lead to a regression of LVH, whereas others that also effectively reduce arterial pressure do not. One factor that may significantly influence LVH is sympathetic nervous activity, and there are indications that cardiac sympathetic activity is increased in many forms of experimental hypertension.[8] Thus, attention has been focused on those antihypertensive drugs that exert their action through antiadrenergic mechanisms or that reflexively stimulate the adrenergic system.

Centrally Acting Antihypertensives

Methyldopa is a centrally acting antihypertensive drug that, through its metabolite alpha-methylnorepinephrine, stimulates alpha-adrenergic receptors in the nucleus tractus solitarius, thereby decreasing adrenergic drive to the cardiovascular system.[9,10] It has been widely studied and has been shown to be efficacious in lowering arterial pressure and regressing LVH, both in animal studies and in essential hypertension. Sen and co-workers[11-14] have demonstrated that methyldopa administered to SHR over a prolonged period will result in a decrease of arterial pressure, regression of LVH, and normalization of DNA and RNA concentrations. Their observations on ventricular connective tissue varied, reflecting possible variations in age and duration of drug treatment.[12,14]

Recently, we have reported on the systemic and regional hemodynamic changes that occur in 23-week-old SHR and WKY that have received methyldopa (400 mg/kg/day orally) for 3 weeks (Fig. 1A). Following treatment, mean arterial pressure (MAP) was significantly lower and heart rate significantly higher in SHR. Heart weights in both WKY and SHR and heart weight to BW (HW/BW) ratio in SHR were also significantly decreased (Fig. 1B). Myocardial blood flow per gram of tissue as well as that to other organs was not compromised by methyldopa treatment under resting conditions.[15] Similar changes in MAP and LV/BW have also been observed in renovascular hypertensive rats treated for 2 weeks with methyldopa.[16]

Electron microscopic studies have also indicated that prolonged treatment with methyldopa can decrease cell size.[17] Spontaneously hypertensive rats treated for 12 weeks (4 to 16 weeks of age) with methyldopa at a dose that did not significantly reduce systolic pressure nevertheless significantly decreased mean cell area in both subepicardium and subendocardium when compared with untreated SHR. Mean cell area in the subepicardium of treated SHR was similar in size to corresponding cells in untreated WKY, but those in the subendocardium, although smaller than in untreated SHR, were still significantly larger than in untreated WKY. Similar changes in capillary density in those myocardial areas were also noted. A recent report on hypertensive patients also suggests that cardiac hypertrophy may regress after methyldopa treatment in the absence of a concomitant decrease in arterial pressure.[18]

Another centrally acting antihypertensive drug that stimulates alpha-adrenergic receptors in the nucleus tractus solitarius is clonidine.[9] Studies analogous to those conducted with methyldopa on systemic and regional hemodynamics were performed in SHR and WKY following treatment with clonidine.[15] The MAP was significantly reduced (equipotent with that observed with methyldopa), as was heart rate in SHR following 3 weeks of treatment with clonidine (0.1 mg/kg/day) (Fig. 2A). No significant changes, however, were found in heart weight or HW/BW ratio (Fig. 2B). Tripling the dose of clonidine resulted in a significantly lower heart rate in WKY and SHR, but other systemic hemodynamic parameters were unchanged compared with controls. Interestingly, the HW/BW ratio was significantly de-

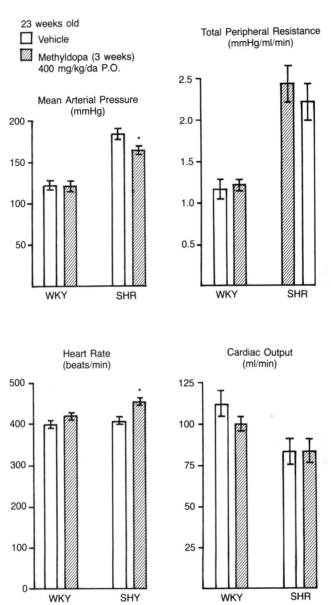

Figure 1A. *Effect of prolonged (3 weeks) treatment with methyldopa on systemic hemodynamics and cardiac mass in Wistar-Kyoto (WKY) and spontaneously hypertensive rats (SHR). See text for details. Mean ± SE; *p < 0.05. (Adapted with permission from Pegram et al.[15])*

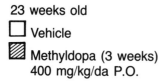

23 weeks old

☐ Vehicle

▨ Methyldopa (3 weeks)
400 mg/kg/da P.O.

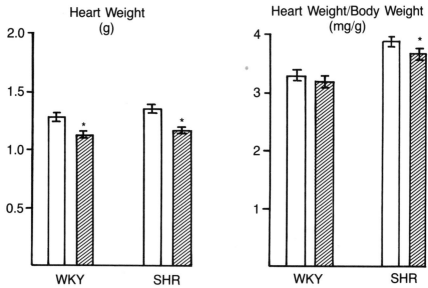

Figure 1B. *Effect of prolonged (3 weeks) treatment with methyldopa on cardiac mass in Wistar-Kyoto (WKY) and spontaneously hypertensive rats (SHR). See text for details. Mean ± SE; *p < 0.05. (Adapted with permission from Pegram et al.[15])*

creased in SHR (Fig. 2B). Blood flow to the myocardium was maintained under both treatment regimens. At the lower dose, blood flow to the splanchnic organs and to muscle was increased in WKY.

Beta-Adrenergic Receptor Blockers

Another widely used group of antihypertensive drugs are the beta-adrenergic receptor blockers. Administration of either propranolol or timolol to WKY and SHR parents and then to the offspring until they were 12 weeks of age resulted in a significant decrease in heart rate and no change in the LV/BW ratio in either male WKY or SHR when compared with their respective controls.[19] Only timolol treatment significantly decreased MAP. Interestingly, sibling female WKY and SHR responded differently to the same drug treatment. Female SHR receiving beta-adrenergic blocking drugs had significantly lower LV/BW ratios despite the fact that arterial pressure was unchanged. These data illustrate in this instance the importance that other factors, such as sex, can have on hemodynamic parameters after drug treat-

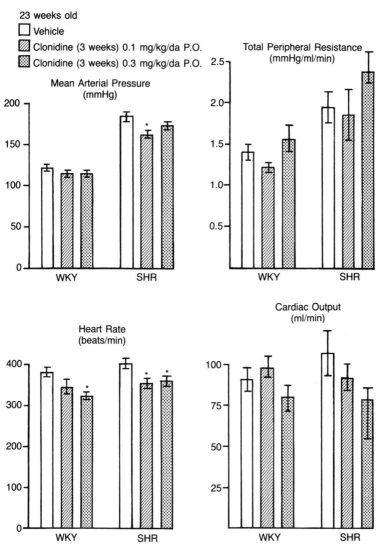

Figure 2A. *Effect of prolonged (3 weeks) treatment with clonidine on systemic hemodynamics in Wistar-Kyoto (WKY) and spontaneously hypertensive rats (SHR). See text for details. Mean ± SE; *p < 0.05. (Adapted with permission from Pegram et al.[15])*

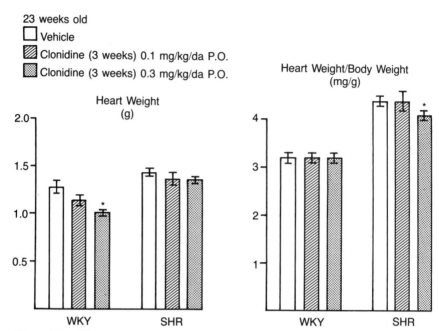

Figure 2B. *Effect of prolonged (3 weeks) treatment with clonidine on cardiac mass in Wistar-Kyoto (WKY) and spontaneously hypertensive rats (SHR). See text for details. Mean ± SE; *p < 0.05. (Adapted with permission from Pegram et al.[15])*

ment. Blood flow changes in animals receiving beta-adrenergic blocking agents were more widespread than those observed with methyldopa or clonidine. Both propranolol and timolol decreased myocardial and muscle blood flow, whereas timolol increased blood flow to the kidneys in SHR and WKY and to skin in SHR.[20]

Not all investigators concur with regard to the effect of beta-adrenergic blocking agents on arterial pressure. Many investigators have reported that administration of either propranolol, timolol, or sotalol had no effect on arterial pressure.[13,19,21–23] Others, however, have reported that propranolol reduced arterial pressure in SHR.[24,25] Richer and colleagues[26] treated male SHR from age 5 to 20 weeks with atenolol. When compared with untreated SHR, there was a decrease in arterial pressure and HW/BW ratio. Yet others have reported that approximately 9 months of treatment with propranolol or metoprolol resulted in a lower arterial pressure in treated SHR, but reduced LV weight only about 10% and did not fully prevent vascular structural changes.[27,28] No clear-cut explanation is available for the disparate effect of beta-adrenergic blockers on arterial pressure and cardiovascular structural changes observed by the various investigators.

Vasodilators

Substantial reductions in arterial pressure can also be elicited by vasodilators. Prolonged treatment (3 weeks) with hydralazine resulted in significant decreases in arterial pressure and TPR in SHR[11,15] and significant increases in cardiac output (CO) in both SHR and WKY[24] (Fig. 3A). Heart weight remained unchanged, but the HW/BW ratio was elevated in treated WKY (Fig. 3B). A similar effect of minoxidil in normotensive rats has also been reported.[13] Blood flow to muscle almost doubled in both WKY and SHR treated with hydralazine and there was a significant increase in myocardial blood flow in WKY.[15]

Vasodilators, then, such as hydralazine or minoxidil, have no direct inhibitory effects on the sympathetic nervous system, but decrease arterial pressure via a reduction in TPR. This in turn leads to reflex responses that stimulate adrenergic drive to the cardiovascular system. Under certain circumstances these agents may actually aggravate LVH[13,15] despite significant reductions in arterial pressure.

Combination Therapy

Several studies have investigated the effect of multiple drug therapy on arterial pressure and the regression of LVH. A combination of reserpine, hydrochlorothiazide, and hydralazine significantly reduced arterial pressure and HW/BW ratio in SHR treated for 6 months.[14] Minoxidil plus propranolol reduced arterial pressure in SHR, but the HW/BW ratio increased.[13] A combination of minoxidil and methyldopa effectively reduced arterial pressure and HW/BW ratio in SHR.[13] More recently, it has been suggested that it may be necessary to use a combination of propranolol and hydralazine in doses that do not increase ventricular catecholamines in order to effect a reduction in arterial pressure as well as a decrease in the HW/BW ratio.[29]

Ventricular Function Following Reversal of LVH

The initial development of cardiac hypertrophy represents a physiologic adaptation enabling the heart to maintain a normal CO in the presence of an increased afterload, but in hypertension of long standing pump functions appear to deteriorate.[30,31] Ultimately, untreated hypertension leads to cardiac dilatation and failure. How, then, does a reduction in arterial pressure and regression of hypertrophy affect ventricular function? This question has been studied recently in SHR[32] and renovascular hypertensive (2K1C) rats[16] that have been treated with methyldopa or unclipping of the renal artery.[16] In both studies assessment of ventricular function was by a rapid-volume infusion of blood or saline in an anesthetized rat preparation in which arterial and LV pressures and aortic flow were monitored. The data

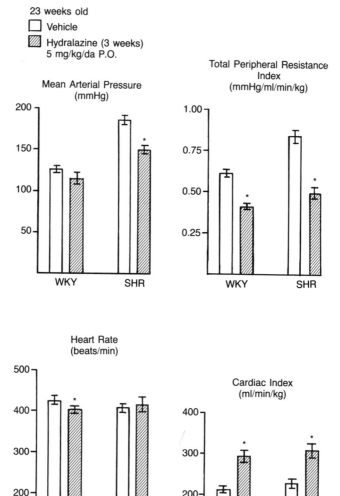

Figure 3A. *Effect of prolonged (3 weeks) treatment with hydralazine on systemic hemodynamics and in Wistar-Kyoto (WKY) and spontaneously hypertensive rats (SHR). See text for details. Mean ± SE; *p < 0.05. (Adapted with permission from Pegram et al.[15])*

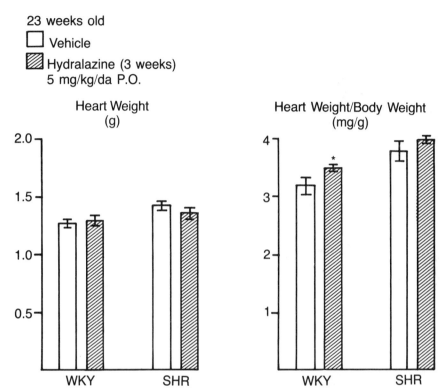

23 weeks old

☐ Vehicle

▨ Hydralazine (3 weeks)
5 mg/kg/da P.O.

Figure 3B. *Effect of prolonged (3 weeks) treatment with hydralazine on cardiac mass in Wistar-Kyoto (WKY) and spontaneously hypertensive rats (SHR). See text for details. Mean ± SE; *p < 0.05. (Adapted with permission from Pegram et al[15])*

from these studies indicate that reduction of arterial pressure and regression of hypertrophy, be it by pharmacologic or surgical means, improves ventricular performance. If, however, arterial pressure was elevated in methyldopa-treated SHR, peak CO in these rats was depressed and was then not different from that of untreated SHR.[32]

Summary

The growing body of data relative to antihypertensive agents and the control of arterial pressure clearly indicate that hemodynamic changes per se cannot be used to predict a change in LV mass. Many factors, including the adrenergic nervous system, interact to influence the course of LVH. However, administration of an antiadrenergic antihypertensive drug alone will not necessarily regress LVH. Current data indicate that methyldopa is efficacious in reducing arterial pressure and in regressing LVH, the latter perhaps independent of significant changes in arterial pressure. Methyldopa-treated animals with reduced arterial pressure and regression of LVH show an improvement in ventricular function when compared with untreated hypertensive animals; however, that function, at least in treated SHR, may still be impaired if the afterload is markedly elevated.

The use of vasodilators alone may exacerbate the problem of cardiac hypertrophy despite a substantial reduction in arterial pressure. There is, however, growing evidence that when vasodilators and beta-adrenergic blockers are administered concomitantly in the proper ratio, both arterial pressure and LVH may be decreased.

References

1. FROHLICH ED, TARAZI RC: Is arterial pressure the sole factor responsible for hypertensive cardiac hypertrophy? Part II. Am J Cardiol 1979; 4: 959–963.

2. CAMBOTTI SL, COLE FE, GERALL AA, FROHLICH ED, MacPHEE AA: Neonatal gonadal hormones and blood pressure in the spontaneously hypertensive rat. Am J Physiol 1984; 247: E258–E264.

3. FROHLICH ED: Hemodynamics and other determinants in development of left ventricular hypertrophy: conflicting factors in its regression. Fed Proc 1983; 42: 2709–2715.

4. GROSSMAN W: Cardiac hypertrophy: useful adaptation or pathologic process? Am J Med 1980; 69: 576–584.

5. TRIPPODO NC, FROHLICH ED: Controversies in cardiovascular research: similarities of genetic (spontaneous) hypertension. Man and rat. Circ Res 1981; 48: 309–319.

6. OKAMOTO K, AOKI K: Development of a strain of spontaneously hypertensive rats. Jpn Circ J 1963; 27: 282–293.

7. FROHLICH ED, PFEFFER MA, PFEFFER JM: Systemic hemodynamics and cardiac function in the spontaneously hypertensive rat: similarities with essential hypertension. In: Strauer BE, ed. The heart in hypertension. Berlin: Springer-Verlag, 1981; 53–71.

8. OESTMAN-SMITH I: Cardiac sympathetic nerves as the final common pathway in the induction of adaptive cardiac hypertrophy. Clin Sci 1981; 61: 265–272.

9. VAN ZWIETEN PA: Antihypertensive drugs with a central action. In: Progress in pharmacology. Stuttgard: Gustaf Fisher Verlag, 1975.

10. HENNING M, RUBENSON A: Evidence that the hypotensive action of α-methyldopa is mediated by central actions of methylnoradrenaline. J Pharm Pharmacol 1971; 23: 407.

11. SEN S, TARAZI RC, KHAIRALLAH PA, BUMPUS FM: Cardiac hypertrophy in spontaneously hypertensive rats. Circ Res 1974; 35: 775–781.

12. SEN S, TARAZI RC, BUMPUS FM: Biochemical changes associated with development and reversal of cardiac hypertrophy in spontaneously hypertensive rats. Cardiovasc Res 1976; 10: 254–261.

13. SEN S, TARAZI RC, BUMPUS FM: Cardiac hypertrophy and antihypertensive therapy. Cardiovasc Res 1977; 11: 427–433.

14. SEN S, BUMPUS FM: Collagen synthesis in development and reversal of cardiac

hypertrophy in spontaneously hypertensive rats. Am J Cardiol 1979; 44: 954–958.

15. PEGRAM BL, ISHISE S, FROHLICH ED: Effect of methyldopa, clonidine, and hydralazine on cardiac mass and hemodynamics in Wistar-Kyoto and spontaneously hypertensive rats. Cardiovasc Res 1982; 16: 40–46.

16. KUWAJIMA I, KARDON MB, PEGRAM BL, SESOKO S, FROHLICH ED: Regression of left ventricular hypertrophy in two-kidney, one clip Goldblatt hypertension. Hypertension 1982; 4 (suppl II): 113–118.

17. TOMANEK RJ, DAVIS JW, ANDERSON SC: The effects of alpha-methyldopa on cardiac hypertrophy in spontaneously hypertensive rats: ultrastructural, stereological, and morphometric analysis. Cardiovasc Res 1979; 13: 173–182.

18. FOUAD FM, NAKASHIMA Y, TARAZI RC, SALCEDO EE: Reversal of left ventricular hypertrophy in hypertensive patients treated with methyldopa. Am J Cardiol 1981; 49: 795–801.

19. PFEFFER MA, PFEFFER JM, WEISS AK, FROHLICH ED: Development of SHR hypertension and cardiac hypertrophy during prolonged beta blockade. Am J Physiol 1977; 232: H639–H644.

20. NISHIYAMA K, NISHIYAMA A, PFEFFER MA, FROHLICH ED: Systemic and regional flow distribution in normotensive and spontaneously hypertensive young rats subjected to lifetime β-adrenergic receptor blockade. Blood Vessels 1978; 15: 333–347.

21. PFEFFER MA, FROHLICH ED, PFEFFER JM, WEISS AK: Pathophysiological implications of the increased cardiac output of young spontaneously hypertensive rats. Circ Res 1974; 34 (suppl 1): 235–244.

22. YAMORI Y: Interaction of neural and non-neural factors in the pathogenesis of spontaneous hypertension. In: Julius S, Ester MD, eds. The nervous system in arterial hypertension. Springfield, IL: Charles C Thomas 1975; 17–50.

23. FORMAL BH, MULROW PJ: Effect of propranolol on blood pressure and plasma renin activity in the spontaneously hypertensive rat. Circ Res 1974; 35: 215–221.

24. VAVRE I, TOM H, GRESELIN E: Chronic propranolol treatment in young spontaneously hypertensive and normotensive rats. Can J Physiol Pharmacol 1973; 51: 727–732.

25. WEISS L, LUNDGREN Y, FOLKOW B: Effects of prolonged treatment with adrenergic receptor antagonists on blood pressure, cardiovascular design and reactivity in spontaneously hypertensive rats (SHR). Acta Physiol Scand 1974; 91: 447–457.

26. RICHER C, BOISSIER JR, GIUDICELLI JF: Chronic atenolol treatment and hypertension development in spontaneously hypertensive rats. Eur J Pharmacol 1978; 47: 393–400.

27. WEISS L, LUNDGREN Y: Left ventricular hypertrophy and its reversibility in young spontaneously hypertensive rats. Cardiovasc Res 1978; 12: 635–638.

28. WEISS L, LUNDGREN Y: Chronic antihypertensive drug treatment in young spontaneously hypertensive rats: effects on arterial blood pressure, cardiovascular reactivity and vascular design. Cardiovasc Res 1978; 12: 744–751.

29. SEN S, TARAZI RC, BUMPUS FM: Reversal of myocardial hypertrophy and influence of adrenergic system. Circulation 1980; 60: 111–121.

30. PFEFFER MA, PFEFFER JM, FROHLICH ED: Pumping ability of the hypertrophying left ventricle of the spontaneously hypertensive rat. Circ Res 1976; 38: 423–429.

31. AVERILL DB, FERRARIO CM, TARAZI RC, SEN S, BAJBUS R: Cardiac performance in rats with renal hypertension. Circ Res 1976; 38: 280–288.

32. SPECH MM, FERRARIO CM, TARAZI RC: Cardiac pumping ability following reversal of hypertrophy and hypertension in spontaneously hypertensive rats. Hypertension 1980; 2: 75–82.

33

Cardiovascular Effects of Autonomic Blockade

EDWARD D. FREIS, M.D.

This chapter is concerned with the hemodynamic effects of generalized autonomic blockade of both the heart and the peripheral blood vessels. Such blockade obviously represents a more complex response than beta-adrenergic blockade per se, which affects the heart primarily. Not only does generalized autonomic blockade affect the heart and the blood vessels, but it also affects both sides of the systemic circulation, that is, both the arterial and the venous sides. Drugs that produce such widespread autonomic blockade have been known for many years. They are the ganglion blocking agents, the classic representative of which is hexamethonium, or C6.

Completeness of Blockade with C6

C6 was introduced by Paton and Zaimis[1] in 1948 and was soon used for the treatment of severe hypertension.[2,3] Despite effective and often marked reduction of blood pressure, hexamethonium was not useful for the treatment of any but the most severe cases of hypertension. This was due to frequent and disturbing side effects as well as the need to inject the drug parenterally. Despite these therapeutic limitations, C6 proved to be of great value as a pharmacologic tool in exploring the effects of generalized autonomic blockade on the heart and circulation.

A surprisingly complete degree of sympathetic blockade was obtained following C6, using various tests of sympathetic blocking activity. The Valsalva overshoot was completely prevented.[4] The same was true for the cold pressor test. In semiclad subjects exposed to cool environmental temperatures, toe skin temperature increased to umbilical temperature after the administration of C6. At the same time, plethysmographic recordings of the big toe showed a marked increase in toe blood flow and pulse volume after C6. Neither tetramethylammonium, another ganglion blocking agent, nor intraarterial tolazoline produced nearly this degree of blockade.

The most conclusive demonstration of the completeness of sympathetic blockade after C6 was provided by a direct comparison between the effects of intravenous C6 on foot blood flow, measured plethysmographically, and lumbar intrathecal or extradural block.[5] Despite the fact that it was given systemically, the degree of increase in foot blood flow was as great as after local blockade of the sympathetic nerves.

Although C6 blocked both parasympathetic as well as the sympathetic nervous system, the former has few circulatory effects, the most important being bradycardia. Therefore, it seemed reasonable to consider that the circulatory changes observed after C6 were almost entirely due to blockade of the sympathetic nervous system.

Adrenergic Blockade and Venous Capacity

Our initial hemodynamic studies with C6 on the resistance and capacitance vessels were in dogs with an open chest.[6] The left ventricle was replaced with a pump, the output of which remained constant despite marked changes in afterload. Blood returning to the left atrium was drained into a reservoir and from there was pumped into the thoracic aorta. By recording the level of blood in the reservoir, it was possible to determine changes in vascular capacity. For example, a decrease in vascular (primarily venous) capacity would transfer blood from the animal to the reservoir, thereby increasing the reservoir level, whereas an increase in venous capacity would lower the reservoir level.

Intravenous injection of C6 into this pump-dog preparation resulted in a prompt reduction in systemic blood pressure. Because the pump output was constant, the reduction of blood pressure must have been due entirely to a decrease in total peripheral resistance (TPR). This was followed by a more slowly developing relaxation of the veins, as was evident from a decrease in pulmonary arterial pressure, a temporary decrease in pulmonary blood flow, and a decrease in the level of blood in the reservoir. The latter indicated that the vasculature of the dog was taking up more blood after C6. The amount so transferred was 150 ml, which in the dog represents about one sixth of the total blood volume. Venodilation should result in a decrease in right heart filling pressure (preload) and a decrease in right heart pressures, which was, in fact, the case.

When norepinephrine, the adrenergic agonist, was administered in physiologic doses to the pump-dog, exactly opposite effects were observed. Systemic blood pressure and pulmonary arterial pressure increased. The level of blood in the reservoir also increased. These observations were interpreted as follows: sympathetic stimulation resulted in constriction not only of the resistance vessels, but also of the capacitance vessels. This resulted in an integrated response that included venous contraction. The latter transferred more of the blood volume into the central circulation, which increased preload and thereby increased cardiac output and pulmonary arterial pressure. Systemic blood pressure increased from the effects of increased TPR. The net result is an increase in systemic and pulmonary blood pressures and of cardiac output (CO). It was the exact opposite of adrenergic blockade after C6, which resulted in dilation rather than constriction of both the arterial and venous sides of the circulation and a decrease in pulmonary blood flow.

Hemodynamic Effects of Adrenergic Blockade in Man

We also examined the hemodynamic effects of C6 in hypertensive patients.[7] Blood pressure decreased after C6, the reduction being associated primarily with a decrease in cardiac output. Right heart pressures decreased simultaneously, suggesting that the reduced CO was secondary to a decreased preload, which in turn resulted from venodilation, as had been seen in the pump-dog.

Another observation emphasizing the importance of the veins in cardiovascular integration was made at this time.[8] Adrenergic blockade was induced with intravenous C6 in volunteer subjects. While they were lying supine, blood was removed from an arm vein as in a usual phlebotomy. After the phlebotomy was completed, the collecting bottle was pressurized and the blood reinfused. During adrenergic blockade, the blood pressure that was recorded in the opposite arm decreased as a direct linear function of the amount of blood withdrawn. Removal of as little as 50 ml of blood resulted in definite reduction of blood pressure. In some subjects total withdrawal of as little as 350 ml of blood resulted in blood pressure decreases to collapse levels. Rapid reinfusion of blood led to a stepwise increase of blood pressure, mirroring the previous decrease, with return of blood pressure to prephlebotomy levels as the reinfusion of blood was completed.

This study demonstrated the marked sensitivity of the sympathetically mediated vascular response to changes in blood volume. Following blockade of the sympathetic system with C6, the blood pressure became a direct function of the blood volume. Thus, when the adrenergic nervous system is functionally intact, it must respond to adjust the resistance and capacitance vessels to even minor changes in blood volume in order to prevent decreases in blood pressure.

The hemodynamic changes resulting from C6 are markedly different in hypertensive patients with congestive heart failure than in patients with compensated hearts. In patients with heart failure the decrease in systemic and right heart pressures was associated with an increase rather than a decrease in CO. Also, instead of remaining unchanged, as in patients with compensated hearts, TPR decreased significantly.

We interpreted these findings to indicate that adrenergic blockade was interrupting a vicious cycle in patients with heart failure.[9] Because of the low CO in congestive heart failure, there was activation of baroreceptor reflexes and other mechanisms that in turn produce both arterial and venous constriction mediated over the adrenergic nervous system. The arteriolar constriction increases TPR, which in turn adds to the workload of the failing heart, thereby further depressing its output (vicious cycle 1). In addition, the venous constriction mobilizes blood in the peripheral circulation, shunting it toward the large central veins and the right heart. The resulting increase in preload may be greater than the failing myocardium can handle, leading again to further depression of CO (vicious cycle 2). We commented that these reflex responses, which were designed to protect the person who has had trauma and acute blood loss, were, in fact, deleterious in the patients who had heart failure.

The improvement in congestive heart failure resulting from C6 was not limited to patients with hypertensive disease. We also assessed the effects of such adrenergic blockade in patients with other forms of heart disease, including valvular heart disease, coronary artery disease, and myocarditis.[9] C6 was effective in reducing the manifestations of congestive heart disease in these conditions. Venous pressure decreased, circulation time shortened, heart rate decreased, and there was improvement in dyspnea and orthopnea. The only condition that did not improve was mitral stenosis. This was not surprising, since this condition may require a higher than normal atrial filling pressure.

We postulated that the beneficial effects of adrenergic blockade were due to interrupting the vicious cycle that is present in heart failure at two sites. By dilating the venous side of the circulation, the blood volume was redistributed away from the engorged central circulation to the peripheral veins, thereby reducing the increased filling pressure toward normal. This principle had been applied in the past in the form of venous tourniquets and phlebotomy.

The second principle, however, was new at the time. Quoting directly from our 1953 article,[9] we stated as follows: "Up to the present time there have been no recognized methods of lowering the peripheral resistance, thereby reducing the workload of the failing heart. By decreasing the total peripheral resistance the work demand on the left ventricle is lessened and by reducing the filling of the right heart the right ventricle is able to contract more effectively."

Our conclusion was, therefore, that in treating congestive heart failure, reductions in both preload and afterload were important. Reduction of preload had long been recognized as an effective approach to the treatment of congestive heart failure, but the importance of afterload reduction was essentially unknown at the time of our report.[9] The only other observation of this type was in the Czech literature and was made by Brod and Fejfar[10] who used alpha-adrenergic blockade with dibenzylchlorethamine to reduce preload and afterload.

It is apparent that both preload and afterload are decreased by alpha- or general adrenergic blockade and that reductions in both are important in the treatment of congestive heart failure. Of the two, however, it seems probable that reduction in afterload is more important than decreasing preload. For example, such drugs as hydralazine, which act only on resistance vessels and not on capacitance vessels, also are effective in the treatment of congestive heart failure.[11] In heart failure patients Cohn et al[12] induced comparable reductions in left ventricular (LV) filling pressure first by phlebotomy or tourniquets and then by afterload reduction using infusion of nitroprusside. The former resulted in a reduction of CO and the latter was followed by an increase. Nevertheless, extensive clinical experience testifies to the value of reducing preload, particularly in patients with overdistended hearts and high filling pressures. Adrenergic blocking agents such as C6 are highly effective in treating heart failure because they favorably influence both the arterial and venous sides of the circulation.

Although this discussion has been concerned with a drug that induces both alpha- and beta-adrenergic blockade, the effects of pure alpha blockade also should be considered. The two principal classes of alpha-adrenergic blocking drugs are the alpha$_1$ blockers, of which prazosin is the leading representative, and drugs that block both alpha$_1$ and alpha$_2$ receptors, such as phentolamine and phenoxybenzamine.

The hemodynamic effects of prazosin are characterized by no change or a slight decrease in CO, a decrease in TPR, and a decrease in right heart pressure.[13] There is a tendency toward orthostatic hypotension, particularly after the initial dose consistent with inhibition of reflex, sympathetically mediated vasoconstriction. In patients with heart failure, CO increases and right and left ventricular pressures decrease.[14,15] These beneficial effects have been ascribed to reduction in cardiac impedance and in preload,[14] similar to our findings with C6. Prazosin has at least a theoretical advantage over C6, however, in that it does not inhibit beta-adrenergic effects on the heart. During long-term treatment, there may be some attenuation of the therapeutic effect of prazosin in patients with heart failure.

The alpha$_1$ and alpha$_2$ blockers, phenoxybenzamine and phentolamine, differ in their hemodynamic effects from prazosin, principally with respect to heart rate change. Norepinephrine may be released in increased amounts after nonselective alpha-adrenergic blockade and can then enter the circulation and stimulate the sinus node to increase heart rate. The increased heart rate as well as greater ventricular inotropism result in an increased cardiac output.[16] This is probably the reason why alpha$_1$ and alpha$_2$ blockers increase CO even in patients with compensated hearts, whereas prazosin does not. Prazosin does not cause a significant increase in heart rate, although the reason for the difference remains speculative. The nonselective alpha$_1$ and alpha$_2$ blockers have not been widely used clinically, largely because of such side effects as tachycardia, palpitations, and orthostatic hypotension.

There are currently available three fundamental approaches to the drug treatment of congestive heart failure: to increase the contractility of the ventricle using inotropic drugs, such as digitalis, or one of the various adrenergic agonists; to administer drugs that relax resistance and capacitance vessels using alpha- or general adrenergic blocking agents or certain vasodilator drugs; or stimulate the heart directly. Although the last has received the most attention, it is apparent that treatment directed toward the peripheral vessels also has important therapeutic effects in heart failure.

Summary

The effects of drugs producing generalized adrenergic blockade are exemplified by the ganglion blocking agent, hexamethonium, or C6. Early studies indicated that C6 produced a high degree of blockade of alpha-adrenergic activity comparable to sympathectomy or spinal anesthesia. Hemodynamic studies in dogs with pump replacement of the left ventricle demonstrated considerable increase in venous capacitance after C6. Studies in patients indicated reduction in right heart pressures and CO consistent with an increase in venous capacitance. Patients with congestive heart failure due to various causes showed an increase rather than a decrease in CO and a decrease in TPR. The beneficial effects in the treatment of congestive heart failure were probably due to a reduction in both preload and afterload.

References

1. PATON WD, ZAIMIS EJ: Clinical potentialities of certain bisquaternary salts causing neuromuscular and ganglionic block. Nature 1948; 162: 810.
2. ARNOLD P, ROSENHEIM ML: Effect of pentamethonium iodide on normal and hypertensive persons. Lancet 1949; 2: 321.
3. RESTALL PA, SMIRK FH: The treatment of high blood pressure with hexamethonium iodide. N Z Med J 1950; 49: 206.
4. FINNERTY FA JR, FREIS ED: Experimental and clinical evaluation in man of hexamethonium (C6), a new ganglionic blocking agent. Circulation 1950; 2: 828–836.
5. SCHNAPER HW, JOHNSON RL, TUOHY EB, FREIS ED: The effect of hexamethonium as compared to procaine or metycaine lumbar block on the blood flow to the foot of normal subjects. J Clin Invest 1951; 30: 786–791.
6. ROSE JC, FREIS ED: Alterations in systemic vascular volume of the dog in response to hexamethonium and norepinephrine. Am J Physiol 1957; 191: 283–286.
7. FREIS ED, ROSE JC, PARTENOPE EA, et al: The hemodynamic effects of hypotensive drugs in man. III. Hexamethonium. J Clin Invest 1953; 32: 1285–1297.
8. FREIS ED, STANTON JR, FINNERTY FA JR, SCHNAPER HW, JOHNSON RL, RATH CE, WILKINS RW: The collapse produced by venous congestion of the extremities or by venesection following certain hypotensive agents. J Clin Invest 1951; 30: 435–443.
9. KELLY RT, FREIS ED, HIGGINS TF: The effects of hexamethonium on certain manifestations of congestive heart failure. Circulation 1953; 7: 169–173.
10. BROD J, FEJFAR Z: Mechanism of transient increase of the cardiac output in adrenergic blockade with Dibenamine. Sb Lek 1951; 53: 154–160.
11. FRANCIOSA JA, PIERPONT G, COHN JN: Hemodynamic improvement after oral hydralazine in left ventricular failure. Ann Intern Med 1977; 86: 388–393.
12. COHN JN, BRODER M, FRANCIOSA JA, GUIHA HN, LIMAS CJ: Relative importance of preload. The influence of impedance on left ventricular performance. Circulation 1973; 48: 5–8.
13. LUND-JOHANSEN P: Hemodynamic changes at rest and during exercise in long term prazosin therapy of essential hypertension. In: Catton DWK, ed. Prazosin: evaluation of a new antihypertensive agent. Amsterdam: Excerpta Medica. 1974; 43.

14. MILLER RR, AWAN NA, MAXWELL KS, MASON DT: Sustained reduction of cardiac impedance and preload in congestive heart failure with the antihypertensive vasodilator prazosin. N Engl J Med 1977; 297: 303–307.

15. CALUCCI WS: Alpha adrenergic receptor blockade with prazosin. Consideration of hypertension, heart failure and potential new applications. Ann Intern Med 1982; 97: 62–77.

16. FOWLER NO, HOLMES JC, GAFFNEY TE, et al: Hemodynamic effects of phenoxy-benzamine in anesthelized dogs. J Clin Invest 1970; 49: 2036–2050.

34

Antiadrenergic Drugs and the Heart: Hemodynamic and Cardiac Effects

HECTOR O. VENTURA, M.D., and FRANZ H. MESSERLI, M.D.

The adrenergic nervous system has been shown to participate in the development and maintenance of an elevated arterial pressure in several forms of experimental and human arterial hypertension. Hence, some drugs that interfere with the function of the adrenergic nervous system have been shown to be useful for the treatment of arterial hypertension. This group of agents, denominated by adrenergic blocking drugs, comprise: centrally acting drugs: clonidine, methyldopa, guanabenz; postganglionic adrenergic blocking drugs: guanethidine, bethanidine, debrisoquin, guanadrel, reserpine; alpha$_1$-adrenoreceptor antagonists: prazosin; and beta-adrenoreceptor antagonists. This report will focus on the hemodynamic and cardiac effects of all the adrenergic blocking drugs with the exception of the beta-adrenoreceptor antagonists (Table I).

Centrally Acting Drugs

Clonidine: Hemodynamic effects. Clonidine reduces centrally mediated sympathetic nervous system activity by its interaction with alpha adrenoreceptors in the brain.[1,2] It has been reported that clonidine administered intravenously to man produces a transient increase in blood pressure followed by a more prolonged decrease. The initial pressure response has been shown to be the result of stimulation of peripheral alpha$_1$ adrenorecep-

TABLE I **Cardiac Effect of Antiadrenergic Drugs**

	Preload	Heart Rate	Contractility	Afterload	Cardiac Mass
Clonidine	↓	↓	↔ ↓	↓	↓ ↔
Methyldopa	↓	↓	↔ ↓	↓	↓
Guanabenz	↓	↓	↔ ↓	↓	?
Reserpine	↓	↓	↔ ↓	↓	↓
Guanethidine	↓	↓	↓	↓	↓
Guanadrel	↓	↓	↔ ↓	↓	↓ ↔
Prazosin	↓	↑	↔ ↑	↓	?

↓ : decrease; ↔: no change; ↑ : increase; ?: not known.

tor, since the prior administration of an alpha blocker, such as phentolamine, prevents this transient hypertensive effect.[3,4] Brod et al[5] have reported that the decrease in arterial pressure is associated with a decrease in cardiac output (CO) and an unchanged peripheral resistance in normotensive subjects and in patients with essential hypertension.

Acute oral administration of clonidine produces an acute decrease in blood pressure that is due to a decrease in both CO and heart rate.[5] In addition, a further decrease in CO and total peripheral resistance (TPR) has been observed during 45° head-up tilt. Therefore, clonidine not only abolishes the usual compensatory vasoconstriction associated with changes of posture, but also causes a moderate further decrease in CO.[6] Chronic treatment with clonidine has been shown to decrease blood pressure through a reduction in both CO and TPR, both in supine or sitting position.[7] However, postural hypotension was not observed. Moreover, clonidine does not alter normal hemodynamic responses to exercise.[7] With long-term administration, CO tends to recover, and the antihypertensive effects seem to be mediated predominantly by a decrease in TPR.

Left ventricular structure. Experimental studies in spontaneously hypertensive rats have shown that clonidine in doses that produce a sustained decrease in blood pressure and heart rate does not alter heart weight or heart weight to body weight ratio.[8] When subsequently the dose of clonidine is tripled, a decrease in heart weight to body weight ratio has been observed, even in the absence of a further decrease in blood pressure. Moreover, under both treatment regimens, the blood flow to the myocardium is maintained.[8] In clinical studies, clonidine has been shown to cause regression of cardiac muscle mass in patients with arterial hypertension.[9]

Methyldopa: Hemodynamic effects. Although it has been a matter of debate, there is sufficient evidence that alpha-methyldopa has a central mode of action.[10] Methyldopa through its metabolite alpha-norepinephrine seems to stimulate alpha-adrenergic receptors in the nucleus tractus solitarius, thereby decreasing adrenergic drive to the cardiovascular system.[2,11] The antihypertensive effect of methyldopa is mainly mediated by a decreased TPR with a small inconsistent reduction in CO and heart rate.[12,13]

The reduction in peripheral resistance has been found to be distributed in the skin and in the coronary circulation.[14] Renal blood flow does not seem to be well preserved, and parenchymal function remains intact.[12,15,16] Thus, as blood pressure decreases, renal vascular resistance also decreases.[15] It has also been shown that alpha-methyldopa increases cerebral blood flow and decreases cerebral vascular resistance.[17]

In the rat, arterial atrial pressure decreases within 6 hours after the administration of alpha-methyldopa, due to a decrease in TPR and possibly a slightly reduced output.[12,15,18–20] In addition, heart rate may be reduced, but the decrease in heart rate is relatively small when compared with the bradycardia resulting from guanethidine.[21]

In contrast to other investigators, Lund-Johansen[22] reported that the antihypertensive effect of methyldopa was related to a decreased cardiac output in patients with mild essential hypertension who were followed for a long-term period.

Unlike ganglion-blocking drugs, methyldopa produces a greater decrease of arterial pressure in the supine position, and postural hypotension is not usually a problem.[23,24] However, large doses of methyldopa, particularly when given in combination with a diuretic, can be associated with postural and exercise hypotension, although this occurs still less often than with bethandine or guanethidine.[25,26]

Left ventricular structure. Alpha-methyldopa has been widely studied and shown to be efficacious in not only lowering arterial pressure, but also in producing a regression of left ventricular hypertrophy (LVH) in animal studies as well as in patients with essential hypertension. Sen and co-workers[27–29] demonstrated that the administration of methyldopa to spontaneously hypertensive rats over a prolonged period will result in a decreased arterial pressure, regression of LVH, and normalization of DNA and myocardial RNA concentrations. Studies from our laboratory have shown that methyldopa in doses of 400 mg/kg/day orally for a 3-week period reduces heart weight in both normotensive Wistar-Kyoto and spontaneously hypertensive rats.[8] A reduction in heart weight was also reported in renovascular hypertensive rats treated for 5 weeks with alpha-methyldopa.[30] The reduction in heart weight was not accompanied by a decrease in myocardial blood flow per gram of tissue.[8]

Electron microscopic studies have indicated that prolonged treatment with alpha-methyldopa can decrease cell size.[31] In spontaneously hypertensive rats treated with alpha-methyldopa for 12 weeks at a dose that did not significantly reduce systolic pressure, mean cell area in both superepicardia and subendocardium was decreased when compared with that in the untreated group.[31]

Several clinical studies have also confirmed the efficacy of alpha-methyldopa in reducing LV mass.[32–37] Reichek et al[33] have shown reductions in LV mass, posterior wall, and septal thickness in patients with essential hypertension. Fouad et al[35] have indicated that the reduction in ventricular mass produced by methyldopa does not always parallel the reduction in arterial mass. Methyldopa has been shown to reduce ventricular mass not only in patients with LVH, but also in patients with normal cardiac mass.[36]

Guanabenz: Hemodynamic effects. Guanabenz is a new antihypertensive agent that acts through stimulation of alpha-adrenoreceptors centrally.[38,39] Noninvasive studies utilizing M-mode echo have shown that guanabenz lowers blood pressure without a consistent change in heart rate, CO, and TPR.[40] Others have shown that the decrease in blood pressure is associated with a decreased renal vascular resistance with no change in renal plasma flow and glomerular filtration rate.[41,42]

In patients with congestive heart failure, guanabenz (4 mg) produces an immediate decrease in blood pressure and heart rate associated with an unchanged CO.[43] In addition, a decrease in TPR and pulmonary wedge pressure was also observed.[43]

Postganglionic Adrenergic Blocking Drugs

Reserpine: Hemodynamic effects. Reserpine depletes stores of catecholamines and 5-hydroxytryptamine in brain, myocardium, blood vessels, and adrenergic nerve endings.[44-46] During chronic therapy with reserpine, both CO, peripheral resistance, and heart rate have been found to be decreased.[47]

Left ventricular structure. Reserpine has been shown to decrease ventricular mass in experimental animal studies.[48] Because of the depletion of catecholamines in myocardium, reserpine can cause heart failure.

Guanethidine, Bethanidine, and Debrisoquin: Hemodynamic effects. This group of drugs lowers arterial pressure through a reduction in both CO and TPR.[49-51] For guanethidine, it appears that initially the decrease in pressure is associated with a decreased CO.[51] After long-term therapy, blood pressure reduction is caused by a decreased peripheral resistance.[52] Postganglionic blocking agents also lower arterial pressure more during upright than in supine positions. This reduced pressure in the upright position is mainly due to an inhibition of the usual compensatory increase in venous tone and in TPR.[49,51,53] There is also a slight decrease in CO that does not seem to result from a direct action on the heart[54] because guanethidine increases CO during dynamic exercise,[51,55] even in subjects with large decreases in blood pressure. Debrisoquin and bethanidine differ from guanethidine only in that they have a faster onset and a shorter duration of action.[56,57]

Left ventricular structure. Guanethidine associated with a thiazide diuretic has been shown to decrease LVH and strain (electrocardiographically) as well as to reduce cardiomegaly as seen on chest radiographic films of patients with essential hypertension.[58]

Guanadrel: Hemodynamic effects. Guanadrel orally has been shown to decrease blood pressure through a decrease in peripheral resistance without changes in CO or heart rate in the supine position.[59-61] Moreover, a greater reduction in blood pressure associated with an inability to increase TPR was reported also in the erect position.[59,61]

A transient pressor response has been reported after the initial dose of guanadrel, which has been ascribed to an initial depletion of catecholamine stores.[61]

Left ventricular structure. The combination of guanadrel and hydrochlorothiazide has been shown to decrease LV mass after 5 weeks of treatment; however, at 12 weeks, LV mass was not significantly reduced.[62] Moreover, this reduction in LV mass was not associated with changes in myocardial contractility as measured by echo indices.[62]

Alpha$_1$-Adrenoreceptor Antagonist

Prazosin: Hemodynamic effects. Prazosin reduces arterial pressure by decreasing TPR through selective blockade of postsynaptic alpha$_1$-adrenergic receptors.[63] Experimental evidence in favor of this mechanism of action indicates that the hypotensive effect of prazosin could be abolished by prior alpha-adrenoreceptor blockade with phentolamine, whereas prazosin does not modify the pressor effect of angiotensin II, serotonin, and vasopressin.[64,65] In addition, prazosin produces vasodilation in isolated vascular beds only when sympathetic innervation is intact.[64,65]

Despite the reduced peripheral resistance, prazosin produces a lesser increase of plasma norepinephrine than phenoxybenzamine or phentolamine because of its receptor selectivity.[63] Acute oral administration of prazosin produces an immediate increase in plasma norepinephrine, heart rate, and plasma renin activity.[66] However, these changes are attenuated during long-term therapy. Cardiac output remains unchanged in essential hypertension and may even increase in patients with congestive heart failure (due to a reduction in preload and afterload). Whether or not prazosin has any effect on LV mass is not known at present.

References

1. FINCH L: The central hypotensive action of clonidine and Bay 1470 in cats and rats. Clin Sci Mol Med 1975; 48 (suppl): 273s–278s.

2. VAN ZWIETEN PA: Antihypertensive drugs with a central action. In: Progress in pharmacology. Stuttgart: Gustaf Fischer Verlag, 1975.

3. KINCAID-SMITH P: Management of severe hypertension. Am J Cardiol 1973; 32: 575–581.

4. SCHMITT H, SCHMITT H: Localization of the hypotensive effect of 2-(2-6-dichlorophenylamino)-2-imidazoline hydrochloride (ST 155, Catapresan). Eur J Pharmacol 1979; 6: 8.

5. BROD J, HORBACH L, JUST H, ROSENTHAL J, NICOLESCU R: Acute effects of clonidine on central and peripheral hemodynamics and plasma renin activity. Eur J Clin Pharmacol 1972; 4: 107–114.

6. ONESTI G, SCHWARTZ AB, KIM KE, SWARTZ C, BREST AN: Pharmacodynamic effects of a new antihypertensive drug, catapres (ST-155). Circulation 1969; 39: 219–228.

7. LUND-JOHANSEN P: Hemodynamic changes at rest and during exercise in long-term prazosin therapy of essential hypertension. In: Cotton DWK, ed. Prazosin—evaluation of a new antihypertensive agent. Amsterdam: Excerpta Medica, 1979; 43–53.

8. PEGRAM BL, ISHISE S, FROHLICH E: Effect of methyldopa, clonidine and hydralazine on cardiac mass and haemodynamics in Wistar-Kyoto and spontaneously hypertensive rats. Cardiovasc Res 1982; 16: 40–46.

9. DRAYER JIM, WEBER MA, GARDIN JM: Mediators of changes in left ventricular mass during antihypertensive therapy. In: TerKeurs HE, Schipperheyn JJ, eds. Cardiac left ventricular hypertrophy. Martinus Nijhoff Netherlands. 1983; 225–235.

10. FROHLICH ED: Methyldopa—mechanism and treatment 25 years later. Arch Intern Med 1980; 140: 954–959.

11. HENNING M, RUBENSON A: Evidence that the hypotensive action of α-methyldopa is mediated by central actions of methylonuradrenaline. J Pharm Pharmacol 1971; 23: 407–411.

12. ONESTI G, BREST AN, NOVACK P, KASPARIN H, MOYER JH: Pharmacodynamic effects of alpha-methyldopa in hypertensive subjects. Am Heart J 1964; 67: 32–38.

13. KIRKENDALL WM, WILSON WR: Pharmacodynamics and clinical use of guanethidine, bretylium and methyldopa. Am J Cardiol 1952; 9(1): 107.

14. COLIEN A, MAXMEN JS, RAGHEB M, et al: Effects of alpha-methyldopa on the myocardial blood flow, utilizing coincidence counting method. J Clin Pharmacol 1967; 7: 77–83.

15. SANNERSTEDT R, VARNAUSKAS E, WERKO L: Hemodynamic effects of methyldopa (Aldomet) at rest and during exercise in patients with renal hypertension. Acta Med Scand 1962; 171: 75–82.

16. MOHAMMED S, HANENSON IB, MAGENHEIM HG, et al: The effects of alpha methyldopa on renal function in hypertensive patients. Am Heart J 1968; 76: 21–27.

17. MEYER JS, SAVADA T, KITAMURA A, et al: Cerebral blood flow after control of hypertension in stroke. Neurology (Minneap) 1968; 18: 772–781.

18. WILSON WR, FISHER FD, KIRKENDALL WM: The acute hemodynamic effects of α-methyldopa in man. J Chron Dis 1962; 15: 907–913.

19. VINCENT WA, KASHEMSANT U, CUDDY RP, et al: The acute hemodynamic effects of α-methyldopa. Am J Med Sci 1963; 246: 558–568.

20. DOLLERY CT, HARINGTON M, HODGE JV: Haemodynamic studies with methyldopa: effect on cardiac output and response to pressor amines. Br Heart J 1963; 25: 670–676.

21. CHAMBERLAIN DA, HOWARD J: Guanethidine and methyldopa: a hemodynamic study. Br Heart J 1964; 26: 528–536.

22. LUNG-JOHANSEN P: Haemodynamic changes in long term α-methyldopa therapy in essential hypertension. Acta Med Scand 1972; 192: 221–226.

23. MESSERLI FH, DRESLINSKI GR, HUSSERL FE, et al: Antiadrenergic therapy. Hypertension 1981; 3 (suppl II): 226–229.

24. FROHLICH ED: Inhibition of adrenergic function in the treatment of hypertension. Arch Intern Med 1974; 133: 1033–1048.

25. PRICHARD BNC, JOHNSTON AV, HILL ID, ROSENHEIM ML: Bethanidine, guanethidine and methyldopa in the treatment of hypertension. A within-patient comparison. Br Med J 1968; 1: 135–144.

26. OATES JA, SELIGMANN AW, CLARK MA, ROUSSEAU P, LEE RE: The relative efficacy of guanethidine, methyldopa and paragyline as antihypertensive agents. N Engl J Med 1965; 273: 729–734.

27. SEN S, TARAZI RC, BUMPUS FM: Biochemical changes associated with development and reversal of cardiac hypertrophy in spontaneously hypertensive rats. Cardiovasc Res 1976; 10: 254–261.

28. SEN S, TARAZI RC, KHAIRALLAH PA, BUMPUS FM: Cardiac hypertrophy in spontaneously hypertensive rats. Circ Res 1974; 35: 775–781.

29. SEN S, TARAZI RC, BUMPUS FM: Cardiac hypertrophy and antihypertensive heart. Cardiovasc Res 1977; 11: 427–433.

30. KUWAJIMA I, KARDON MB, PEGRAM BL, SESOKO S, FROHLICH ED: Regression of

left ventricular hypertrophy in two-kidney, one clip Goldblatt hypertension. Hypertension 1982; 4 (suppl II): 113–118.

31. TOMANEK RJ, DAVIS JW, ANDERSON SC: The effects of alpha-methyldopa on cardiac hypertrophy in spontaneously hypertensive rats: ultrastructural, sterological and morphometric analysis. Cardiovasc Res 1979; 13: 173–182.

32. COREA L, BENTIVOGLIO M, VERDECCHIA P: Reversal of left ventricular hypertrophy in essential hypertension by early and long-term treatment with methyldopa. Clin Trials J 1981; 18: 380–394.

33. REICHEK N, FRANKLIN BB, CHANDLER T, MUHAMMAD A, PLAPPERT T, ST. JOHN-SUTTON M: Reversal of left ventricular hypertrophy by anti-hypertensive therapy. Eur Heart J 1982; 3 (suppl A): 165–169.

34. WOLLAM GL, HALL DW, PORTER VD, DOUGLAS MB, et al: Time course of regression of left ventricular hypertrophy in treated hypertensive patients. Am J Med 1983; 75: 100–109.

35. FOUAD FM, NAKASHIMA Y, TARAZI RC, SALCEDO EE: Reversal of left ventricular hypertrophy in hypertensive patients treated with methyldopa. Lack of association with blood pressure control. Am J Cardiol 1982; 49: 795–801.

36. DRAYER JIM, WEBER MA, GARDIN JM, LIPSON JL: The effect of chronic antihypertensive therapy on cardiac anatomy in patients with essential hypertension. Am J Med 1983; 75: 116–120.

37. WEINSTEIN M, HILEWITZ H, PAGE S: The effects of single-dose methyldopa and diuretics on blood pressure and left ventricular mass. Arch Intern Med 1984; 144: 1629–1633.

38. WALKER BR, HARE LE, DKEITCH MV: Comparative antihypertensive effects of guanabenz and clonidine. J Int Med Res 1982; 10: 6–14.

39. BAUM T, SHROPSHIRE AT: Studies of the antrally mediated hypotensive activity of guanabenz. Eur J Pharmacol 1976; 37: 31–44.

40. SNAH RS, WALKER BR, VANOV SK: Guanabenz effects on blood pressure and noninvasive parameters of cardiac performance in patients with hypertension. Clin Pharmacol Ther 1976; 19: 732–737.

41. BOSANAC P, DUBB T, WALKER BR, GOLDBERG M, AGUR Z: Renal effects of guanabenz, a new antihypertensive. J Clin Pharmacol 1976; 16: 631–636.

42. WARREN SE, COHEN IM, BONG AP, O'CONNOR DT: Guanabenz and hydrochlorothiazide for the treatment of essential hypertension: enhanced renal perfusion. Curr Ther Res 1980; 28: 530–534.

43. OLIVARI MT, LEVINE BT, CARLYLE P, COHN JN: Hemodynamic and neurohumoral effects of central vs peripheral sympathetic inhibition in heart failure (abstr). Circulation 1983; 68 (suppl III): 132.

44. IGGO A, WOGT M: Preganglionic sympathetic activity in normal and in reserpine-treated cats. J Physiol (London) 1960; 150: 114–133.

45. ARIDSEY CA, BRAUNWALD E, MORROW AG, MASON DT: Myocardial norepinephrine concentration in man. N Engl J Med 1963; 269: 653.

46. COHEN SJ, YOUNG MW, LAU SH, HAFT JI, DAMATO AN: Effects of reserpine therapy on cardiac output and atrioventricular conduction during rest and controlled heart rates in patients with essential hypertension. Circulation 1968; 37: 738–746.

47. MOYER JH: Cardiovascular and renal hemodynamic response to reserpine. Ann

NY Acad Sci 1954; 59: 82–94.

48. SEN S: Regression of cardiac hypertrophy experimental animal model. Am J Med 1983; 75: 87–93.

49. VILLAREAL H, EXAVIE JS, RUBIO V, DAVILA H: Effect of guanethidine and betylium tosilate on systemic and renal hemodynamics in essential hypertension. Am J Cardiol 1964; 14: 633–640.

50. CHRYSANT SG, ADAMOPOULOS PN, NISHIYAMA K, FROHLICH ED: Hemodynamic effects of bethanidine: a new sympatholytic antihypertensive drug (abstr.). Circulation 1974; 50 (suppl 3): 105.

51. RICHARDSON DW, WYSO EM, MCGEE JH, et al: Circulatory effects of guanethidine: clinical, renal and cardiac responses to treatment with a novel antihypertensive drug. Circulation 1960; 22: 184–190.

52. KISIN F, YURHAKOU S: Effects of reserpine, guanethidine and methyldopa on cardiac output and its distribution. Eur J Pharmacol 1976; 35: 253–258.

53. HANSSON L, PASCUAL A, JULIUS S: Comparison of guanadrel and guanethidine. Clin Pharmacol Ther 1973; 14: 204–208.

54. MOSER M: Guanethidine and bethanidine in the management of hypertension. Am Heart J 1969; 77: 423–427.

55. DOLLERY CT, EMSLIE-SMITH D, SHILLINGFORD JP: Haemodynamic effects of guanethidine. Lancet 1961; 2: 331–334.

56. JOHNSON AW, PRICHARD BNC, ROSENHEIM ML: The use of bethanidine in the treatment of hypertension. Lancet 1964; 2: 659–661.

57. KITCHIN AH, TURNER RWD: Studies on debrisoquine sulfate. Br Med J 1966; 2: 728–731.

58. LEWIS JA, KAVELMAN DA: Longterm follow-up of patients with hypertensive heart disease treated with guanethidine. Can Med Assoc J 1963; 88: 1010–1013.

59. CANZIANO JL, BLOOMFIELD DK: Hemodynamic effects of a new antihypertensive agent, guanadrel sulfate. Curr Ther Res 1969; 11: 736–744.

60. BLOOMFIELD DK, CANZIANO JL: Guanadrel and guanethidine in hypertension. Clin Pharmacol Ther 1969; 11: 200–204.

61. PASCUAL AV, JULIUS S: Short-term effectiveness and hemodynamic actions of guanadrel, a new sympatholytic drug. Curr Ther Res 1972; 14: 333–342.

62. DEQUATRO V, ALLEN JW: The comparative antihypertensive and cardiac effects of guanadrel and propranolol. Health Sci Rev 1984; 1: 17–20.

63. OKUN R: Effectiveness of prazosin as initial antihypertensive therapy. Am J Cardiol 1983; 51: 644–650.

64. BROGDEN RN, HEEL RC, SPEIGHT JM, AVERY GS: Prazosin: a review of its pharmacological properties and therapeutic efficacy in hypertension. Drugs 1977; 14: 163–197.

65. GRAHAM RM, OATES HF, STOKER LM, STOKES GS: Alpha blocking action of the antihypertensive agent prazosin. J Pharmacol Exp Ther 1977; 201: 747–752.

66. RUBIN PC, BLASCHKE TF: Studies on the clinical pharmacology of prazosin I: Cardiovascular, catecholamine and endocrine changes following a single dose. Br J Clin Pharmacol 1980; 10: 23–32.

35

Beta Blockade and Cardiac Function

B. SILKE M.D.
S.H. TAYLOR M.D.

Cardiac pumping activity is maintained through two distinct mechanisms. The intrinsic ability to respond to increased stretch with increased force of contraction is a fundamental biologic property of the healthy sarcomere (that is, the Frank-Starling mechanism). The value of this mechanism is restricted to maintaining cardiac pumping integrity at basal or near basal levels, but its usefulness is impaired in cardiac disease. The second mechanism is entirely dependent on the sympathetic nervous system; stimulation of the latter through the beta-adrenoceptor pathway is the only source by which cardiac pumping function can be rapidly adjusted over the wide range of demands encountered in normal ambulant man. Again, the efficiency of such stimulation is reduced in the damaged heart. It is, therefore, to be expected that drugs that attenuate such sympathetic stimulation will depress the mechanical activity of the heart, particularly in established cardiac disease. Despite the breadth of knowledge of the mechanisms controlling left ventricular (LV) pumping performance, and the well-documented pharmacodynamic effects of beta-adrenoceptor blocking drugs both in animals and man, there is a relative paucity of data concerning the influence of these drugs on those hemodynamic variables that describe LV pumping function in the conditions for which they are usually prescribed, namely, hypertension, angina pectoris, and myocardial infarction (MI). Therefore, this review is devoted to describing the quantitative effects of such blockade on cardiac pumping activity in these pathologic conditions.

Measurement of Left Ventricular Pumping Function in Intact Man

It is important to define those measurements that most reliably and precisely describe the pumping activity of the ventricle in man. Clues to the integrity of such pumping function in intact man may be derived from a wide range of noninvasive techniques. However, without exception, each of these techniques measures mechanical variables that are ancillary to the precise determinants of LV pumping performance, namely, the response of the pumped output to a change in filling load. Ancillary methods of study are not without value, for example, radionuclide measurement of ejection fraction. However, these methods are incapable of describing the global mechanical

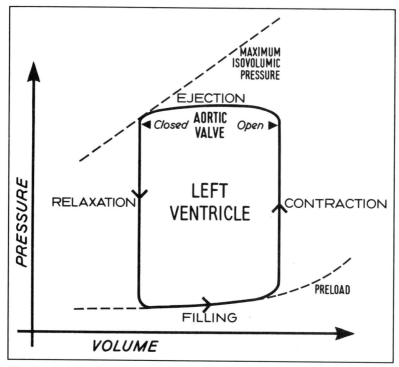

Figure 1. *Cardiac function as defined by the pressure-volume loop throughout a complete cardiac cycle.*

performance of the ventricle, particularly under a wide range of filling loads. The wide variability of many noninvasive methods also invalidates their use in the measurement of the relatively small changes that usually result from drug therapy.[1] How then can the mechanical performance of the ventricle be measured in man?

The pumping function of the left ventricle is ideally described by its pressure-volume relationships (Fig. 1). Although conceptually exact when applied to the pumping activity of the normal ventricle, description of its pressure volume characteristics suffers from a number of imponderables when applied to the contractile events in the diseased heart. Dyskinetic contraction due to regional pathologic lesions in the ventricular wall distorts the systolic component. This situation is aggravated by splinting of the sarcomeres by interstitial fibrosis and by atherosclerotic narrowing of the coronary vessels. As a consequence, the predicted changes induced by blockade of beta adrenoceptors, which may be apt in the normal heart, are inappropriate as a measure of its systolic performance when the ventricle is diseased and dilated. Diastolic relaxation of the diseased heart is also distorted. Hypertrophy, fibrosis, and other factors reduce the compliance of the ventricular wall, thus impeding interpretation of the influence of attenuation of sympathoadrenal stimulation. These restrictions hinder estimates of the efficiency of the heart as a pump; moreover, the influence of heart rate and preload is likely to be far more critical to the shape of the pressure volume loop in pathologic myocardial conditions than in the normal ventricle. The pressure volume loop may indeed afford an appropriate model to describe the effects of drugs on the mechanical performance of the left ventricle in the normal heart of the experimental animal, but even in this situation inferences may be invalid unless certain obligatory criteria are satisfied. It is essential that the reduction in myocardial contractility is not accompanied by changes in systemic arterial impedance, preload, or heart rate. Clearly, such exacting criteria are rarely achieved even in the experimental animal. Moreover, the distortion of the physical relationships induced by disease renders analysis of the influence of such a potent therapeutic intervention as beta-adrenoceptor blockade on such an idealized system open to impossible errors. Due to such considerations, we must be content with less ideal measurements of LV performance, particularly in evaluating the effects of beta-blocking therapy on the heart.

The most universally accepted measure of LV pumping performance is the filling pressure-pumped output relationship of the left ventricle. Sole dependence on this relationship has some disadvantages. It is a relationship that measures only work against pressure during ejection and it assumes linear influences of heart rate and preload on its performance. It ignores the proportion of blood expelled per stroke, that is, the ejection fraction, a prime measure of LV contractile competence. It is also far more sensitive in describing some therapeutic interventions than others; for example, it is more sensitive in reflecting interventions that result in direct changes in preload or afterload than interventions that are only indirectly represented, as with positive or negative inotropic drugs. Despite these serious shortcomings, this relationship is still the most commonly employed to describe the results of pharmacodynamic interventions, and the majority of published data pertains to this single relationship. We propose, therefore, to use this relationship to compare the influence of the beta-adrenoceptor antagonists on LV function in normal man and in patients with hypertension and coronary heart disease.

The studies to be considered will fulfil the following criteria: (1) Measurements of LV end-diastolic pressure or left heart filling pressure (pulmonary wedge pressure, pulmonary artery occluded pressure, or pulmonary artery diastolic pressure) measured directly; (2) cardiac output (CO) measured by a validated technique (Fick, indicator dilution) and its variability under the conditions of use stated; and (3) simultaneous measurements of systemic arterial pressure and heart rate documented.

Effect of Beta-Adrenoceptor Antagonists on Left Ventricular Performance in Normal Subjects

The relationship between the left heart filling pressure and the cardiac output following beta blockade in normal subjects has been defined in 6 healthy volunteers. Propranolol (10 mg intravenously) resulted in an increase in the

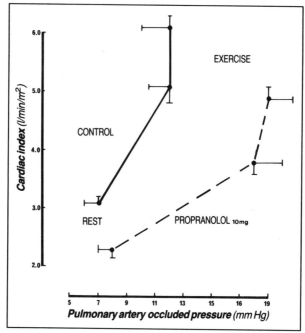

Figure 2. *Effect of propranolol (10 mg intravenously) on the relationship between CO and LV filling pressure, from rest to exercise and at 2 bicycle workloads in 6 normal volunteers.*

right atrial pressure and a reduction in the heart rate, CO, and stroke volume (SV) at rest without consistent effect on the pulmonary artery occluded pressure (Fig. 2). During constant load supine bicycle exercise (750 to 1000 kpm), the heart rate, SV, and CO were significantly less and the pulmonary artery occluded pressure significantly greater than that measured at similar levels of exercise in the control study. The right atrial pressure was also increased during exercise, significantly more than in the control study. These changes suggest that at low sympathetic states at rest, propranolol induced a small reduction in cardiac performance, but in a ventricle with adequate pumping reserve the hemodynamic consequences of beta blockade were clearly unmasked by exercise. Other data agree with these findings. Chamberlain[2] has previously documented that beta-blockade increases cardiac size in normal subjects, but the CO reduction in these subjects was clearly demonstrated only during exercise.[3] Data on practolol showed little effect on resting cardiac performance both at rest and during dynamic exercise in subjects with little evidence of cardiac disease.[4] However, during maximal and submaximal exercise, evidence of depression of CO and exercise capacity were clearly demonstrated following intravenous propranolol.[5]

Coronary Artery Disease

Effects of Beta Blockade in Angina Pectoris: The interpretation of impact of beta-blocking drugs in angina is complicated by the frequency with which acute LV decompensation is induced by exercise. Thus recognition that exercise-induced increase in LV end-diastolic pressure[6,7] and volume[8,9] are associated with the onset of symptoms is necessary when interpreting effects of beta blockade. The dose-response effects of beta blockade on resting cardiac performance in angina have been studied in detail; there are dose-related reductions in CO and dose-related increases in pulmonary artery occluded pressure. These findings are consistent for the different beta-blocking drugs.[10,11] The hemodynamic profile appears influenced by the presence or absence of the ancillary pharmacologic property of intrinsic sympathomimetic activity (ISA), and such hemodynamic differences may persist at the light levels of exercise that induce angina in coronary artery disease (Fig. 3). These results are in general agreement for data on practolol,[12,13] metoprolol,[14] oxprenolol,[15,16] and propranolol.[17–19] Apart from the ISA of beta-blocking drugs, concurrent vasodilation, with simultaneous reduction in LV afterload, can improve cardiac pumping function. The alpha- and beta-blocking drug labetalol resulted in lesser depression of cardiac pumping compared with an equivalent beta-blocking dose of propranolol;[20] addition of the calcium antagonist nifedipine to the cardioselective beta-blocking agent metoprolol induced less cardiodepression compared with beta-blocking monotherapy.[21]

Effects of Beta Blockade in Myocardial Infarction: Although beta blockade is increasingly recommended for use in MI, the hemodynamic impact on cardiac performance and possible differences between agents in MI have been poorly characterized. Propranolol (2 to 8 mg), in uncomplicated MI, induced greater reductions in pumped CO compared with similar doses in patients with stable angina.[22] This may be ascribable to reflex sympathetic activation following infarction[23] with increased circulatory plasma catecholamines.[24] Interestingly, despite the greater effects on CO, the increase in LV filling pressure was lower in MI. In a high sympathetic state, it might be predicted that the relevance of ISA in maintaining cardiac performance would be attenuated. This is, indeed, the case; a comparison of pindolol and propranolol, in equivalent beta-blocking doses, showed no clear separation of the effects of each drug on CO and LV filling pressure.[25]

Effects in Hypertension: Despite the wealth of hemodynamic data on beta blockade in hypertension,[26,27] the majority of studies have been accomplished using the dye dilution technique, and simultaneous assessment of CO and LV filling pressure is consequently unavailable. The effect of propranolol and oxprenolol on cardiac performance in 12 patients with uncomplicated hypertension has been assessed; the acute intravenous effects were compared with the long-term (3 months) effects of sustained oral medication. Studies were undertaken at rest and during supine bicycle exercise (Fig. 4). In the control studies the increases in CO were associated with increases in LV filling pressure; however, these increases appeared less marked than the

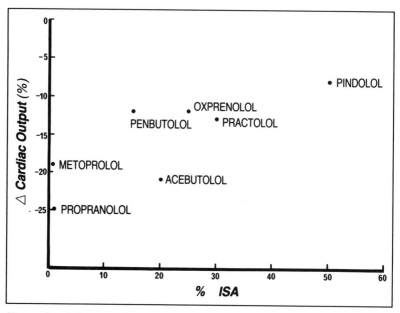

Figure 3. *Influence of the ISA of 7 beta-blocking drugs on exercise CO, (n = 53). Comparison with a control exercise period at the same workload following equivalent beta-blocking doses of each drug.*

increase seen during the reversible LV failure of angina. Following the administration of both propranolol and oxprenolol, the increase in resting LV filling pressure was of a similar order to that in patients with angina; however, during exercise, there was further additional depression of cardiac function (that is, the increment of LV filling pressure increased further). During sustained oral therapy, there were no significant differences in the relationship between CO and LV filling pressure compared with that following acute intravenous administration of either drug. This was despite a substantial (40/20 mmHg) reduction in blood pressure. These data suggest that the acute hemodynamic impact of beta-blocking drugs, with particular respect to CO and systemic vascular resistance, will not be modified during sustained therapy.

Lund-Johansen[28] has compared the acute and long-term effects of many beta-blocking drugs on the circulation in essential hypertension. The long-term data on atenolol, metoprolol, bunitrolol, penbutolol, and timolol support this hypothesis; the acute increase in systemic vascular resistance and reduced exercise CO is maintained during chronic therapy. Interestingly, the addition of prazosin to tolamolol[29] or the combination of alpha and beta blockade[30] substantially attenuated the adverse effects of beta blockade on systemic vascular resistance. Man in 'T Veld and Schalekamp[31] have demonstrated that both during the acute and sustained therapy of hypertension there is an inverse relationship between the change in systemic vascular resistance and the percentage of ISA resident in a beta-blocker compound; a

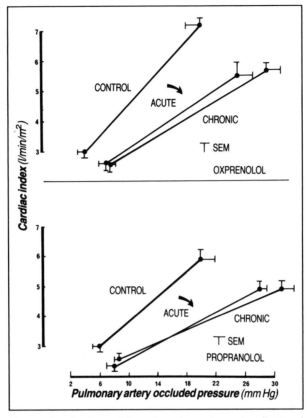

Figure 4. *Acute and long-term hemodynamic effects of propranolol and oxprenolol on cardiac pumping function in essential hypertension.*

long-term increased systemic vascular resistance persists for agents without ISA (propranolol, timolol, atenolol, metoprolol), is unchanged for agents with ISA in the 10% to 25% range (penbutolol, acebutolol, oxprenolol, alprenolol), and decreases with ISA greater than 25% (practolol, pindolol). The relevance of the continued disorder of systemic vascular resistance during the sustained therapy of hypertension is uncertain; however, it is probable that it reflects a continuing depression of central cardiac pumping function.

Summary

Beta blockade results in dose-related attenuation of sympathetic stimulation at cardiac beta-adrenoceptors; the hemodynamic consequences reflect global cardiac depression and are present in normal subjects and patients with coronary artery disease and hypertension. The CO is reduced and LV filling pressure increased. Although these changes are evident in normal subjects, they are particularly apparent in the stressed ventricle or when the cardiac reserve is impaired by the disease process. Factors modifying the hemodynamic response to beta blockade include the level of sympathetic nervous tone, the presence or absence of ISA in the beta-blocking compound, and the compliance of the left ventricle. In low sympathetic conditions the decrease in resting CO can be effectively prevented by a moderate degree of ISA. Conversely, in high sympathetic states, a reduction in CO may occur even in compounds possessing a substantial degree of ISA. Beta blockade usually induces dose-related increases in LV filling pressure; however, in high sympathetic states (MI, heart failure), the expected increase may not occur and on occasion the LV pressure may be reduced, due to improvement in myocardial compliance.

The immediate hemodynamic impact of beta blockade would not appear to be substantially modified during sustained therapy; hemodynamic differences between drugs with respect to central and peripheral effects during long-term beta blockade can be correlated with the ISA of the drug. The concurrent use of alpha-receptor or slow-channel blocking compounds can improve the hemodynamic profile during chronic beta blockade due to the reduction in LV afterload.

References

1. JOHNSON BF, MEERAN MK, FRANK A, TAYLOR SH: Systolic time intervals in measurement of inotropic drugs. Br Heart J 1981; 46: 513–521.

2. CHAMBERLAIN D: Effects of beta-adrenergic blockade on heart size. Am J Cardiol 1966; 18: 321–328.

3. CHAMBERLAIN DA, HOWARD J: The haemodynamic effects of beta-sympathetic blockade. Br Heart J 1964; 2: 213–217.

4. GIBSON D, SOWTON E: Effects of ICI 50172 in man during erect exercise. Br Med J 1968; 1: 213–215.

5. EPSTEIN SE, ROBINSON BF, KAHLER RL, BRAUNWALD E: Effects of beta-adrenergic blockade in the cardiac response to maximal and submaximal exercise in man. J Clin Invest 1965; 44: 1745–1753.

6. TAYLOR SH, SILKE B, LEE PS: Intravenous beta-blockade in coronary heart disease: is cardioselectivity or intrinsic sympathomimetic activity hemodynamically useful? N Engl J Med 1981; 306: 631–635.

7. SVENDSEN T, HARTLING OJ, TRAP-JENSEN J, MCNAIR A, BLIDDAL J: Adrenergic beta-receptor blockade: haemodynamic importance of intrinsic sympathomimetic activity. Clin Pharmacol Ther 1981; 29: 711–718.

8. DEHMER GJ, FALKOFF M, LEWIS SE, HILLIS LD, PARKEY RW, WILLERSON JT: Effect of oral propranolol on rest and exercise left ventricular ejection fraction, volumes and segmental wall motion in patients with blood angina pectoris. Assessment with equilibrium gated blood pool imaging. Br Heart J 1981; 45: 656–666.

9. COLTART DJ, ALDERMAN EL, ROBINSON SC, HARRISON DC: Effect of propranolol on left ventricular function, segmental wall motion and diastolic pressure-volume relation in man. Br Heart J 1975; 37: 357–364.

10. TAYLOR SH, SILKE B, LEE PS, HILAL A: Haemodynamic dose-response effects of intravenous beta-blocking drugs with different ancillary properties in patients with coronary heart disease. Eur Heart J 1982; 3: 564–569.

11. REALE A, NIGRI A, GIOFFRE PA, MOTOLESE M: Acute influence of different beta-blocking agents upon left heart haemodynamics at rest and during exercise in patients with coronary heart disease. Eur J Cardiol 1979; 2: 101–109.

12. GIBSON DG: Haemodynamic effects of practolol. Postgrad Med J 1971; 47 (suppl): 16–21.

13. SOWTON E, BALCON R, CROSS D, FRICK H: Haemodynamic effects of ICI 50,172 in patients with ischaemic heart disease. Br Med J 1968; 1: 215–216.

14. HENDRY WG, SILKE B, TAYLOR SH: Haemodynamic dose-response effects of intravenous metoprolol in coronary heart disease. Eur J Clin Pharmacol 1981; 19: 323–327.

15. BENSAID J, SCEBAT L, LENEGRE J: Haemodynamic effects of intravenous oxprenolol. Postgrad Med J 1970; 46 (suppl): 49–56.

16. SILKE B, HILAL A, TAYLOR SH: Haemodynamic dose-response effects of intravenous oxprenolol in coronary heart disease. J Cardiovasc Pharmacol 1981; 3: 716–727.

17. COLTART DJ: Haemodynamic effects of beta-blockade in patients with angina pectoris. Postgrad Med J 1976; 52 (suppl 4): 47–55.

18. GRANDJEAN T, RIVIER JL: Cardiocirculatory effects of beta-adrenergic blockade in organic heart disease. Comparison between propranolol and Ciba 39,089 Ba. Br Heart J 1968; 30: 50–59.

19. PARKER JO, WEST RO, DI GIORGI S: Hemodynamic effects of propranolol in coronary heart disease. Am J Cardiol 1968; 21: 11–19.

20. SILKE B, NELSON GIC, AHUJA RC, TAYLOR SH: Comparative haemodynamic dose-response effects of propranolol and labetalol in coronary heart disease. Br Heart J 1982; 48: 364–371.

21. NELSON GIC, SILKE B, AHUJA RC, HUSSAIN M, FORSYTH D, TAYLOR SH: The effect on left ventricular performance of nifedipine and metoprolol singly and together in exercise-induced angina pectoris. Eur Heart J 1984; 5: 67–79.

22. SILKE B, NELSON GIC, VERMA SP, et al: Enhanced haemodynamic effects of propranolol in acute myocardial infarction. Eur Heart J 1984; 5: 366–373.

23. KARLSBERG RP, PENKOSKE PA, CRYER PE, CORR PB, ROBERTS R: Rapid activation of the sympathetic nervous system following coronary artery occlusion: relation to infarct size, site and haemodynamic impact. Cardiovasc Res 1979; 13: 523–531.

24. VALORI C, THOMAS M, SHILLINGFORD J: Free noradrenaline and adrenaline excretion in relation to clinical syndromes following myocardial infarction. Am J Cardiol 1967; 20: 605–617.

25. SILKE B, VERMA SP, AHUJA RC, et al: Is the sympathomimetic activity (ISA) of beta-blocking drugs relevant in acute myocardial infarction? Eur J Clin Pharmacol 1984; 27: 509–515.

26. HANSSON L: Beta-adrenergic blockade in essential hypertension. Acta Med Scand [Suppl] 1973; 550: 7–40.
27. TARAZI RC, DUSTAN HP: Beta-adrenergic blockade in hypertension. Am J Cardiol 1972; 29: 633–640.
28. LUND-JOHANSEN P: Central haemodynamic effects of beta-blockers in hypertension. Eur Heart J 1983; 4 (suppl D): 1–12.
29. LUND-JOHANSEN P: Haemodynamic long-term effects of prazosin plus tolamolol in essential hypertension. Br J Clin Pharmacol 1977; 4: 141–145.
30. LUND-JOHANSEN P, BAKKE OM: Haemodynamic effects and plasma concentrations of labetalol during long-term treatment of essential hypertension. Br J Clin Pharmacol 1979; 7: 169–174.
31. MAN IN 'T VELD AJ, SCHALEKAMP MADH: Haemodynamic consequents of intrinsic sympathomimetic activity and cardioselectivity in beta-blocker therapy for hypertension. Eur Heart J 1983; 4 (suppl D): 31–41.

36

Cardiac Effects of Direct-Acting Vasodilators

JOSEPH A. FRANCIOSA, M.D.

The hemodynamic hallmark of hypertension is inappropriate elevation of the systemic vascular resistance. Because systemic vascular resistance may be within the absolute normal range in some patients, elevation of blood pressure in such cases has been attributed to increased cardiac output (CO).[1] However, for any given CO, systemic vascular resistance is usually elevated in patients with hypertension compared with normotensive subjects (Fig. 1). Interventions that reduce systemic vascular resistance are therefore useful in the management of hypertension. Vasodilator drugs can be defined as those agents that reduce systemic vascular resistance by directly relaxing vascular smooth muscle. Vasodilation can also be the result of indirect action on vascular smooth muscle by inhibition of sympathetic nervous activity or antagonism of circulating neurohumoral vasoconstrictor substances. This discussion will be concerned primarily with direct-acting vasodilator drugs.

Vasodilator Effects on Cardiac Function

The primary hemodynamic action of vasodilators is to lower the systemic blood pressure. This hypotensive effect in turn triggers compensatory physiologic responses intended to restore blood pressure, and usually consists of tachycardia with an increase in CO.[2,3] These compensatory responses are frequently effective, so that direct-acting vasodilators have not been very useful for long-term antihypertensive monotherapy. The hemodynamic response patterns to vasodilators are not uniform, but vary due to inherent differences in properties of specific drugs and to differences in patient characteristics. Site of primary action is an important drug-specific property. Vasodilators that tend to localize more in systemic arterial tissue, such as hydralazine and minoxidil, dilate primarily resistance vessels, resulting in marked reduction of systemic arterial pressure with significant tachycardia and increased CO, and little change in systemic venous or pulmonary arterial pressures.[4-7] Agents that act primarily on capacitance vessels, such as nitroglycerin and nitrates, markedly reduce systemic venous and pulmonary arterial pressures, with a tendency to lower CO because of venous pooling and re-

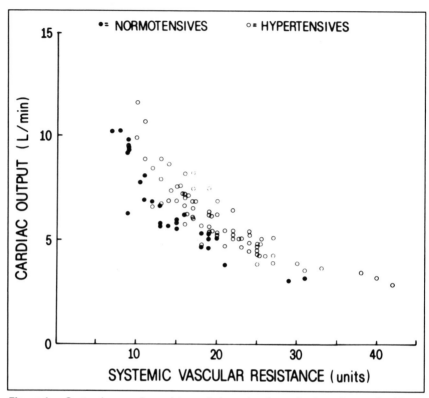

Figure 1. *Systemic vascular resistance in hypertensive patients and normal subjects. Patients with hypertension generally fall to the right, that is, along the higher resistance axis, compared with normal subjects.*

duced cardiac preload.[8] The modest decrease in systemic blood pressure may be a result of lower stroke volume (SV) as well as arterial dilation. Vasodilators with balanced arterial and venous activity, such as nitroprusside, reduce venous and pulmonary arterial as well as systemic arterial pressures with varying effects on CO, depending on the net effects of concomitant reduction in cardiac preload and afterload.[9]

A major determinant of hemodynamic response to vasodilators is the status of ventricular function. Output of the normal ventricle is largely dependent on cardiac preload as the normal heart operates on a steep preload curve. Changes in afterload are well compensated for by the normal ventricle and the afterload function curve is relatively flat.[10] The converse applies to the failing ventricle, which operates on a depressed flattened preload curve. Instead, the failing ventricle operates on a steep curve inversely related to afterload.[11,12] Thus, CO response to a vasodilator will depend on the interplay of specific drug effects on preload and afterload and of the status of ventricular dependence on the specific loading conditions. An example of this interplay

TABLE I   **Hemodynamic Responses to Nitroprusside***

Subjects	Blood Pressure	Left Ventricular Filling Pressure	Cardiac Output	Heart Rate
		Change (%)		
Normal	−15	−45	−15	+15
Hypertensive without heart failure	−20	−50	−25	+25
Congestive heart failure	−20	−40	+55	− 5

*Used with permission from Franciosa.[9]

is provided by observing hemodynamic responses to the balanced preload and afterload reducer, sodium nitroprusside (Table I). When normal subjects or hypertensive patients without heart failure and patients with heart failure are given an infusion of nitroprusside to reduce blood pressure comparably, left ventricular (LV) filling pressure decreases similarly in all groups. In the preload-dependent normal subjects or patients with hypertension without heart failure, CO declines slightly and heart rate increases reflexly. In afterload-dependent patients with LV failure, CO increases and heart rate actually decreases slightly.[3,9,12] These hemodynamic effects of vasodilators in patients with heart failure are of considerable therapeutic value and should be useful in relieving symptoms due to increased ventricular filling pressures or inadequate CO. Sodium nitroprusside is now widely used to treat acute LV failure of various causes.[13–17]

This short-term efficacy of vasodilators in acute left heart failure has generated considerable interest in extending their use to the long-term management of chronic congestive heart failure. A number of vasodilators have been tested for this purpose and include nitrates, hydralazine, prazosin, minoxidil, captopril, and slow-channel calcium blockers.[18] All these agents are capable of reducing ventricular filling pressures and raising CO to varying degrees. Quantitative differences between them probably reflect their different sites of action in large part. Their hemodynamic effects are generally sustained although tolerance may occasionally develop.[3,9,18] The sustained hemodynamic improvement is often associated with amelioration of symptoms and increased exercise capacity of patients with chronic heart failure.[18] Despite these encouraging results to date, the ultimate role of long-term vasodilator therapy for chronic heart failure is yet to be established pending the outcome of ongoing trials aimed at assessing efficacy on morbidity and mortality. In the meantime vasodilators are considered adjunctive to standard digitalis and diuretic therapy.

Other factors may also determine the cardiac and hemodynamic effects of vasodilators. The hypotensive effect of vasodilators, occasionally associated with a decrease in SV, can reflexly stimulate baroreceptors with consequent sympathoadrenal activation. As a result, circulating catecholamines and plasma renin activity usually increase.[19,20] This leads to increased sympathetic drive to the heart with augmentation of heart rate and contractility. Certain vasodilators, especially hydralazine, may directly stimulate the heart. Intracoronary infusion of hydralazine in nonsystemic doses increases heart rate and enhances contractility in experimental animals.[3] Whether such direct cardiac stimulation occurs at clinically employed doses of hydralazine is unclear.[21] Effects of vasodilators on regional vascular beds may also influence cardiac performance. Renal vasodilation can reduce tone of the afferent arterioles, thereby decreasing glomerular filtration pressure. In addition, reflex stimulation of the renin-angiotensin system may occur, and this combination of events can lead to significant salt and water retention with elevation of cardiac filling pressures.[6,22] Most vasodilators act on coronary arteries and increase total coronary blood flow.[9] Regional distribution of flow within the myocardium may vary, however, among drugs and underlying pathophysiology.[23] Despite this increase in coronary blood flow, vasodilators are well-known precipitators of myocardial ischemia and angina pectoris, primarily due to their effects on heart rate and contractility, which combine to increase myocardial oxygen demand disproportionate to any increase in blood flow and oxygen delivery. Myocardial ischemia can depress ventricular function and offset the beneficial hemodynamic effects of vasodilation and reduced afterload.

It is apparent from the foregoing discussion that vasodilators may improve hemodynamics and cardiac performance, but the interaction of direct and indirect cardiovascular effects of these agents may account for the nonuniform responses and seemingly paradoxical effects sometimes produced by these agents. For example, minoxidil, a potent predominantly arterial dilator, lowers systemic vascular resistance and increases CO without changing ventricular filling pressures in patients with heart failure.[7] Minoxidil also significantly increases LV ejection fraction in these patients, but despite these apparently beneficial effects, patients do not experience an increase in exercise capacity and may even worsen clinically because of concomitant fluid retention, arrhythmias, and angina.[24]

Vasodilator Effects on Cardiac Structure

Left ventricular hypertrophy (LVH) commonly develops during the course of hypertension and congestive heart failure, and treatment of these disorders can eliminate or prevent the hypertrophy. In the spontaneously hypertensive rat, vasodilator drugs have reduced blood pressure more than antiadrenergic drugs, but only the latter agents prevented hypertrophy.[25] This suggests an important role of the adrenergic nervous system in the genesis of cardiac hypertrophy. Prolonged sympathetic stimulation of the heart can produce myocardial damage and cellular hypertrophy.[26,27] Vasodilator-induced reflex sympathetic stimulation may therefore account for inability of these agents to prevent or eliminate LVH in hypertension. In contrast, long-term vasodilator therapy has reduced myocardial cell size in patients with chronic heart failure.[28] This apparent paradox may relate to the fact that circulating catecholamines are already quite high in heart failure and vasodilator-mediated improvement in hemodynamics may result in withdrawal of sympathetic tone. It has been observed that plasma catecholamine levels increase little during minoxidil administration in heart failure, and they may even decrease significantly during nitroprusside infusion in some patients with heart failure.[7,29] Our concepts regarding the significance of cardiac hypertrophy are currently being reassessed. Although prevention or regression of cardiac hypertrophy has generally been regarded as a favorable outcome, it is possible that hypertrophy represents an important compensatory response for the overburdened ventricle. Reversal of hypertrophy could precipitate heart failure in the presence of an acute increase in cardiac load, such as might be imposed by recurrent hypertension or acute cardiac injury.[30] Thus, vasodilators with their complex hemodynamic and neurohumoral actions can play a pivotal role in influencing cardiac structure.

Conclusions

Direct-acting vasodilators appear to be useful agents in the management of hypertension and heart failure. Because of their direct and rapid onset of action, they are especially valuable in the treatment of acute hypertensive emergencies and acute LV failure. The role of vasodilators for long-term therapy of heart failure or hypertension needs further definition. The hemodynamic effects of these agents appear to produce sustained clinical benefits, but the other indirect reflex and neurohumoral responses to vasodilators may result in complex, potentially harmful alterations of cardiac structure and function over the long-term. Perhaps newer vasodilator drugs, such as the renin-angiotensin antagonists or slow-channel calcium entry blockers, will be less potent activators of the sympathetic nervous system and be better suited to prolonged administration.

References

1. MESSERLI FH, VENTURA HO, REISEN E, et al: Borderline hypertension and obesity: two prehypertensive states with elevated cardiac output. Circulation 1982; 66: 55–60.
2. JUDSON WE, HOLLANDER W, WILKINS RW: The effects of intravenous apresoline (hydralazine) on cardiovascular and renal function in patients with and without congestive heart failure. Circulation 1956; 13: 664–674.
3. FRANCIOSA JA, PIERPONT G: Cardiovascular clinical pharmacology of impedance reducing agents. J Chron Dis 1981; 34: 341–352.
4. MOORE-JONES D, PERRY HM JR: Radioautographic localization of hydralazine-1-C_{14} in arterial walls. Proc Soc Exp Biol Med 1966; 122: 576–579.
5. ABLAD B, JOHNSSON G: Comparative effects of intra-arterially administered hydralazine and sodium nitrite on the blood flow and the volume of forearm. Acta Pharmacol Toxicol (Copenh) 1963; 20: 1–15.
6. KLOTMAN PE, GRIM EC, WEINBERGER MH: The effects of minoxidil on pulmonary and systemic hemodynamics in hypertensive man. Circulation 1977; 55: 394–400.

7. FRANCIOSA JA, COHN JN: Effects of minoxidil on hemodynamics in patients with congestive heart failure. Circulation 1981; 63: 652–657.

8. FRANCIOSA JA, BLANK RC, COHN JN: Nitrate effects on cardiac output and left ventricular outflow resistance in chronic congestive heart failure. Am J Med 1978; 64: 207–213.

9. FRANCIOSA JA, COHN JN: Hemodynamic responsiveness to short- and long-acting vasodilators in left ventricular failure. Am J Med 1978; 65: 126–133.

10. SARNOFF SJ, MITCHELL JH: Control of function of heart. In: Hamilton WF, Dow P, eds. Handbook of physiology. Washington, DC: American Physiological Society, 1962; 489–532.

11. ROSS J JR: Afterload mismatch and preload reserve: a conceptual framework for the analysis of ventricular function. Prog Cardiovasc Dis 1976; 18: 255–264.

12. FRANCIOSA JA: Outflow resistance as a regulator of left ventricular performance. Angiology 1978; 29: 393–401.

13. COHN JN, FRANCIOSA JA: Vasodilator therapy of cardiac failure. N Engl J Med 1977; 297: 27–31, 254–258.

14. FRANCIOSA JA, GUIHA NH, RODRIGUERA E, et al: Improved left ventricular function during nitroprusside infusion in acute myocardial infarction. Lancet 1972; 1: 650–654.

15. COHN JN, FRANCIOSA JA, FRANCIS GS, et al: Effect of short-term infusion of sodium nitroprusside on mortality rate in acute myocardial infarction complicated by left ventricular failure. Results of a Veterans Administration Cooperative Study. N Engl J Med 1982; 306: 1129–1135.

16. GUIHA NH, COHN JN, MIKULIC E, et al: Treatment of refractory heart failure with infusion of nitroprusside. N Engl J Med 1974; 291: 587–592.

17. FRANCIOSA JA, SILVERSTEIN SR: Hemodynamic effects of nitroprusside and furosemide in left ventricular failure. Clin Pharmacol Ther 1982; 32: 62–69.

18. FRANCIOSA JA: Effectiveness of long-term vasodilator administration in the treatment of chronic left ventricular failure. Prog Cardiovasc Dis 1982; 24: 319–330.

19. BRUNNER H, HEDWALL PR, MEIER M: Influence of adrenergic beta-receptor blockade on the acute cardiovascular effects of hydralazine. Br J Pharmacol 1967; 30: 123–133.

20. LIN M, McNAY JL, SHEPHERD AMM, KEETON TK: Effects of hydralazine and sodium nitroprusside on plasma catecholamines and heart rate. Clin Pharmacol Ther 1983; 34: 474–480.

21. KOCH-WESER J: Myocardial inactivity of therapeutic concentrations of hydralazine and diazoxide. Experientia 1974; 30: 170–171.

22. PIERPONT GL, BROWN DC, FRANCIOSA JA, COHN JN: Effect of hydralazine on renal function in patients with congestive heart failure. Circulation 1980; 61: 323–327.

23. CHIARELLO M, GOLD HK, LEINBACH RC, et al: Comparison between the effects of nitroglycerin and nitroprusside on ischemic injury during acute myocardial infarction. Circulation 1976; 54: 766–773.

24. FRANCIOSA JA, JORDAN RA, WILEN MM, LEDDY CL: Minoxidil in patients with chronic left heart failure: contrasting hemodynamic and clinical effects in a controlled trial. Circulation 1984; 70: 63–68.

25. SEN S, TARAZI RC, KAIRALLAH PA, BUMPUS FM: Cardiac hypertrophy in spontaneously hypertensive rats. Circ Res 1974; 35: 775–781.

26. OESTMAN-SMITH I: Cardiac sympathetic nerves as the final common pathway in
the induction of adaptive cardiac hypertrophy. Clin Sci 1981; 61: 265–272.

27. TARAZI RC, SEN S: Catecholamines and cardiac hypertrophy. In: Mezey KC,
Caldwell ADS, eds. Catecholamines and the heart. London: Academic Press
and Royal Society of Medicine, 1979; 48–57.

28. UNVERFERTH DV, MEHEGAN JP, MAGORIEN RD, UNVERFERTH BJ, LEIER CV: Regression of myocardial cellular hypertrophy with vasodilator therapy in
chronic congestive heart failure associated with idiopathic dilated cardiomyopathy. Am J Cardiol 1983; 51: 1392–1398.

29. OLIVARI MT, LEVINE TB, COHN JN: Abnormal neurohumoral response to nitroprusside infusion in congestive heart failure. J Am Coll Cardiol 1983; 2: 411–
417.

30. FERRARIO CM, SPECH MM, TARAZI RC, DOI Y: Cardiac pumping ability in rats
with experimental renal and genetic hypertension. Am J Cardiol 1979; 44: 979–
985.

37

Calcium Channel Blockers in Hypertension: The Role of Their Cardiac Effects

ALAN T. HIRSCH, M.D.
BARRY M. MASSIE, M.D.
ISAO K. INOUYE, M.D.
JULIO F. TUBAU, M.D.

The development of calcium channel blocking agents has provided us with drugs with demonstrated efficacy in the therapy of coronary artery vasospastic disease, exertional angina, and supraventricular arrhythmias. During early trials for these applications, it became apparent that they also held promise as antihypertensive drugs, with a profile of actions unique among presently available agents. During the past decade, European and Japanese studies have further defined their antihypertensive effects. Theoretical considerations suggest that their unique cardiac effects may increase their value in the long-term treatment of hypertension, particularly in certain subsets of patients. Verapamil and nifedipine have undergone extensive clinical trials; diltiazem has been less well studied, but because of its relatively more benign side effects, it deserves more attention. Many newer agents of this class are also under investigation. However, the ultimate role of the calcium blockers in essential hypertension, although promising, requires further delineation and rigorous confirmation.

Mechanism of Action

An increase in peripheral vascular resistance is the most common hemodynamic abnormality in essential hypertension.[1] Thus, a reduction of peripheral resistance is the most direct way to correct pharmacologically the underlying pathophysiology. A potential role for calcium channel blockers is suggested by the dependence of vascular smooth muscle on the role of Ca^{++} in the regulation of vasomotor tone.[2]

The cell membrane participates in regulating the flux of Ca^{++} from extracellular to intracellular sites, both in the cytosol and in the sarcoplasmic reticulum and mitochondria. Several mechanisms are involved and are repre-

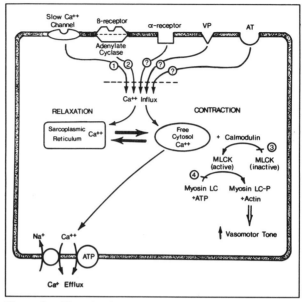

Figure 1. *The role of calcium and calcium channel blocking drugs in the regulation of vascular smooth muscle tone. Major routes of calcium influx and efflux are schematically depicted. These agents decrease transmembrane calcium influx by blocking influx at the slow-calcium channel and by decreasing alpha-adrenergic receptor-associated influx. The relative importance of inhibited calcium influx associated with vasopressin (VP) and angiotensin (AT) receptor stimulation is unknown. Secondary effects include inhibition of myosin light chain kinase (MLCK) activation and decreased phosphorylation of myosin light chains. Crossbridge formation and vasomotor tone are thus decreased. LC-P = phosphorylated light chain.*

sented schematically in Figure 1. Influx may occur via either voltage or receptor-mediated membrane Ca^{++} channels; alpha receptors are thought to mediate a small calcium influx, but a larger influx enters through the slow-calcium channels. Free intracellular Ca^{++} increases further as the sarcoplasmic reticulum releases its sequestered Ca^{++} stores. Efflux from the cells may be coupled to sodium or occur via a separate energy-dependent process. Inside the cell, Ca^{++} regulation is a pivotal factor in vascular muscle contraction and relaxation. As a terminal step required for actin-myosin interaction, the free intracellular Ca^{++} concentration must increase at least 100-fold toward 10^{-6} M. As intracellular Ca^{++} concentration increases, a series of biochemical events leads to vasoreactivity. A small cytoplasmic protein, calmodulin, selectively binds Ca^{++} and activates myosin light chain kinase.

These events induce phosphorylation of myosin from adenosine triphosphate (ATP); actin and myosin then interact and produce smooth muscle contraction.

Catecholamine-induced vasoconstriction, and likely that produced by angiotensin and vasopressin, is dependent on receptor-mediated Ca^{++} influx. Ca^{++} entry blockers are structurally heterogeneous compounds, originally classified together due to their common property of inhibition of cellular Ca^{++} influx. In addition to Ca^{++} entry blockade, verapamil and, possibly, diltiazem may also cause a noncompetitive inhibition of peripheral alpha$_2$ receptors, thereby modulating additional vasodilation.[3] Since Ca^{++} transport is involved in many physiologic processes related to hypertension, including nerve terminal secretion of norepinephrine, adrenal secretion of aldosterone and transmembrane Na^+ transports, Ca^{++} entry blockade may lower blood pressure by multiple mechanisms, but the clinical significance of these actions remains to be elucidated.

Experimental models of hypertension support the concept that pathologic calcium regulation may be a feature of the essential hypertensive state.[4] Calcium itself has a direct vasoconstrictor action on vascular smooth muscle in vitro. In vivo, epidemiologic studies offer conflicting results: lower serum ionized Ca^{++} concentrations were noted in a small group of hypertensive patients compared with controls,[5] but a study of a larger Belgian population noted a positive correlation between total plasma calcium levels and systemic blood pressure.[6] In a well-defined experimental model of hypertension, the spontaneously hypertensive rat, Ca^{++} binding by the vascular cell membrane, mitochondrial handling of Ca^{++}, and Ca^{++} fluxes in other cell membranes are disturbed, again suggesting a role for Ca^{++} in the pathogenesis of hypertension.[4]

In addition to its effect on vascular smooth muscle tone, Ca^{++} may alter the cardiac contribution to arterial pressure. Inhibition of myocardial cell Ca^{++} fluxes produces negative inotropic and chronotropic responses. In vitro, all available agents produce directionally similar cardiac effects and all relax vascular smooth muscle. Verapamil produces greater direct depression of contractility than nifedipine, and diltiazem may have a lesser negative inotropic effect than either. All three agents alter the action potentials of the slow-channel dependent cells of the sinus and atrioventricular nodes, reducing their automaticity and rate of depolarization.

In vivo, these direct effects are variably balanced by reflex sympathetic mechanisms; thus, clinically relevant in vivo effects are not always those that would be predicted from the experimental studies. These are also summarized in Table I. Cardiac performance is not usually impaired. In fact, in both canine and human hemodynamic studies, nifedipine use is often associated with an increase in cardiac index (CI), and verapamil is associated with a stable or decreased CI, whereas diltiazem causes the least change from baseline.[7] Similarly, the negative chronotropic effect of nifedipine is often superseded by a sympathetic-mediated increase in heart rate. Heart rate is not significantly altered by verapamil and diltiazem in most patients, although small decreases at rest and larger reductions during exercise may occur.

TABLE I   In Vivo Effects of Calcium Entry Blocking Drugs

	Nifedipine	Verapamil	Diltiazem
Systemic resistance	↓↓↓	↓↓	↓↓
Coronary resistance	↓↓	↓	↓↓
Cardiac output*	↑↑	↔ or ↓	↔
Heart rate	↑ or ↔	↔ or ↓	↔ or ↓
Atrioventricular conduction	↔	↓	↔ or ↓

↑, ↑↑, ↑↑↑, and ↓, ↓↓, ↓↓↓ = mild, moderate, or marked increase or decrease; ↔ = no change.
*In patients with normal left ventricular function. All three agents may depress ejection fraction and cardiac output in patients with poor left ventricular function.

Antihypertensive Effects

Many studies describing the efficacy of verapamil and nifedipine as primary antihypertensive agents have been published. Detailed recent reviews of these data have also appeared.[4,8,9]

Despite their variable direct effects on the myocardium, all presently available and investigational calcium blockers reversibly inhibit vascular smooth muscle tone. This effect is heightened in direct proportion to pretreatment systemic vascular resistance and arterial pressure.[10,11] Thus, when verapamil or nifedipine are administered to normotensive humans, only a minimal decrease in blood pressure occurs. This contrasts rather dramatically with the response in a hypertensive cohort. In this situation, verapamil (180 to 360 mg/day) or nifedipine (20 to 80 mg/day) produces a prompt 15% to 20% decrease in arterial pressure.[12,13] Nifedipine, in particular, has been utilized with a generally good result in the acute therapy of accelerated hypertension and hypertensive emergencies.[14] A 10% to 20% decrease in systolic and diastolic pressures persists during chronic drug therapy. In addition to their similar hypotensive potencies, both agents have been found to produce a greater antihypertensive effect in individuals with low plasma renin activity.[10,15] Early suggestions that verapamil is particularly effective in elderly patients remain unconfirmed, but may represent a promising application.

Long-term studies of calcium blockers in hypertension are limited and controlled trials are even rarer. Table II summarizes selected English language studies that have evaluated therapy with these agents for a minimum of 3 weeks. In general, the studies support the efficacy of these drugs, but the frequency of side effects and lack of pharmacologic tolerance during chronic therapy remain to be documented in more rigorous trials.

Previously available direct-acting vasodilators, such as hydralazine, minoxidil, and diazoxide, stimulate the potent coexisting homeostatic regulators of arterial pressure, which are often responsible for both diminished long-term pharmacologic efficacy and for the development of adverse effects. Calcium channel blockers, if they are to be more effective during

TABLE II The Results of Selected Trials of Oral Nifedipine, Verapamil, and Diltiazem in the Primary Therapy of Hypertension.

Reference	Drug	No.	Duration of Therapy	BP ↓ (s/d mmHg)*	HR Δ (bpm)*	Other Findings
Kiowski et al[11]	N, 20 mg tid	11	6 weeks	21/13	—	NE & PRA unchanged
McLeay et al[16]	N, 10 mg q8h	9	16 weeks	35/25	—	PRA unchanged
Olivari et al[13]	N, 10 mg q6h	27	3 weeks	33/25	—	GFR & PRA unchanged
Lederballe Pedersen and Mikkelson[17]	N, 30–60 mg/day	10	6 weeks	24/19	+9	SE, peripheral flushing only
Lederballe Pedersen et al[18]	N, 30–60 mg/day	18	4 weeks	25/17	+7	22% SE dropout rate
Gould et al[19]	V, 120–160 mg tid	16	6 weeks	22/17	−10	Blunted BP increase with exercise
Lewis et al[20]	V, 80–120 mg tid	21	4 weeks	27/22	—	10% SE dropout rate
Lewis[21]	V, 80–120 mg tid	75	52 weeks	28/19	—	19% total dropout rate
Lederballe Pedersen[22]	V, 320–640 mg/day	5	7 weeks	14/12	−10	Atrioventricular conduction stable
Buhler et al[15]	V, 240–720 mg/day	43	13 week mean treatment	19/15	—	BP decrease maximum with ↑ age & ↓ PRA
Inouye et al[23]	D, 120 mg tid	14	8 weeks	18/16	—	PRA unchanged; NE increased
Klein et al[24]	D, 180–270 mg/day	23	8 weeks	11/14	—	SE less than with N treatment

N = nifedipine; V = verapamil; D = diltiazem; BP = blood pressure; HR = heart rate; s/d = systolic/diastolic; NE = plasma norepinephrine concentration; PRA = plasma renin activity; GFR = glomerular filtration rate; SE = side effects; tid = three times a day; q8h = every 8 hours.
*BP and HR findings are those recorded with chronic use.

chronic therapy, would have to avoid these pitfalls. In fact, nifedipine has been noted to produce an initial increase in circulating catecholamines and plasma renin activity;[25] as a result, heart rate and cardiac output (CO) increase. With continued use, however, levels of both circulating catecholamines and renin, as well as heart rate and CO, tend to return toward baseline values.[13,16] Chronic nifedipine therapy has been moderately well tolerated, with the most common adverse reactions being headache (5%), flushing (3%), palpitations (5%), and occasional gastrointestinal complaints.[26] Pedal edema has been reported but, in association with unaltered renin and aldosterone levels, true volume expansion is rare.

Verapamil administration, compared with nifedipine, produces more pronounced direct depression of both pacemaker cells and contractility. Both acute and chronic use are associated with relatively stable heart rates and

CO. Again, circulating catecholamine concentrations remain near baseline. Although renin production may be mildly stimulated, verapamil decreases the release of aldosterone from adrenal zona glomerulosa cells.[27] Side effects reported during chronic verapamil use are similar to those noted with nifedipine, perhaps with fewer headaches but more common gastrointestinal complaints, particularly constipation. Acute parenteral use may prolong atrioventicular conduction.[22] With long-term oral therapy, atrioventricular conduction is unchanged or is only slightly depressed.[28] Nonspecific central nervous system side effects and altered sexual performance have received little mention in the trials performed to date.

Multiple studies with calcium blocking drugs suggest that renal function is either unchanged or improved when total body weight, urine flow, or sodium balance is measured in humans or experimental animals.[29,30] Therefore, it seems that in contrast to previous vasodilators, hydralazine and minoxidil, calcium channel blocking drugs are effective vasodilators with negligible stimulatory effects on the best-studied homeostatic mechanisms.

There is a relative paucity of information regarding the use of diltiazem in hypertension, but it also appears to be effective. Studies in three genetically distinct hypertensive rat models have demonstrated a uniform antihypertensive action.[31] Recent experience at our institution has demonstrated that patients with mild to moderate hypertension (mean sitting blood pressure, $153 \pm 16/100 \pm 4$), treated for 8 weeks with diltiazem 180 to 360 mg/day, exhibited a 18 mmHg decrease in sitting systolic blood pressure and a 16 mmHg decline in sitting diastolic blood pressure.[23] These changes were comparable to those produced by hydrochlorothiazide 100 mg/day in the same patients. As in previous reports,[24,32] a high percentage of patients responded to therapy, and adverse effects were minimal. Despite a significant increase in circulating norepinephrine levels, heart rate remained unchanged. Plasma renin activity was also unaffected.

Advantages of Calcium Channel Blockers in Patients with Accompanying Cardiac Disease

Historically, the earliest reports of significant cardiovascular benefits of the then-new calcium blocking drugs demonstrated impressively decreased coronary vascular resistance and increased coronary flow. The relaxation of coronary vascular tone is due to the selective inhibition of transmembrane Ca^{++} fluxes. Coronary responsiveness to circulating vasoactive hormones is diminished, and alpha-adrenergic and angiotensin receptor sensitivity is decreased when calcium entry blockers are present. This direct action on the coronary circulation is responsible for the favorable results in vasospastic angina.[33] Although the number of patients with variant angina and hypertension is small, there are data to suggest that coronary blood flow per unit mass and coronary reserve are limited in subjects with left ventricular hypertrophy (LVH).[34] Any advantage for calcium channel blockers in antihypertensive therapy based on coronary vasodilation will have to be supported by careful studies, and this will be an important area for further investigation.

As either primary or adjunctive therapy, calcium channel blockers are also effective in the management of exertional angina pectoris. This benefit is achieved primarily by favorable changes in the major determinants of myocardial oxygen consumption. During exertion, blood pressure is lowered, LV size and wall tension may decrease, contractility may be reduced, and heart rate is often slower. Thus, in the patient with coexisting hypertension and coronary artery disease, treatment with calcium blockers may be especially appropriate.[35]

There is growing interest in the use of calcium blockers in decompensated hypertensive heart failure; drug-induced peripheral vasodilation reduces afterload, with a resulting improvement in cardiac performance. A recent report demonstrated that nifedipine reduces both preload and afterload and improved LV performance as assessed by acute hemodynamic measurements.[36] In contrast, although systemic vascular resistance was decreased, LV performance was little changed or worsened when verapamil was utilized; this was presumed to be due to its greater negative inotropic and less potent vasodilator effects. However, it should be noted that all calcium channel blockers may depress contractility. A recent preliminary report suggests that this concern is warranted in the setting of severe left ventricular dysfunction; the improvement in cardiac performance with nifedipine was significantly less than that obtained with hydralazine, with equivalent degrees of arteriolar vasodilation.[37]

Verapamil may have a special role in the treatment of patients with hypertension and concomitant supraventricular arrhythmias. Since atrial fibrillation is a common accompanying problem in hypertensive patients, single drug therapy may both control blood pressure and the ventricular response rate.

Other Potentially Important Cardiac Effects of Calcium Channel Blockers in Hypertension

Besides the previously discussed situations in which hypertension coexists with conditions that are especially amenable to therapy with calcium blockers, these agents may have other, as yet unproved, advantages as a result of their actions on the cardiovascular system. The clinical importance of potential myocardial preservation when calcium blockers are administered before experimental infarction is under active investigation.[33,38] Protection from ischemia may be secondary to decreased coronary artery spasm, improved collateral coronary blood flow, or to their negative inotropic effects. Also, the potentially toxic reperfusion shifts of Ca^{++} from extracellular to intracytoplasmic and mitochondrial sites after ischemic injury may be prevented by pretreatment with calcium blockers.

In the few reports available, long-term calcium channel blocker therapy has not been associated with altered levels of serum lipoproteins; thus the long-term atherogenic risk is probably not increased. Lipoprotein fractions and total cholesterol were unchanged after therapy with verapamil[28,39] and diltiazem.[40] In fact, rabbits fed high cholesterol diets demonstrated decreased atherogenesis when either nifedipine[41] or verapamil[42] were concomitantly administered.

Left ventricular hypertrophy is a well-recognized response to poorly controlled hypertension.[43] However, if appropriate antihypertensive treatment is delivered during the early, adaptive phase of myocardial hypertrophy, then perhaps late clinical cardiac failure may be prevented. Inasmuch as hypertensive LVH is associated with an eight fold increase in late cardiovascular mortality,[44] the prevention and regression of hypertrophy may be considered an important goal. Studies of experimental hypertension in the spontaneously hypertensive rat have shown that drug regimens that produce similar decreases in systemic arterial pressure may have variable effects on LV mass.[45] Vasodilators, in particular, may be less effective in preventing hypertrophy relative to their ability to reduce arterial pressure.

Via their unique mechanism of action, calcium channel blocking drugs are presently the most promising vasodilators to reduce hypertensive LVH. Spontaneously hypertensive rats treated with nifedipine show markedly less cardiac hypertrophy than appropriate controls.[46,47] We have recently noted a prevention of LVH progression in spontaneously hypertensive rats treated with diltiazem. This was accompanied by a preservation of LV function and reversal of coronary flow abnormalities.[48] A reduction in LVH was demonstrated in a 2-kidney, 1-clip Goldblatt rat model when treated with nitrendipine, a long-acting congener of nifedipine.[49] In a small series of 9 patients followed by McLeay et al[16] utilizing nifedipine 30 mg/day for a total of 4 months, posterior LV wall and septal thicknesses defined by M-mode echo were decreased, as was calculated LV mass.

The hemodynamic consequences of LVH are notable even before systolic dysfunction ensues. Alterations in ventricular wall thickness, abnormalities in active diastolic relaxation, and later changes in the myofibril and collagen matrix of the left ventricle are likely responsible for an increase in chamber stiffness. Left atrial enlargement, which is often an early electrocardiographic sign of LVH, is probably an early consequence of the resulting increases in diastolic LV pressures.[50] Equilibrium blood pool radionuclide measurements demonstrate impairment of LV filling in hypertensive patients, even while resting and exercise ejection fraction are normal.[51,52] The severity of these abnormalities appears to be correlated with the degree of LVH. Calcium channel blocking drugs appear to reverse the diastolic filling abnormalities associated with both coronary artery disease and hypertrophic cardiomyopathy.[53,54] Early evidence from our laboratory suggests that diltiazem may also improve LV diastolic filling in patients with hypertension whose blood pressure is controlled.[55] Whether calcium blocker-mediated improvement in diastolic filling will be translated into reduced symptoms in patients with hypertension with dyspnea related to "noncompliant" left ventricles also remains to be determined.

Summary

Over the past decade, multiple lines of research have implicated trans-membrane Ca^{++} fluxes as the final cellular mediator of the heightened systemic vascular resistance that characterizes the majority of hypertensive states. Calcium channel blockers exhibit a potent vasodilating effect by directly relaxing vascular smooth muscle. In contrast with previous vasodilators, reflex stimulation of heart rate, catecholamines, and the renin-aldosterone system appear to be minimal. Numerous, but as yet predominantly uncontrolled, studies indicate that these agents effectively lower blood pressure in hypertensive subjects. They appear to have a more pronounced antihypertensive effect when administered to patients who are older and have low renin and high vascular resistance.

Because of the unique spectrum of pharmacologic effects of the calcium channel blockers and their actions on the cardiovascular system in particular, these agents have potentially important advantages in several groups of patients, including those with coexisting coronary disease, variant angina, supraventricular arrhythmias, and perhaps in those with mild degrees of LV dysfunction. Whether their actions on the coronary circulation and on diastolic LV dysfunction, and their ability to prevent or delay the progression of LVH and atherogenesis will prove to be of clinical significance remains to be elucidated.

In contrast to patients with ischemic heart disease, who may tolerate minor adverse effects in exchange for antianginal efficacy of a drug, symptom-free patients with hypertension may report a higher incidence of side effects and tolerate drug therapy less well. Thus, the final role of calcium channel blockers will await the delineation of their toxic to therapeutic ratio in controlled, long-term studies.

Acknowledgment

This work was supported in part by training grant GM 07546 of the NIGMS, grant number HL 28146 of the NHLBI, and by the Veterans Administration Research Service.

References

1. KOCH-WESER J: Vasodilator drugs in the treatment of hypertension. Arch Intern Med 1974; 133: 1017–1027.
2. COHN JN: Calcium, vascular smooth muscle, and calcium entry blockers in hypertension. Ann Intern Med 1983; 98: 806–809.
3. VAN ZWEITEN PA, VAN MEEL JCA, TIMMERMANS PBMWM: Pharmacology of calcium entry blockers: interaction with vascular alpha-adrenoreceptors. Hypertension 1983; 5 (suppl II): 8–17.

4. LEDERBALLE PEDERSEN O: Calcium blockade as a therapeutic principle in arterial hypertension. Acta Pharmacol Toxicol (Copenh) 1981; 49 (suppl 2): 1–31.

5. MCCARRON DA: Low serum concentrations of ionized calcium in patients with hypertension. N Engl J Med 1982; 307: 226–228.

6. KESTELKOOT H, GEBOERS J, VAN HOOF R: Epidemiologic study of the relationship between calcium and blood pressure. Hypertension 1983; 5 (suppl II): 52–56.

7. MILLARD RW, LATHROP DA, GRUPP G, et al: Differential cardiovascular effects of calcium channel blocking agents: potential mechanisms. Am J Cardiol 1982; 49: 499–506.

8. SPIVACK C, OCKEN S, FRISHMAN WH: Calcium antagonists; clinical use in the treatment of systemic hypertension. Drugs 1983; 25: 154–177.

9. HEIDLAND A, HEIDBREDER E, HORL WH, SCHAFER R: Calcium antagonists in the treatment of hypertension. Contrib Nephrol 1982; 33: 254–269.

10. ERNE P, BOLLI P, BERTEL O, et al: Factors influencing the hypotensive effects of calcium antagonists. Hypertension 1983; 5 (suppl II): 97–102.

11. KIOWSKI W, BERTEL O, ERNE P, et al: Hemodynamic and reflex responses to acute and chronic antihypertensive therapy with the calcium entry blocker nifedipine. Hypertension 1983; 5 (suppl I): 70–74.

12. BONADUCE D, PETRETTA M, POSTIGLIONE M, CONDORELLI M: Hemodynamic study of nifedipine administration in hypertensive patients. Am Heart J 1983; 105: 865–867.

13. OLIVARI MT, BARTORELLI C, POLESE A, et al: Treatment of hypertension with nifedipine, a calcium antagonistic agent. Circulation 1979; 59: 1056–1062.

14. BERTEL O, CONEN D, RADU EW, et al: Nifedipine in hypertensive emergencies. Br Med J 1983; 286: 19–21.

15. BUHLER FR, HULTHEN UL, KIOWSKI W, et al: The place of the calcium antagonist verapamil in antihypertensive therapy. J Cardiovasc Pharmacol 1982; 4: S350–S357.

16. MCLEAY RAB, STALLARD TJ, WATSON RDS, LITTLER WA: The effect of nifedipine on arterial pressure and reflex cardiac control. Circulation 1983; 67: 1084–1090.

17. LEDERBALLE PEDERSEN O, MIKKELSON E: Acute and chronic effects of nifedipine in arterial hypertension. Eur J Clin Pharmacol 1978; 14: 375–381.

18. LEDERBALLE PEDERSEN O, CHRISTENSEN CK, et al: Relationship between the antihypertensive effect and steady-state plasma concentration of nifedipine given alone or in combination with a beta-adrenoreceptor blocking agent. Eur J Clin Pharmacol 1980; 18: 287–293.

19. GOULD BA, MANN S, KIESO H, et al: The 24-hour ambulatory blood pressure profile with verapamil. Circulation 1982; 65: 22–27.

20. LEWIS GRJ, MORLEY KD, LEWIS BM, BONES PJ: The treatment of hypertension with verapamil. NZ Med J 1978; 87: 351–354.

21. LEWIS GRJ: Verapamil in the management of chronic hypertension. Clin Invest Med 1980; 3: 175–177.

22. LEDERBALLE PEDERSEN O: Does verapamil have a clinically significant antihypertensive effect? Eur J Clin Pharmacol 1978; 13: 21–24.

23. INOUYE IK, MASSIE BM, SIMPSON P, et al: Antihypertensive therapy with diltiazem and comparison with diuretic. Am J Cardiol 1984; 53: 1588–1592.

24. KLEIN W, BRANDT D, VRECKO K, HARRINGER M: Role of calcium antagonists in the treatment of essential hypertension. Circ Res 1983; 52 (suppl I): 174–181.

25. AOKI K, KONDO S, MOCHIZUKI A, YOSHIDA T, et al: Antihypertensive effect of cardiovascular calcium antagonist in hypertensive patients in the presence and absence of beta-adrenergic blockade. Am Heart J 1978; 96: 218–226.
26. LEWIS JG: Adverse reactions to calcium antagonists. Drugs 1983; 25: 196–222.
27. FAKUNDING JL, CATT KJ: Dependence of aldosterone stimulation in adrenal glomerulosa cells on calcium uptake: effects of lanthanum and verapamil. Endocrinology 1980; 107: 1345–1353.
28. MIDTBO K, HALS O, VAN DER MEER J: Verapamil compared with nifedipine in the treatment of essential hypertension. J Cardiovasc Pharmacol 1982; 4: S363–S368.
29. LEONETTI G, SALA C, BIANCHINI C, et al: Antihypertensive and renal effects of orally administered verapamil. Eur J Clin Pharmacol 1980; 18: 375–382.
30. YOKOYAMA S, KABURAGI T: Clinical effects of intravenous nifedipine on renal function. J Cardiovasc Pharmacol 1983; 5: 67–71.
31. TAKATA Y, HOWES LG, HUTCHINSON JS: Antihypertensive effect of diltiazem in young or adult rats of genetically hypertensive strains. Clin Exp Hypertens 1983; A5: 455–468.
32. MAEDA K, TAKASUGI T, TSUKANO Y, et al: Clinical study on the hypotensive effect of diltiazem hydrochloride. Int J Clin Pharm Ther Toxicol 1981; 19: 47–55.
33. STONE PH, ANTMAN EM, MULLER JE, BRAUNWALD E: Calcium channel blocking agents in the treatment of cardiovascular disorders. Part II: hemodynamic effects and clinical applications. Ann Intern Med 1980; 93: 886–904.
34. STRAUER BE: Performance, wall dynamics and coronary function of the left ventricle in hypertensive heart disease. In: Strauer BE, ed. The heart in hypertension. Berlin: Springer-Verlag, 1981; 251–284.
35. FRISHMAN WH, KLEIN NA, KLEIN P, et al: Comparison of oral propranolol and verapamil for combined systemic hypertension and angina pectoris. Am J Cardiol 1982; 50: 1164–1172.
36. GUAZZI MD, CIPOLLA C, SGANZERLA P, et al: Clinical use of calcium channel blockers as ventricular unloading agents. Eur Heart J 1983; 4 (suppl A): 181–187.
37. ELKAYAM U, WEBER L, ROSE J, et al: Nifedipine versus hydralazine in the treatment of severe heart failure: an evidence for a negative inotropic effect of nifedipine (Abstr) Circulation 1983; 68(4): III-8.
38. NAYLER PG, FERRARI R, WILLIAMS A: Protective effect of pretreatment with verapamil, nifedipine and propranolol on mitochondrial function in the ischemic and reperfused myocardium. Am J Cardiol 1980; 46: 242–248.
39. LEWIS GRJ: The longterm management of hypertension with verapamil. Clin Exp Pharmacol Ther 1982; 6 (suppl): 107–112.
40. WADA S, NAKAYAMA M, MASAKI K: Effects of diltiazem hydrochloride on serum lipids: comparison with beta-blockers. Clin Ther 1982; 5: 163–173.
41. HENRY PD, BENTLEY KI: Suppression of atherogenesis in cholesterol-fed rabbit treated with nifedipine. J Clin Invest 1981; 68: 1366–1369.
42. ROULEAU JL, PARMLEY WW, STEVENS J, et al: Verapamil suppresses atherogenesis in cholesterol-fed rabbits. J Am Coll Cardiol 1983; 1: 1453–1460.
43. MASSIE BM: Myocardial hypertrophy and cardiac failure: a complex interrelationship. Am J Med 1983; 68 (suppl 3A): 67–74.

44. KANNEL WB, SORLIE P: Left ventricular hypertrophy in hypertension: prognostic and therapeutic implications (the Framingham Study). In: Strauer BE, ed. The heart and hypertension. Berlin: Springer-Verlag, 1981; 223–242.

45. SEN S, TARAZI RC, BUMPUS FM: Cardiac hypertrophy and antihypertensive therapy. Cardiovasc Res 1977; 11: 427–433.

46. KAZDA S, GARTHOFF B, KNORR A: Nitrendipine and other calcium entry blockers (calcium antagonists) in hypertension. Fed Proc 1983; 42: 196–200.

47. MOTZ W, PLOEGER M, RINGSGWANDL G, et al: Influence of nifedipine on ventricular function and myocardial hypertrophy in spontaneously hypertensive rats. J Cardiovasc Pharmacol 1983; 5: 55–61.

48. TUBAU JF, WIKMAN-COFFELT J, MASSIE BM, et al: Diltiazem prevents hypertrophy progression, preserves systolic function, and normalizes myocardial O$_2$ utilization in the spontaneously hypertensive rat. Clin Res; in press.

49. KOBAYASHI K, TARAZI RC: Effect of nitrendipine on coronary flow and ventricular hypertrophy in hypertension. Hypertension 1983; 5 (suppl II): 45–51.

50. FROHLICH ED, TARAZI RC, DUSTAN HP: Clinical-physiologic correlations in the development of hypertensive heart disease. Circulation 1971; 44: 446–455.

51. FOUAD FM, TARAZI RC, GALLAGHER JH, et al: Abnormal left ventricular relaxation in hypertensive patients. Clin Sci 1980; 59: 411s–414s.

52. INOUYE IK, MASSIE BM, LOGE D, et al: Abnormal left ventricular filling: an early finding in mild to moderate systemic hypertension. Am J Cardiol 1984; 53: 120–126.

53. BONOW RO, LEON MB, ROSING DR, et al: Effects of verapamil and propranolol on left ventricular systolic function and diastolic filling in patients with coronary artery disease: radionuclide angiographic studies at rest and during exercise. Circulation 1981; 65: 1337–1350.

54. BONOW RO, ROSING DR, BACHARACH SL, et al: Effects of verapamil on left ventricular systolic function and diastolic filling in patients with hypertrophic cardiomyopathy: assessment with radionuclide cineangiography. Circulation 1981; 64: 787–796.

55. INOUYE IK, MASSIE BM, LOGE D, et al: Failure of antihypertensive therapy with diuretic, beta-blocking and calcium channel-blocking drugs to consistently reverse left ventricular diastolic filling abnormalities. Am J Cardiol 1984; 53: 1583–1587.

38

Calcium Antagonists and Pathophysiologic Mechanisms of Hypertension

WOLFGANG KIOWSKI, M.D.
FRITZ R. BÜHLER, M.D.
PETER BOLLI, M.D.
U. LENNART HULTHÉN, M.D.
PAUL ERNE, M.D.

Essential hypertension, in its established phase, is hemodynamically characterized by increased peripheral vascular resistance. Intracellular free calcium concentration is the main determinant of the excitation contraction coupling mechanisms of vascular smooth muscle cells and, thereby, importantly determines the extent of tension development and the height of vascular resistance.[1,2] Therefore, from a theoretical point of view, arterial vasodilators should be ideally suited to correct this hemodynamic abnormality. However, their use for treatment of hypertension has been limited by baroreflex stimulation and consecutive sympathetic nervous system activation and volume retention.[3] Both effects counter or even abolish their antihypertensive effects. The possibility has been considered that a cellular defect of cation handling leads to elevated cellular free calcium concentration and increased peripheral vascular resistance in hypertension.[2] Evidence both from studies in man and animals supports this contention. Intra-arterial infusions of the calcium antagonists verapamil and nifedipine produced marked vasodilation in humans.[4,5] Systemic administration of both drugs caused a decrease of blood pressure in hypertensive but not in normotensive subjects.[6] Finally, a greater relaxation in the presence of verapamil and nifedipine has been demonstrated in blood vessels from spontaneously hypertensive compared with normotensive rats.[7,8] Therefore, if cellular calcium handling were indeed disturbed in human essential hypertension, calcium antagonists might specifically influence or normalize this abnormality, be it primary or secondary. Early experience with these drugs in hypertension also suggested that volume retention may not occur during therapy,[9] a characteristic rendering calcium antagonists an attractive addition to already available drugs for treatment of hypertension.

Greater Calcium-Dependent Vasoconstriction in Hypertensive Subjects

The study of specific mechanisms in the regulation of vascular resistance in man often utilizes the assessment of the effects of drugs with a known mechanism of action on the cardiovascular system. The systemic administration of drugs, such as intravenous verapamil, however, is almost inevitably accompanied by reflexly mediated cardiovascular changes. Measurement of changes of flow or flow resistance, therefore, usually represents a mixture of drug and counterregulatory effects and does not allow an exact differentiation between the two. In contrast, the regional administration of drugs, such as intra-arterial verapamil, avoids these problems. Drug dosages can be kept sufficiently small to avoid systemic actions while still providing high local concentrations. We employed the regional approach, using the forearm vascular bed and brachial artery infusions of verapamil to investigate the dependency of arteriolar tone of calcium influx in patients with essential hypertension and in normotensive subjects. Since vessels from hypertensive subjects may also have an altered structure with an increased wall to lumen ratio that may affect the response to vasoactive drugs, the forearm vascular response after calcium entry blockade was compared with that following nonspecific vasodilation by sodium nitroprusside.

Eleven normotensive women (21 to 29 years old; mean, 49) and 11 women with essential hypertension (WHO I–II; 38 to 62 years old; mean, 49) were studied. Details of these investigations have been published.[10]

Basal hemodynamic data are given in Table I. Heart rate was somewhat but not significantly higher in patients with hypertension compared with normotensive subjects, as was forearm blood flow. Infusion of verapamil induced a stepwise increase in forearm blood flow in both groups. The increase in forearm blood flow to verapamil at all dosages was greater in patients with hypertension compared with normal subjects, whereas there was no significant difference with sodium nitroprusside (Fig. 1). To adjust for the response to sodium nitroprusside, the increase in forearm flow for all dosages of verapamil was divided by the increase in forearm flow for sodium nitroprusside in each subject. Even after this adjustment, the vasodilatory response to verapamil was significantly greater in patients compared with normotensive subjects (F = 3,5, p = 0.025, profile analysis). In patients but not in normotensive subjects, mean blood pressure was reduced 3 minutes after starting the two highest dosages of verapamil (basal, 114 ± 3 mmHg; verapamil 40 μg/min/100 ml of forearm tissue, 109 ± 4 mmHg, p < 0.01; verapamil 75 μg/100 min/ml of forearm tissue, 106 ± 4 mmHg, p < 0.001) but not after infusion of sodium nitroprusside.

The findings of this study suggest a functional abnormality in essential hypertension, with increased dependency of arterial tone on calcium influx. This concept is in agreement with observations on the spontaneously hypertensive rat[7,8] and with a recent report using a similar approach in human essential hypertension.[11] The finding of a decrease in blood pressure in hypertensive but not normotensive subjects after administration of the two

TABLE I Blood Pressure, Heart Rate, Forearm Blood Flow, Plasma Norepinephrine, Plasma Epinephrine, Plasma Renin Activity, and Plasma Angiotensin II Under Basal Conditions in Normotensive and Hypertensive Women*

Intra-arterial Blood Pressure (mm Hg)		Heart rate	Forearm Flow (ml/min/100 ml)		PNE	PE	PRA	PAII
S	D	(bpm)	Right	Left	(pg/ml)	(pg/ml)	(ng/ml/3 hr)	(pg/ml)
Normotensive								
125 ± 4	64 ± 1	61 ± 2	1.8 ± 0.3	1.8 ± 0.2	195 ± 24	61 ± 15	1.5 ± 0.6	14 ± 3
(n = 11)	(n = 11)	(n = 11)	(n = 7)	(n = 11)	(n = 9)	(n = 9)	(n = 6)	(n = 6)
Hypertensive								
164 ± 6	89 ± 2	68 ± 2	2.5 ± 0.2	2.1 ± 0.2	288 ± 41	65 ± 19	1.7 ± 0.4	11 ± 3
(n = 11)	(n = 11)	(n = 11)	(n = 11)	(n = 11)	(n = 11)	(n = 11)	(n = 11)	(n = 11)
p								
< 0.001	<0.001	ns	ns	ns	ns	ns	ns	ns

*The values are given as means ± SEM.
S = systolic; D = diastolic
PNE = plasma norepinephrine; PE = plasma epinephrine; PRA = plasma renin activity II; PAII = plasma angiotensin II.

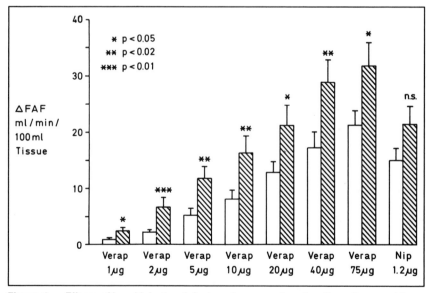

Figure 1. *Effects of brachial artery infusion of verapamil and sodium nitroprusside on forearm blood flow in normotensive (open bars) and hypertensive (crosshatched bars) subjects. The levels of significance between normotensive and hypertensive subjects are indicated.*

highest dosages of verapamil would also be compatible with this contention and confirms previous reports.[6] Although our studies were performed in the human forearm, which may not be representative of other vascular beds, our observations demonstrate an abnormality in calcium entry-dependent mechanisms in essential hypertension, a finding that offers the possibility that this mechanism can be disrupted through the use of calcium antagonists for the treatment of hypertension.

Antihypertensive Mechanisms of Calcium Antagonists and Counterregulation

The hemodynamic response to a vasodilator drug represents a mixture of immediate drug effects and counterregulatory mechanisms. Depending on the magnitude of the latter, blood pressure will decrease more or less. Since counterregulation varies considerably between individuals, the relevance of homeostatic reflex mechanisms of antihypertensive response to the calcium antagonist nifedipine was investigated in 13 Caucasian men aged 20 to 60 years (mean, 42.2) with newly diagnosed essential hypertension (WHO I-II). Details of the study have been published.[12] Patients were given placebo tablets three times daily for 2 weeks followed by 6 weeks of therapy with nifedipine 20 mg in slow release form three times daily. Hemodynamic investigations were carried out on the last day of the placebo and active treatment period. Thirty minutes after placement of all catheters, blood volume, systemic and forearm hemodynamics, and baroreflex sensitivity were measured and arterial blood was drawn for determination of plasma norepinephrine and epinephrine concentrations and renin activity. Next, nifedipine was infused into a brachial artery in four dosages (2.5, 10, 20, 40 μg) over a period of 3 minutes each and forearm blood flow was measured before and during the third minute of each infusion. Patients then received nifedipine 10 mg sublingually and hemodynamic measurements were repeated. Repeat measurements of baroreflex sensitivity and blood for hormone determinations were obtained again after 30 minutes. For the second hemodynamic investigation, patients were instructed to take a morning dose of nifedipine at 7 a.m. and hemodynamic and hormone measurements were performed approximately 2½ hours later.

Intra-arterial administration of nifedipine resulted in a dose-dependent vasodilation (Fig. 2) without affecting arterial blood pressure. Acutely, nifedipine, 10 mg sublingually, caused a decrease in blood pressure within 15 minutes (Fig. 3). This was associated with an increase in heart rate and cardiac index (CI), and a decrease in systemic and forearm vascular resistance. With chronic treatment, blood pressure decreased further compared with the acute effects, but systemic vascular resistance did not change. Heart rate and CI were no longer different from control values. Again, forearm hemodynamic responses paralleled those of the systemic circulation. Blood volume did not change during chronic treatment. Plasma norepinephrine concentrations and plasma renin activity increased 30 minutes after administration of

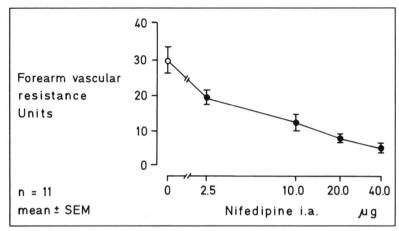

Figure 2. *Decrease of forearm vascular resistance after brachial artery infusions of nifedipine in 11 subjects with essential hypertension.*

10 mg of nifedipine (Fig. 4); at 6 weeks, values tended to return toward control levels. Plasma epinephrine concentrations remained unchanged. The acute decrease of blood pressure was correlated inversely with pretreatment baroreflex sensitivity ($r = -8.03$, $p < 0.01$) which did not change throughout the study (Fig. 5). Among the factors that predicted changes of blood pressure during chronic therapy, the decrease of blood pressure correlated with pretreatment blood pressure ($r = 0.63$, $p < 0.05$) and was inversely related to chronic changes of heart rate (percent mean pressure versus percent heart rate, $r = 0.75$, $p < 0.01$). Moreover, chronic changes of systemic vascular resistance correlated directly with pretreatment values and changes of forearm vascular resistance after intra-arterial infusions of the two highest dosages of nifedipine correlated directly with chronic changes of systemic vascular resistance (Fig. 6).

Our results confirm the potent and rapid vasodilator and antihypertensive properties of nifedipine.[13] Although the hemodynamic pattern indicated vasodilation as the main hemodynamic action underlying the blood pressure lowering effects, the lack of correlation between changes of blood pressure and systemic vascular resistance indicates that factors other than vasodilation per se were important for the blood pressure lowering response. There is evidence that the acute blood pressure lowering effect of nifedipine was counteracted by baroreflex-mediated sympathetic stimulation. Thus, acutely reduced systemic vascular resistance was accompanied by increased heart rate and thereby increased cardiac index and plasma norepinephrine concentrations. The importance of counterregulatory mechanisms is also emphasized by the correlation between baroreflex sensitivity and the acute changes of blood pressure.

At six weeks of nifedipine therapy, there was no longer hemodynamic or biochemical evidence of sympathetic stimulation, even though systemic

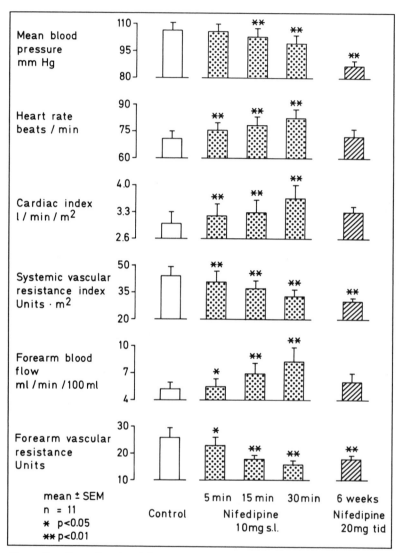

Figure 3. *Central and peripheral hemodynamic effects of acute sublingual and chronic oral therapy with nifedipine in 11 patients with essential hypertension.*

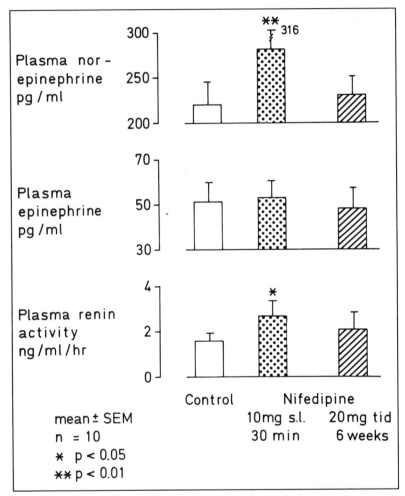

Figure 4. *Effects of acute and chronic therapy with nifedipine on plasma catecholamine concentrations and plasma renin activity in 11 patients with essential hypertension.*

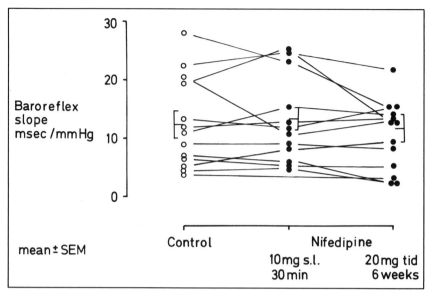

Figure 5. *Lack of effect of nifedipine therapy on arterial baroreflex sensitivity in essential hypertension.*

vascular resistance was still reduced. It appears that a reduction of acutely increased sympathetic activity during chronic therapy accounts for the additional blood pressure lowering effect seen during chronic therapy, a view supported by the inverse correlation between changes of heart rate and blood pressure. Thus, patients with mild chronic heart rate elevation had the poorest blood pressure response, and vice versa. This suggests a small degree of sympathetic stimulation that persists in nonresponders to chronic nifedipine therapy. Blood volume was unchanged during chronic therapy. Therefore, nifedipine is different from many other vasodilators that act directly on smooth muscle cells, since these drugs when given alone cause marked tachycardia, increases of plasma norepinephrine and renin activity, and marked volume retention.[3] Moreover, baroreflex sensitivity was unchanged during acute and chronic therapy, indicating a normal cardiovascular reflex control. The latter findings are in keeping with a resetting of arterial baroreflexes toward the level of the pharmacologically lowered blood pressure. This effect may be more pronounced in responders than in nonresponders.

Besides elucidating the hemodynamic mechanisms of action of nifedipine in hypertension, our data provide information on the role of calcium for the control of vascular resistance in hypertension. The greater the blood pressure decreased, the higher the pretreatment pressure. In analogy, the greater the decrease of systemic vascular resistance, the higher the pretreatment vascular resistance. Changes of forearm vascular resistance after brachial artery infusions of nifedipine were also directly correlated with chronic changes in

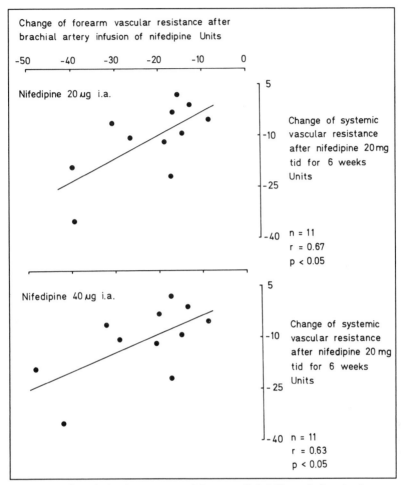

Figure 6. *Correlation between arteriolar vasodilatability and chronic changes of systemic vascular resistance during nifedipine therapy. Arteriolar vasodilator response was assessed as changes of forearm vascular resistance after brachial artery infusions of 20 and 40 μg nifedipine infused over 3 minutes each.*

systemic vascular resistance. Thus, chronic systemic vasodilation correlated with a measure of nifedipine-induced arteriolar dilatability. Inasmuch as correlations can be taken as evidence of cause and effect, these findings might suggest that the antihypertensive and vasodilator effects of nifedipine resulted from the reversal of a calcium-dependent vasoconstrictor mechanism, the importance of which seems to increase as blood pressure and vascular resistance increase.

The hemodynamic studies performed suggest an enhanced calcium-dependent vasoconstrictor mechanism or mechanisms in essential hypertension and an important role for sympathetic activation, particularly during an early phase of treatment, whereas a small degree of sympathetic activation appears to be of importance during chronic therapy only in patients with poor blood pressure responses. The overall lack of clinically relevant sympathetic nervous system stimulation and the lack of volume retention make these potent arterial vasodilators feasible for antihypertensive monotherapy, which was shown to be more effective in the older patients with low renin and relatively higher blood pressures[14] and who are known to have blunted cardiovascular reflexes.[15]

Acknowledgment

Supported by the Swiss National Research Fund No. 3.807.80.

References

1. BOHR DF: Vascular smooth muscle updated. Circ Res 1973; 32: 665–672.
2. BLAUSTEIN MP: Sodium ions, calcium ions, blood pressure regulation and hypertension: a reassessment and a hypothesis. Am J Physiol 1977; 232: C165–C173.
3. KOCH-WESER J: Vasodilator drugs in the treatment of hypertension. Arch Intern Med 1974; 133: 1017–1027.
4. SINGH BN, ELLRODT G, PETER CT: Verapamil: a review of its pharmacological properties and therapeutic use. Drugs 1978; 15: 169–197.
5. HENRY PD: Comparative pharmacology of calcium antagonists: nifedipine, verapamil and diltiazem. Am J Cardiol 1980; 46: 1047–1058.
6. McGREGOR GA, ROTELLAR C, MARKANDU ND, SAGNELLA GA: Contrasting effects of nifedipine, captopril and propranolol in normotensive and hypertensive subjects. J Cardiovasc Pharmacol 1982; 4 (suppl 3): S358–S362.
7. LEDERBALLE PEDERSEN O, MIKKELSEN E, ANDERSSON K-E: Effects of extracellular calcium on potassium and noradrenaline induced contractions in the aorta of spontaneously hypertensive rats. Increased sensitivity to nifedipine. Acta Pharmacol Thoxicol (Copenh) 1978; 43: 137–144.
8. MOCHIZUKI A, AOKI K, KONDO S, MIZUNO T, HOTTA K: Specificity of tension development and calcium flux of the arterial smooth muscle in SHR. Jpn Heart J 1979; 20 (suppl I): 225.
9. OLIVARI MT, BARTORELLI C, POLESE A, et al: Treatment of hypertension with nifedipine, a calcium antagonistic agent. Circulation 1979; 59: 1056–1062.
10. HULTHÉN UL, BOLLI P, AMANN FW, KIOWSKI W, BÜHLER FR: Enhanced vasodilation in essential hypertension by calcium channel blockade with verapamil. Hypertension 1982; 4 (suppl II): 26–31.
11. ROBINSON BF, DOBBS RJ, BAYLEY S: Response of forearm resistance vessels to verapamil and sodium nitroprusside in normotensive and hypertensive men: evidence for a functional abnormality of vascular smooth muscle in primary hypertension. Clin Sci 1982; 63: 33–42.

12. Kiowski W, Bertel O, Erne P, Hulthén UL, Bolli P, Ritz R, Bühler FR: Haemodynamic and reflex mechanisms of acute and chronic antihypertensive therapy with the calcium channel blocker nifedipin. Hypertension 1983; 5 (suppl 1): 70.

13. Robinson BF, Dobbs RJ, Kelsey CR: Effects of nifedipine on resistance vessels, arteries and veins in man. Br J Clin Pharmacol 1980; 10: 433.

14. Bühler FR, Hulthén UL, Kiowski W, Bolli P: Greater antihypertensive efficacy of the calcium channel inhibitor verapamil in older and low renin patients. Clin Sci 1982; 63: S439–S442.

15. Bertel O, Bühler FR, Kiowski W, Lütold BE: Decreased beta-adrenoreceptor responsiveness as related to age, blood pressure and plasma catecholamines in patients with essential hypertension. Hypertension 1980; 2: 130–138.

39

Angiotensin Converting Enzyme Inhibitors

FRANZ H. MESSERLI, M.D.
HECTOR O. VENTURA, M.D.
CELSO AMODEO, M.D.

For many years, the extensive studies of the renin-angiotensin-aldosterone system bore little relevance for practicing cardiologists. For them, the renin-angiotensin-aldosterone cascade was a complex endocrine mechanism involved in regulation of arterial pressure, electrolyte homeostasis, and fluid volume regulation that became clinically important only in some rather exotic forms of secondary hypertension. The early experimental and clinical reports of disturbances of the renin-angiotensin-aldosterone axis in congestive heart failure by Davis, Genest, Robertson, and Cohn provided a pathophysiologic explanation of some clinical findings, but were otherwise of mostly academic interest. Nevertheless, these studies clearly indicated that the pressor effect of angiotensin contributes to the systemic vasoconstriction observed in congestive heart failure. Not surprisingly, the introduction of drugs that specifically inhibited enzymatic steps in the renin-angiotensin-aldosterone cascade aroused great enthusiasm among those involved in the treatment of congestive heart failure. Captopril, the first available oral angiotensin-converting enzyme (ACE) inhibitor, soon became a cornerstone in the management of patients with overt or latent congestive heart failure and in patients with severe hypertension who benefited from unloading of the left ventricle. However, recent studies indicated that the vasodilating activity of ACE inhibitors was not solely confined to those patients with increased activity of the renin-angiotensin-aldosterone system. This, together with the introduction of less toxic compounds, allowed the use of these agents as first-line therapy in uncomplicated essential hypertension. It is therefore particularly timely to review the cardiovascular effects of this new promising class of antihypertensive agents.

Classification

According to their chemical structure, ACE inhibitors can be classified as peptides and nonpeptides. Among the peptide inhibitors are the crude extracts of venom from two poisonous Brazilian snakes.[1] These poisons were initially thought to be bradykinin potentiating factors until the first peptides inhibiting ACE were extracted. The nonpeptide SQ20881 (teprotide) was found to have the most potent action in vitro or in vivo[2] and was used to study the role of angiotensin II in arterial hypertension as well as in volume homeostasis.[3,4] Teprotide has to be given parenterally and it therefore was not useful in the treatment of arterial hypertension. Only the synthesis of orally active compounds, such as captopril, enalapril, lisinopril, and pivalopril, has compelled us to think of converting enzyme inhibition as a novel therapeutic approach to the treatment of arterial hypertension and congestive heart failure.

The nonpeptide ACE inhibitors comprise chelating agents such as ethylene diaminetetraacetic acid (EDTA) and heavy metals such as Hg^{2+} and Pb^{2+}.

Mechanism of Action

Since ACE inhibitors competively lower circulating angiotensin levels, their main antihypertensive effect, as can be expected, consists of arteriolar and venous vasodilation as well as decreased aldosterone secretion. However, it soon became evident that ACE inhibitors decreased arterial pressure in a much larger number of hypertensive subjects than initially anticipated. This observation provoked the search for additional mechanisms of action. It was previously demonstrated that angiotensin II had a facilitating action on pre- and postsynaptic adrenergic receptors as well as on baroreceptor reflexes.[5] Conversely, ACE inhibition might lower arterial pressure by interfering with this activity, thereby acting, at least to some extent, as a sympatholytic agent.[6,7] Also, ACE inhibition has been described as having a direct renal tubular action that could be mediated by a decrease in the passive membrane permeability to sodium[8,9] (possibly leading to vasodilation). Moreover, ACE inhibition may potentiate the action of bradykinin and other kinins, thereby further promoting vasodilation.[10] Other findings, such as the release of prostaglandin, are difficult to account for by ACE inhibition alone.[11,12] Finally, the demonstration that angiotensin II is directly involved in protein synthesis opens up the intriguing possibility that ACE inhibitors may interfere with certain intracellular mechanisms as well.[13]

Although certain differences have been described with regard to potency, side effects, toxicity, and endocrine findings among various ACE inhibitors, their cardiovascular properties are remarkably similar.

Essential Hypertension

Hemodynamics: The decrease in arterial pressure associated with converting enzyme inhibition results, acutely and over the long term, from a decrease in total peripheral resistance (TPR) (Tables I and II).[14-24] Systemic flow as measured by cardiac output (CO) remains unchanged, as do heart

TABLE I   **Hemodynamic Effects of Captopril in Arterial Hypertension***

Reference	No. Pt.	Time (mo)	Dose (mg)	HR	MAP	CI	SI	TPR
Acute
14	14		50	0	−16	0	0	−13
15	8		350	−1	−15	5	6	−19
16	10		50	0	−12	−10	−10	−11
17	21		25	−3	−17	1	3	−19
18	14		25	−1	−12	−1	3	−11
19	13		—	6	−14	10	−1	−21
20	6		75	−7	−8	1	9	−13
21	26		25	2.3	−11	−1.3	−3	−10
Mean	14.0		85.7	−0.5	−13.1	+0.59	+0.87	−14.6
Chronic
14	17	1	450	−9	−22	−13	−4	−9
18	11	2	75	0.5	−18	16	15	−30
20	8	0.25	75	−2	−15	2	5	−18
21	18	2	375	0.5	−18	16	16	−29
22	7	6	75	−17	−2	1	22	−2
Mean	12.2	2.25	210	−5.4	−15	4.4	10.8	−17.6

HR = heart rate; MAP = mean arterial pressure; CI = cardiac index; SI—stroke index; TPR = total peripheral resistance.
*Percent change from pretreatment values.

rate and most often pulmonary wedge pressure. The acute and chronic hemodynamic effects may be somewhat different in hypertensive patients. When all the available studies are pooled, however, little difference between the effects of acute and chronic ACE medication can be documented (Tables I and II). The degree of both the acute and chronic reduction of arterial pressure correlates often, but not always, with pretreatment concentration of circulating plasma angiotensin II levels or plasma renin activity. Studies from our laboratories[23,25] have shown that the immediate antihypertensive effect was mediated by a decreased TPR with little change in CO, stroke volume, heart rate, and indices of contractility, as measured by M-mode echo, whereas a slight decrease in heart rate was observed. After 12 weeks of treat-

TABLE II   **Chronic Hemodynamic Effects of Enalapril in Arterial Hypertension***

Reference	Dose (mg)	HR	MAP	CI	SV	TPR
23	20–40	−6	−18	+6	−19	−24
24*	20–40	+8	−17	+16	+8	−28
Mean		+1	−17.5	+11	−5.5	−26

HR = heart rate; MAP = mean arterial pressure; CI = cardiac index; SV—stroke volume; TPR = total peripheral resistance.
*In responders only. Percent change from pretreatment values.

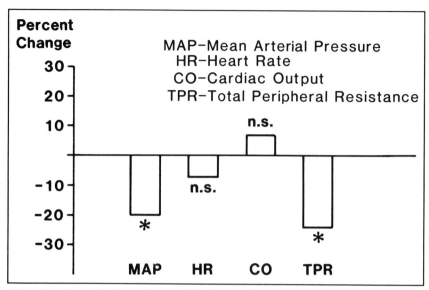

Figure 1. *Percent change in systemic plasma volume and renal hemodynamics after 8 weeks of enalapril treatment. *p < 0.05.*

ment, the decrease in arterial pressure remained unchanged, heart rate had returned to pretreatment levels, and systemic flow remained preserved. Similarly, 3 months of uninterrupted enalapril treatment lowered arterial pressure by a decrease in TPR without significant change in CO and heart rate. No expansion of plasma volume was observed in either study. In our laboratory, 12 weeks of enalapril therapy produced a decrease of arterial pressure by 18% and of TPR by 24% without changes in CO or heart rate (Fig. 1).[23]

The lack of reflexive tachycardia observed with ACE inhibition appears to be a common feature and was also documented with angiotensin receptor blockers.[26–28] Angiotensin-converting enzyme inhibitors may enhance parasympathetic activity and diminish a possible adrenergic effect of angiotensin on the heart or the central nervous system. The absence of reflexive tachycardia cannot be ascribed to baroreceptor dysfunction, since various studies have shown that the response to head-up tilt remains normal and is not significantly affected by ACE inhibition,[29] and orthostatic hypotension is unusual.[30,31]

Renal Circulation

Renal blood flow has been shown to increase with ACE inhibition, whereas glomerular filtration rate did not change.[26,32,33] Accordingly, an impressive decrease in renal vascular resistance could be documented. In our study, enalapril resulted in a decrease of renal vascular resistance of 26% from pretreatment values (Fig. 2).[23] Long-term observations of up to 2 years have shown that renal blood flow may continue to improve throughout treat-

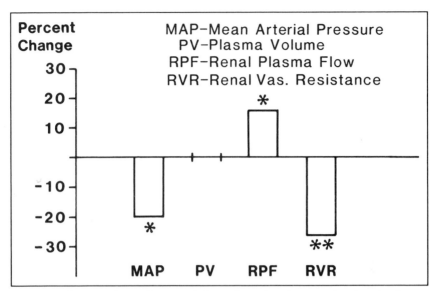

Figure 2. *Percent change in systemic hemodynamics after 8 weeks of enalapril treatment. *p < 0.05; **p < 0.01.*

ment and in a few patients an increase of up to 100% from pretreatment values has been observed.[34]

Venous Circulation: The association of a decrease in TPR without change in CO has been shown to occur with other vasodilating agents exerting an effect on both venous and arteriolar vascular smooth muscle. Evidence that converting enzyme inhibition may have a venous dilatory effect is suggested by studies indicating dilation of hand veins after intravenous ACE inhibition and by an increase of forearm venous distensibility in patients with severe arterial hypertension while they were receiving converting enzyme inhibitory treatment.[35,36]

Cerebral blood flow seems to continue to be maintained by autoregulation despite the decrease in arterial pressure when captopril is given.[37-39] In contrast, a decrease in hepatic blood flow was observed after captopril therapy in patients with essential hypertension.[40] Studies from our laboratory have shown that a single oral dose of captopril reduces vascular resistance uniformly in splanchnic, renal, and skeletal muscle and cutaneous vascular beds, with a selective increase in skeletal muscle flow.[25]

Cardiac Effects: Left ventricular mass has been shown to decrease in parallel with the decrease in arterial pressure during converting enzyme inhibition.[23,41,42] The decrease results from a reduction in both LV dimensions and wall thickness. No difference with regard to this effect is observed among various converting-enzyme inhibitors. In our study, 3 months of enalapril treatment produced a reduction of LV mass by almost 30% from pretreatment values.[23] No change in contractility, such as measured by velocity of circumferential fiber shortening or fractional fiber shortening, was observed. The mechanism by which converting enzyme inhibition reduces LV mass remains speculative. The reduced afterload that occurs in all patients in whom arterial pressure is lowered is certainly a major factor that allows left ventricular hypertrophy (LVH) to regress. However, since angiotensin may increase myocardial protein synthesis, it can be speculated that, in turn, converting enzyme inhibition may inhibit such protein synthesis in the contractile myocyte.[13] Also, ACE inhibition may decrease the adrenergic outflow to the cardiac muscle. A decrease in cardiac adrenergic drive is, in turn, a common feature of several antihypertensive agents that have been shown to permit regression of LVH in animals and in man.

Congestive Heart Failure

The increased activity of the renin-angiotensin-aldosterone system that is commonly observed in patients with decompensated heart failure produces vasoconstriction and sodium retention, both of which potentiate cardiac decompensation as well as resistance to therapy.[14,29,43-59] The ACE inhibitors when given either acutely or chronically as well as angiotensin II receptor inhibitors have been shown to exert a favorable hemodynamic response in patients with congestive heart failure (Tables III and IV). In all patients who show a hemodynamic response, arterial pressure decreases, CO increases, and TPR decreases, whereas heart rate does not usually change (Tables III

TABLE III   Acute Hemodynamic Effects of Captopril in Congestive Heart Failure*

Reference	# Pt.	Time (mo)	Dose (mg)	HR	MAP	CI	SI	TPR
Acute
14	14		50	−9	−29	21	38	−43
43	10		90	0	−8	21	20	−19
44	36		25	−8	−15	18	25	−27
45	11		25	−7	−9	13	20	−22
46	10		50	−13	−18	17	49	−30
47	11		82	−6	−22	19	27	−31
48	18		25	−5	−24	39	48	−46
49	12		25	−10	−13	0	11	−14
50	12		25	−1	−11	29	21	−25
51	14		25	−6	−24	25	36	−35
52	8		25	0	−20	16	16	−24
53	11		100	0	−16	16	15	−26
54	36		25	−7	−16	20	6	−34
Mean	15.6		44.0	−5.5	−17.3	19.5	25.5	−28.9
Chronic
43	8	6	90	0	−16	15	15	−21
46	7	2	150	−6	−24	44	57	−44
49	10	3	75	−4	−15	39	48	−39
50	8	2	99	−5	−11	24	32	−23
55	6	3	300	−10	−4	14	21	−13
Mean	7.8	3.2	142.8	−5.0	−14.0	27.2	34.6	−28.0

HR = heart rate; MAP = mean arterial pressure; CI = cardiac index; SI = stroke index; TPR = total peripheral resistance.
*Percent change from pretreatment values.

TABLE IV   Acute Hemodynamic Effects of Enalapril in Congestive Heart Failure*

Reference	No. Pt	Dose (mg)	HR	MAP	CI	PCW (%)	PAP (%)
29	9	10–40	−4	−9	+16	−19	−6
56	8	5	−9	−18	+15	−23	−17
57	12	10	−8	−17	+24	−20	−5
58	8	5–10	+7	−11	+7	−17	−5
59	6	10	−6	−15	+20	−30	−12
Mean	8.6	11.5	−4.0	−14	16.4	−21.8	−9

HR = heart rate; MAP = mean arterial pressure; CI = cardiac index; SI = stroke index; PAP = pulmonary artery pressure; PCW = pulmonary capillary wedge pressure.
*Modified with permission from Massie.[60]

and IV). Concomitantly, a decrease in right atrial pressure and pulmonary wedge pressure can be seen. Moreover, a significant reduction in cardiopulmonary volume and in cardiopulmonary/total body volume ratio occurs, suggesting distinct venodilation.[43] Since ACE inhibition in congestive heart failure lowers afterload, reduces LV internal diameter, and slightly decreases wall thickness, a distinct reduction of peak systolic wall stress occurs. From a hemodynamic standpoint, this response is similar to the one seen with other vasodilators that affect both arterial and venous vascular smooth muscle. The magnitude of the hemodynamic response is dose dependent, but does not seem to differ from one converting enzyme inhibitor to the other. Intravenous infusion of teprotide and oral administration of captopril or enalapril yield a response of the same magnitude. However, patients with low plasma renin activity often exhibit a small acute effect of the drug, whereas those with elevated plasma renin activity have a distinct decrease in TPR and arterial pressure. Other investigators did not find a significant correlation between pretreatment plasma renin activity and any of the subsequent hemodynamic changes produced by converting enzyme inhibition.[43] Clearly, the beneficial effects of converting enzyme inhibition in congestive heart failure cannot be related to the reduction in peripheral angiotensin levels alone. Conceivably, converting enzyme inhibition may also decrease the adrenergic drive to the cardiovascular system.

Several studies have indicated that the acute hemodynamic effects are sustained over a prolonged period of time (Table IV). The New Zealand studies demonstrated that exercise tolerance almost doubled after 3 months of enalapril treatment, whereas a control group did not exhibit any improvement with regard to functional class of the New York Heart Association or exercise tolerance.[56] Although a decrease in arterial pressure seems to be a prerequisite for the clinical improvement in congestive heart failure, this effect also sharply limits the effectiveness of these drugs under the same circumstances. Symptomatic hypotension may occur in up to 20% of patients and seems to be dose related. However, in these patients hypotension can occasionally lead to transient renal dysfunction and to exacerbation of ischemic heart disease.

References

1. FERRERA SH: A bradykinin potentiating factor (BPF) present in the venom of Bothrops jararaca. Br J Pharmacol 1965; 24: 163–169.
2. CUSHMAN DW, OUDETTI MA: Inhibitors of angiotensin converting enzyme. In: Ellis GP, West GB, eds. Progress in medical chemistry, vol. 17. Elsevier/North-Holland Biomedical Press, 1980; 42–104.
3. BEUGIS RG, COLEMAN TG, YOUNG DB, McCAA RD: Longterm blockade of angiotensin formation in various normotensive and hypertensive rat models using converting enzyme inhibition (80-14225). Circ Res 1978; 43 (suppl I): I-45–I-53.
4. HOLLENBERG N: Pharmacologic interruption of the renin-angiotensin system. Annu Rev Pharmacol Toxicol 1979; 19: 559–582.
5. ZIMMERMAN BG: Adrenergic facilitation by angiotensin: does it serve a physiological function? (editorial review). Clin Sci 1981; 60: 343–348.
6. CLOUGH DP, COLLIS MG, CONWAY J, HATTON R, KEDDIE JR: Interaction of angiotensin-converting enzyme inhibitors with the function of the sympathetic nervous system. Am J Cardiol 1982; 49: 1410–1414.
7. ZIMMERMAN BG, SYBERTZ EJ, WONG PC: Interaction between sympathetic and renin-angiotensin system. J Hypertens 1984; 2: 581–587.
8. MASAKI Z, FERRARIO CM, BUMPUS FM: Effects of SQ 20,881 on the intact kidney of dogs with two-kidney, one clip hypertension. Hypertension 1980; 2: 649–656.
9. McCAA RE, HALL JE, McCAA CS: The effects of angiotensin I converting enzyme inhibitors on arterial pressure and urinary sodium excretion: role of renal renin angiotensin and kallikrein-kinin-system. Circ Res 1978; 43 (suppl I): I-32.
10. JOHNSON CI, CLAPPISON BH, ANDERSON WP, YASUJIMA M: Effect of angiotensin-converting enzyme inhibition on circulating and local kinin levels. Am J Cardiol 1982; 49: 1401–1404.
11. SWARTZ SL, WILLIAMS GH: Angiotensin-converting enzyme inhibition and prostaglandins. Am J Cardiol 1982; 49: 1405–1409.
12. McGIFF TC, TERRAGNO NA, MALIK KU, LONIGRO AJ: Release of a prostaglandin E-like substance from coumine kidney by bradykinin: comparison with eledoisim. Circ Res 1972; 31: 36–43.
13. RE RN: Cellular biology of the renin-angiotensin systems. Arch Intern Med 1984; 144: 2037–2041.
14. WENTING GJ, DEBRAYN JHB, MAN IN'T VELD AJ: Hemodynamic effects of captopril in essential hypertension and cardiac failure: correlations with short- and longterm effects on plasma renin. Am J Cardiol 1982; 49: 1453–1459.
15. DALY P, ROULEAU JL, COUISINEAU D: Acute effects of captopril on the coronary circulation of patients with hypertension and angina. Am J Med 1984; 76: 111–115.
16. HASHIMOTO H, KUNIO H, KOKUBU T: Effects of a single administration of captopril on hemodynamic and serum angiotensin converting enzyme activity, plasma renin activity, and plasma aldosterone concentration in hypertensive patients. Jpn Circ J 1981; 45: 176–180.
17. MOOKHERJEE S, ANDERSON GH, EICH R: Acute effects of captopril on cardiopulmonary hemodynamic and renin-angiotensin-aldosterone and bradykinin

profile in hypertension. Am Heart J 1983; 105: 106–112.

18. FAGARD R, AMERY A, REYBROUCK T: Acute and chronic systemic and pulmonary hemodynamic effects of angiotensin converting enzyme inhibition with captopril in hypertensive patients. Am J Cardiol 1980; 46: 295–305.

19. FOUAD FM, CEIMO JMK, TARAZI RC, BRAVO EL: Contrasts and similarities of acute hemodynamic responses to specific antagonism of angiotensin II (Sar', Thr[8] AII) and to inhibition of converting enzyme (captopril). Circulation 1980; 61: 163–169.

20. CODY RJ JR, TARAZI RC, BRAVO EC, FOUAD MD: Hemodynamics of orally active converting enzyme inhibitor (SQ 14,255) in hypertensive patients. Clin Sci Mol Med 1978; 55: 453.

21. FAGARD R, et al: Haemodynamic effects of captopril in hypertensive patients: comparison with saralasin. Clin Sci 1979; 57: 131s–134s.

22. FOUAD FM, TARAZI RC, BRAVO EL, et al: Long-term control of congestive heart failure with captopril. Am J Cardiol 1982; 49: 1489–1496.

23. DUNN FG, OIGMAN W, VENTURA HO, MESSERLI FH, KOBRIN I, FROHLICH ED: Enalapril improves systemic and renal hemodynamic and allows regression of left ventricular mass in essential hypertension. Am J Cardiol 1984; 53: 105–108.

24. FOUAD FM, TARAZI RC, BRAVO EL, et al: Hemodynamic and antihypertensive effects of the new oral angiotensin-converting enzyme inhibitor MK-421 (enalapril). Hypertension 1984; 6: 167–174.

25. VENTURA HO, FROHLICH ED, MESSERLI FH, KOBRIN I, KARDON BM: Immediate regional blood flow distribution following angiotensin converting enzyme inhibition in patients with essential hypertension. Am J Med 1984; 76 (suppl 5B): 58–61.

26. MOOKHERJEE S, OBEID A, WARNER R, ANDERSON G, EICH R, SMULYAN H: Systemic and pulmonary hemodynamic effects of saralasin infusion in hypertension. Am J Cardiol 1978; 42: 987–992.

27. MILLAR JA, McGRATH BP, MATTHEWS PG, JOHNSTON CE: Acute effects of captopril on blood pressure and circulating hormonal levels in salt replete and depleted normal subjects and essential hypertensive patients. Clin Sci 1981; 61: 75–83.

28. MILLER ED JR, SAMUELS AI: Inhibition of angiotensin conversion in experimental renovascular hypertension. Science 1972; 177: 1108–1109.

29. CODY FS, COUIT AB, SCHAER GL: Evaluation of a long-acting converting enzyme inhibitor (enalapril) for the treatment of congestive heart failure. J Am Coll Cardiol 1983; 1: 1154–1159.

30. BRAVO EL, TARAZI RC: Converting enzyme inhibition with an orally active compound in hypertensive man. Hypertension 1979; 1: 39–46.

31. FROHLICH ED, COOPER RA, LEWIS EJ: Review of the overall experience of captopril in hypertension. Arch Intern Med 1984; 144: 1441–1444.

32. HOLLENBERG NH: Renal hemodynamics in essential and renovascular hypertension. Influence of captopril. Am J Med 1984; 76 (suppl B): 22–28.

33. PESSINA AC, SEMPLICINI A, ROSSI G, et al: Effects of captopril on renal function in hypertensive patients. Am J Cardiol 1982; 49: 1572–1573.

34. BAUER J: Personal communication.

35. COLLIER JG, ROBINSON BF: Comparison of effects of locally infused angiotensin I

and II on hand veins and forearm arteries in man: evidence for converting enzyme activity in limb vessels. Clin Sci 1974; 47: 189.

36. JOHNS DW, AYERS CR, WILLIAMS SC: Dilation of forearm blood vessels after angiotensin-converting enzyme inhibition by captopril in hypertensive patients. Hypertension 1984; 6: 545–550.

37. FERRONE RA, HERAN CL, ANTONACCIO MJ: Comparison of the acute and chronic hemodynamic effects of captopril and guanethidine in spontaneously hypertensive rats. Clin Exp Hypertens 1980; 2: 247–272s.

38. BARRY DI: Cerebrovascular aspects of converting enzyme inhibition. II: blood-brain barrier permeability and effect of intracerebroventricular administration of captopril. J Hypertens 1984; 2: 599–604.

39. BARRY DI, PAULSON OB, JARDEN JO, JUHLER M, GRAHAM DI, STRANDGAARD S: Effects of captopril on cerebral blood flow in normotensive and hypertensive rats. Am J Med 1984; 76: 79–85.

40. GROSSLY R, BIHAU D, GIMSON AES, WESTABY D, RICHARDSON PJ, WILLIAMS R: Effects of converting enzyme inhibitor on hepatic blood flow. Am J Med 1984; 76: 62–65.

41. PFEFFER JM, PFEFFER MA, MURSKY I, BRAUNWALD E: Regression of left ventricular hypertrophy and prevention of left ventricular dysfunction by captopril in the spontaneously hypertensive rat. Proc Natl Acad Sci (USA) 1982; 79: 3310–3314.

42. SEN S, TARAZI RC, BUMPUS FM: Effect of converting enzyme inhibitor (SQ 14225) on myocardial hypertrophy in spontaneously hypertensive rats. Hypertension 1982; 2: 169–176.

43. AWAN NA, MASON DT: Vasodilator therapy of severe congestive heart failure: the special importance of angiotensin-converting enzyme inhibition with captopril. Am Heart J 1982; 104 (part 2): 1127–1136.

44. CREAGER MA, FAXON DP, HALPERIN JL, et al: Determinants of clinical response and survival in patients with congestive heart failure treated with captopril. Am Heart J 1982; 104 (part 2): 1147–1154.

45. KUGLER J, MASKIN CS, FRISHMAN W: Variable clinical response to longterm angiotensin inhibition in severe heart failure: demonstration of additive benefits of alpha-receptor blockade. Am Heart J 1982; 104 (part 2): 1154–1159.

46. ADER R, CHATTERJEE K, PORTS T: Immediate and sustained clinical improvement in chronic heart failure by an oral angiotensin converting enzyme inhibitor. Circulation 1980; 61: 931.

47. LEVINE TB, FRANCIOSA JA, COHN JN: Acute and longterm response to an oral converting-enzyme inhibitor, captopril, in congestive heart failure. Circulation 1980; 62: 35–41.

48. SHARPE DN, COXON R: Hemodynamic effects of captopril in chronic heart failure: efficacy of low-dose treatment and comparison with prazosin. Am Heart J 1982; 104 (part 2): 1164–1171.

49. CODY RJ, COUIT A, SCHAER G: Captopril pharmacokinetics and the acute hemodynamic and hormonal response in patients with severe chronic congestive heart failure. Am Heart J 1982; 104 (part 2): 1180–1183.

50. CODY RJ: The effect of captopril on postural hemodynamics and autonomic responses in chronic heart failure. Am Heart J 1982; 104 (part 2): 1190–1196.

51. MASSIE BM, KRAMER BL, TOPIC N: Acute and long-term effects of captopril on left

and right ventricular volumes and function in chronic heart failure. Am Heart J 1982; 104 (part 2): 1197–1203.

52. POWERS ER, BONNERMAN KS, STONE J: The effects of captopril on renal, coronary and systemic hemodynamics in patients with severe congestive heart failure. Am Heart J 1982; 104 (part 2): 1203–1210.

53. HERMANOVICH J, AWAN NA, LUI H: Comparative analysis of the hemodynamic actions of captopril and sodium nitroprusside in severe chronic congestive heart failure. Am Heart J 1982; 104 (part 2): 1211–1214.

54. PACKER M, MEDINA N, YUSHAK M: Contrasting hemodynamic responses in severe heart failure: comparison of captopril and other vasodilator drugs. Am Heart J 1982; 104 (part 2): 1215–1223.

55. TOPIC N, KRAMER B, MASSIE BM: Acute and longterm effects of captopril on exercise cardiac performance and exercise capacity in congestive heart failure. Am Heart J 1982; 104 (part 2): 1172–1179.

56. FITZPATRICK D, INKRAM H, NICHOLLS MG, et al: Haemodynamic, hormonal, and electrolyte effects of enalapril in heart failure. Br Heart J 1983; 50: 163–169.

57. DICARLO L, CHATTERJEE K, PARMLEY WW, et al: A new angiotension converting enzyme inhibitor in chronic heart failure: acute and chronic hemodynamic evaluations. J Am Coll Cardiol 1983; 2: 1865–1871.

58. DUNKMAN WB, WILEN M, FRANCIOSA JA, et al: Enalapril (MK-421), a new angiotensin converting enzyme inhibitor. Chest 1983; 5: 539–545.

59. TURINI GA, WEBER B, BRUNNER HR: The renin-angiotensin system in refractory heart failure: clinical, hemodynamic and hormonal effects of captopril and enalapril. Eur Heart J 1983; 4: 189–197.

60. MASSIE B: Enalopril: A new CEI for hypertension and heart failure. Cardiol Product News 1984; 13, A: 1–13.

40

Electrocardiographic Changes in the Course of Antihypertensive Treatment

EDWARD D. FREIS, M.D.

As early as 1948 Freis and Stanton[1] reported that treatment of severe hypertension with Veratrum viride often resulted in reversal of electrocardiographic (ECG) changes toward normal. Helmcke et al[2] in 1957 compared the ECG signs of left ventricular hypertrophy (LVH) before and after treatment with antihypertensive drugs. Patients whose blood pressure responded to treatment showed improvement in LVH three times more frequently than those whose blood pressure was not controlled. Dern et al[3] as well as Leishman[4] also found improvement frequently occurred in the ECG of treated patients. The relationship between blood pressure reduction and regression of LVH was not consistent, however. Therefore, a quantitative estimate of benefit was not possible because some patients may show improvement in the ECG spontaneously and also because there was no untreated control group for comparison.

The Veterans Administration Trial

The first control trial was the Veterans Administration Cooperative Study.[5] This study included male patients with diastolic blood pressure measurements in the range of 90 to 114 mmHg before treatment. The patients were randomly assigned on a double blind basis, one group receiving active drugs consisting of a combination of hydrochlorothiazide, reserpine and hydralazine, the other receiving placebos. Average follow-up was about 3 years, and in some cases it was more than 5 years.

Twelve lead ECGs were obtained in 143 of the control patients and 137 of the treated patients before treatment and 1 year after randomization. In some of these patients ECG recordings were obtained also at 2, 3, 4, and 5 years (average, 2.9 years). The average age was 51 years, and 42% of the patients were black. Cardiac enlargement by radiographs was exhibited in 22% of the control patients and 28% of the treated patients. Prerandomization blood pressure (mean of last two clinic visits) averaged 164/104 mmHg in the control patients and 164/105 mmHg in the treated cases. In the treated patients the average blood pressure decreased to 137/87 mmHg after treatment and remained at that level or slightly lower. In the control group the blood pressure remained essentially unchanged.

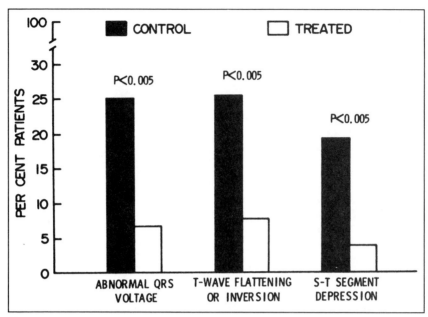

Figure 1. *Percentage of patients developing voltage changes or ST-T abnormalities following randomization who did not exhibit such changes prior to randomization. (Reprinted with permission from Poblete et al.[5])*

All ECGs were read by one person who was blinded as to the clinical features of the patient, including treatment status. The ECG characteristics were classified according to a revised Minnesota code.[6] In addition, the sum of the magnitudes of the S-wave in V_1 and the largest R-wave in V_5 or V_6 was obtained. Left ventricular hypertrophy was diagnosed if the sum exceeded 35 mm in accordance with the criteria of Sokolow and Lyon.[7] The prerandomization ECGs indicated LVH by this criterion in 32% of the treated group and 18% of the control group. Other than this, the prerandomization ECGs were similar in the treated and control groups.

Prevention of Abnormalities: During an average follow-up period of 2.9 years, highly significant ($p < 0.005$) differences developed between the treated and control groups with regard to voltage, T-wave, and ST-segment alterations (Fig. 1). Of the patients who did not exhibit LVH at entry, 25% of the control group compared with only 6.6% of the treated patients developed abnormal voltage. Also, 25.5% of the control patients developed T-wave flattening or inversion compared with 7.5% of the treated group. The incidence of ST-segment depression was 19.3% in the placebo group and 3.8% in the treated patients. There were no differences in the two groups of patients in the incidence of Q and QS patterns, left axis deviation, atrioventricular or ventricular conduction defects, or arrhythmias.

Reversions to Normal: In patients who already exhibited voltage criteria of LVH at entry into the study 74.4% of the treated patients reverted to normal voltage compared with 24.0% of the control group (p < 0.005). A similar trend was seen with respect to flattened or inverted T-waves, with 51.5% of the treated patients and 33.3% of the control group reverting to normal. However, this latter difference was not significant. The difference in normalization of ST-segment depression was significant, however, (p < 0.05) with 57.1% of the treated patients compared with 22.2% of the control group showing this improvement. There were no significant differences in other ECG characteristics, such as conduction defects, arrhythmias, and Q and Q-S patterns.

Fifteen patients in the treated group and 9 of the control subjects exhibited abnormal voltage plus T-wave or ST-segment criteria of LVH before randomization. These abnormalities reverted to normal in 60% of the treated patients compared with none in the control group.

Treatment was effective in preventing or reversing the ECG signs of LVH irrespective of the level of blood pressure before randomization. The effect of the extent of blood pressure reduction during treatment on the ECG changes of LVH also was analyzed. Although there was a trend toward greater reduction of blood pressure in the patients whose voltage abnormalities reverted to normal, the difference from those who did not was not significant. Age also did not appear to influence the effectiveness of treatment.

Other Controlled Studies

The Public Health Service Hospitals Cooperative Study[8] was restricted to patients with pretreatment diastolic blood pressure of 90 to 114 mmHg. Patients with clinically evident end-organ disease, including LVH, were excluded from the trial. The mean age of the patients was only 44 years and both sexes were represented. During a follow-up period of 7 years ECG evidence of LVH developed in 23.1% of control patients compared with 7.3% of the treated group.

The Hypertension Detection and Follow-up Program (HDFP) is the largest of the clinical trials, containing approximately 11,000 patients.[9] The program represents an evaluation of the effectiveness of global medical care as practiced in the community compared with special care in a teaching hospital supplied without cost to the patient. Development of LVH in patients with normal baseline ECGs occurred in 1.5% of the referred care patients compared with 1.2% of the special care patients. Although this is a much smaller difference than was observed in the previous trials, it should be emphasized that many of the referred care or control patients were also treated. Regression of abnormal ECGs was seen in 60% of special care patients and in 49% of referred care.

Although the Oslo trial[10] showed no evidence of benefit of treatment in preventing coronary heart disease, there was a marked effect on prevention of LVH. Seven patients in the control group versus none in the treated patients developed these ECG signs during the follow-up period. Furthermore, 6 of 7 showed progressive increase in blood pressure before the development of these ECG changes.

Comment

The accumulated data indicate that antihypertensive drug treatment has a marked protective effect against the development of LVH. Treatment protected against the development of increased QRS voltage, ST-segment depression and T-wave flattening or inversion. Treatment also was associated with a reversal of these abnormalities when they were present before treatment. There was, however, no significant association of treatment with changes in Q or QS patterns or in conduction defects.

These observations of the effects of treatment on the ECG are consistent with other data,[5,8,10] indicating that antihypertensive treatment favorably influences hypertensive complications. This was manifested in the ECG by the striking benefit in preventing or reversing the signs of LVH as opposed to the lack of prevention or improvement in Q wave, Q-S changes, and conduction defects, which are related to atherosclerosis of the coronary arteries.

The pathogenesis of the ST-T changes in LVH has not been well clarified. They are generally considered to be a reflection of left ventricular strain and of consequent increased myocardial oxygen consumption. If this is indeed the case, it seems likely that the reversal of these changes would reflect a reduction in myocardial oxygen demand due to the decrease in blood pressure. A study correlating hemodynamic findings with ECG changes in hypertensive patients with QRS changes alone compared with QRS changes with ST-T abnormalities revealed no significant differences in cardiac output, total peripheral resistance, or diastolic blood pressure in the two groups.[11] However, systolic blood pressure was significantly higher in the group exhibiting both QRS and ST-T changes. Also in the Veterans Administration trial, untreated patients with systolic elevations above 165 mmHg developed three times more ST-segment depression than those with lower systolic blood pressures.[5] These observations are consistent with the theory that ST-T changes are a reflection of increased myocardial strain during systole.

Summary

Marked improvement in the ECG signs of LVH has been consistently noted since the early trials of antihypertensive drug treatment. In the Veterans Administration study the incidence of abnormal QRS voltage, ST-segment depression or T-wave flattening or inversion occurred only one-fourth as frequently in the treated patients compared with the untreated control group. The patients with ECG evidence of LVH before randomization exhibited reversal of the signs of LVH 2.5 times more frequently in the treated group than in the control patients. Other control trials have obtained similar favorable results with treatment. On the other hand, improvement in ischemic changes associated with coronary heart disease has not been demonstrated following treatment. It is concluded that antihypertensive drug treatment markedly improves the ECG changes related to LVH, but not to coronary heart disease in patients with hypertension.

References

1. FREIS ED, STANTON JR: A clinical evaluation of Veratrum viride in treatment of essential hypertension. Am Heart J 1948; 36: 1–16.
2. HELMCKE JG, SCHNECKLOTH R, CORCORAN AC: Electrocardiographic changes of left ventricular hypertrophy: effects of antihypertensive treatment. Am Heart J 1957; 53: 549–557.
3. DERN PL, PRYOR R, WALKER SH, SEARLS DT: Serial electrocardiographic changes in treated hypertensive patients with reference to voltage criteria, mean QRS vectors, and the QRS-T angle. Circulation 1967; 36: 823–829.
4. LEISHMAN AWD: The electrocardiogram in hypertension. Q J Med 1951; 20: 1–12.
5. POBLETE PF, KYLE MC, PIPBERGER HV, FREIS ED: Effect of treatment on morbidity in hypertension. Veterans Administration Cooperative Study on Antihypertensive Agents. Effect on the electrocardiogram. Circulation 1973; 48: 481–490.
6. ROSE GA, BLACKBURN H: Cardiovascular Survey Methods. WHO Monograph 56, Geneva, 1968.
7. SOKOLOW M, LYON TP: The ventricular complex in left ventricular hypertrophy as obtained by unipolar precordial and limb leads. Am Heart J 1949; 37: 161–186.
8. SMITH WM: Treatment of mild hypertension. Results of a ten-year intervention trial. U.S. Public Health Service Hospitals Cooperative Study Group. Circ Res 1977; 40: I-98–I-105.
9. Hypertension Detection and Follow-up Cooperative Group, U.S.A.: Regression of left ventricular hypertrophy with antihypertensive therapy (abstr). International Society of Hypertension, Mexico City, 1982; 193.
10. HELGELAND A: Treatment of mild hypertension: a five year controlled drug trial. The Oslo study. Am J Med 1980; 59: 725–732.
11. HAMER J, SHINEBOURNE E, FLEMING J: Significance of electrocardiographic changes in hypertension. Brit Med J 1969; 1: 79.

PART VII
SPECIAL CONSIDERATIONS

41

Cardiac Effects of Weight Reduction in Obesity Hypertension

JAMES K. ALEXANDER, M.D.

Although the association of elevated blood pressure with obesity is well known, our insight into this relationship is rather limited. This is due to difficulties in characterizing obesity, on the one hand, and difficulties in defining mechanisms of this hypertension, on the other. Indices of obesity based on height and weight, for example, do correlate to some extent with the degree of adiposity indicated by skin fold thickness and body density, but all of them are imprecise, actually giving poor estimates of obesity, which are reasonably accurate only at the extremes of distribution. Also, it has not been possible clearly to implicate well-recognized factors operative in so-called essential hypertension as important pathogenic mechanisms in obesity hypertension. It is difficult to invoke a relative increase in circulatory volume, for example, since blood volume measurements do not correlate with the presence or absence of hypertension.[1,2] Calculated systemic vascular resistance, presumably an index of arteriolar narrowing, is lower in obese than in lean hypertensive patients.[1,2] In fact, the etiopathogenesis of hypertension with obesity is unknown. A survey of current hypotheses is beyond the scope of this presentation, but it is pertinent to emphasize that mechanisms of hypertension with obesity do not appear to be the same as those in essential hypertension, and some explanation must be found for the fact that not all obese persons are hypertensive. Indeed, in a survey of blood pressure in extremely obese subjects by direct intra-arterial measurement some years ago, we found that one-third were normotensive.[3]

The hemodynamic features of obesity hypertension include increases in blood volume and cardiac output (CO) and stroke volume (SV) paralleling the amount of excess weight. Calculated systemic vascular resistance tends to be normal,[1,4,5] and negatively correlated with blood volume.[5] Left ventricular (LV) work is significantly increased.[6,7] In the absence of frank LV failure, CO response to exercise is within the normal range,[6,8] but LV filling pressure is augmented either at rest or during exercise with secondary pulmonary hypertension.[1,4,8] These hemodynamic alterations are associated with the development of left ventricular hypertrophy (LVH), documented by both postmortem[9] and echo studies.[7,10,11] Because the increase in LV afterload is accompanied by augmented preload as well, hypertrophy is associ-

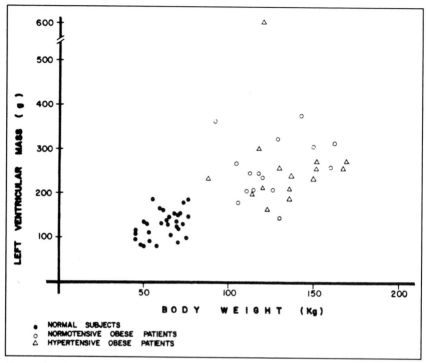

Figure 1. *Relation of echo-determined left ventricular wall mass to body weight in 30 subjects near predicted ideal weight (normal), and in 30 normotensive and hypertensive obese patients. (Reproduced with permission from Cueto et al.[11])*

ated with greater LV end-diastolic dimension. Thus, the ratio of chamber radius to ventricular wall thickness, an index of wall stress, tends to remain within a normal range.[7] When obesity is pronounced, these changes in LV wall mass and dimensions are present, whether hypertension is present or not[7,11] (Fig. 1).

Although weight reduction of the obese hypertensive person does not ensure a favorable effect on blood pressure, decrements to or toward normal may be anticipated in about one half of such subjects, regardless of age or relative weight.[12,13] Decrements in pressure do not necessarily parallel those in weight, so that modest weight reduction may result in significantly lower pressures.[14] Maintenance of lowered weight is likely to be accompanied by a stable decrement in pressure, and return of hypertension usually follows regain of weight.[12]

Although depressed in some cases, LV ejection fraction is generally in a normal range on echo assessment.[11] The magnitude of the EF slope is reduced, and left atrial dimension is increased.[11]

With weight and blood pressure reduction, parallel decrements in circulating blood volume and heart size take place. In a series of severely obese

TABLE I   **Effects of Weight Reduction on Roentgenographic Cardiac Diameter in Very Obese Subjects***

Subject	Sex	Age (yr)	Weight Loss (kg)	% Body Weight	Mean Arterial Blood Pressure (mmHg)		Blood Volume, (liters)	Cardiac Diameter (cm)	Thoracic Diameter (cm)	Cardiothoracic Ratio
2	M	22	74	34	Before:	97	8.8	14.8	35.2	0.42
					After:	92	7.0	13.8	35.2	0.39
5	F	29	53	29	Before:	145	9.2	17.0	30.2	0.56
					After:	104	7.1	14.5	29.3	0.49
4	F	59	59	32	Before:	110	7.1	13.9	30.3	0.46
					After:	98	5.6	12.8	30.3	0.42
1	F	48	48	36	Before:	100	7.0	14.6	29.1	0.51
					After:	78	4.4	12.4	29.2	0.43
7	M	34	46	25	Before:	95	9.5	15.3	35.0	0.44
					After:	79	7.7	13.9	35.0	0.40
6	F	35	46	29	Before:	90	9.4	15.2	32.1	0.47
					After:	71	7.7	13.1	32.1	0.41
3	F	23	39	34	Before:	90	5.9	12.8	27.5	0.46
					After:	75	5.2	9.9	27.0	0.37
Mean			52	31	105 ± 21		8.1 ± 1.4	14.8 ± 1.2	31.3 ± 2.7	0.47 ± 0.04
					85 ± 13		6.4 ± 1.3	12.9 ± 1.4	31.2 ± 2.9	0.41 ± 0.04
p value					0.05		0.05	<0.05	NS	<0.05

NS = not significant.
*Listed in descending order of percent body weight reduction. (Modified with permission from Alexander and Peterson.[15])

subjects achieving 31% reduction in body weight, we found that decrements of 18% and 21% in mean arterial pressure and blood volume, respectively, were accompanied by a 13% reduction in cardiac diameter on chest film (Table I, Fig. 2). As total body oxygen transport decreases with loss of adipose tissue, CO is reduced proportionately, since systemic arteriovenous oxygen difference narrows only modestly. There is usually little change in systemic vascular resistance, since both blood pressure and CO decrease[15,16] (Fig. 3). During exercise at comparable workloads, oxygen consumption, CO, and SV are less following weight loss.[16] Nevertheless, LV diastolic and pulmonary wedge pressures tend to remain elevated at rest or during exercise, even though CO decreases to or toward normal.[15,16] Also, there is no significant change in LV function curves constructed on the basis of rest and exercise data.[15] There appear to be no definitive studies at this time on the reversibility of LVH with weight reduction in obesity hypertension. Persistent elevation of LV filling pressure for as long as 3 years after weight loss suggests that diastolic chamber compliance may remain depressed without alteration of hypertrophic changes.[15]

With regard to dietary therapy, it may be pointed out that postural hypotension and dizziness are often observed with fasting or markedly restricted calorie regimens. Natriuresis and obligatory water loss consequent to excretion of ketones and solutes deriving from catabolism of lean tissue lead to contraction of plasma volume and sometimes hypotension.[17,18] More importantly, experimental and clinical evidence indicates that diminished

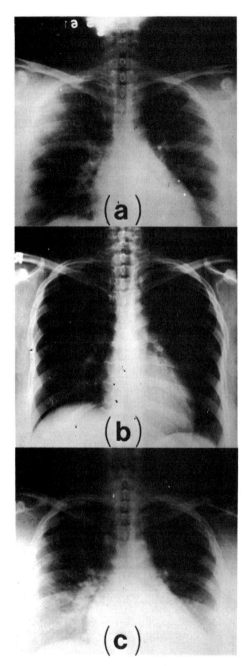

Figure 2. *Sequential chest films of a woman:* (a) at age 29 years, weight 184 kg, blood volume 9.2 liters, blood pressure (intra-arterial) 201/114 mmHg; (b) with weight reduction to 157 kg 2 years later; blood volume was 7.1 liters, blood pressure 125/89 mmHg; (c) at age 36 she had regained weight to 249 kg, with blood volume 10.3 liters and blood pressure 173/108 mmHg.

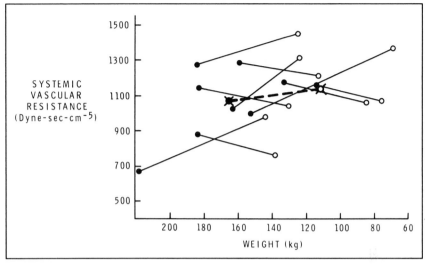

Figure 3. *Effect of weight loss on systemic vascular resistance at rest in nine very obese subjects. (From the data of Alexander and Peterson.[15])*

sympathetic activity plays a significant role.[19–21] The decrement in blood pressure with very low caloric intake is accompanied by reduced urinary catecholamines, plasma renin, and norepinephrine concentrations, and with enhanced aldosterone secretory rates, even though total body sodium is maintained. Thus, in this setting elevated blood volume does not confer immunity to the potential effects of reduced sympathetic activity on vasomotor tone, sometimes effecting drastically reduced LV preload and SV.

Finally, ventricular arrhythmia and fibrillation may complicate fasting regimens as a result of myocardial potassium depletion, associated in some cases with Q-T prolongation, lactic acidosis, or LV systolic dysfunction.[22–25]

Summary

Obesity hypertension is a high-output state with augmentation of both preload and afterload, leading to the development of eccentric LVH. Ventricular diastolic chamber compliance is characteristically reduced, usually, but not always, with well-preserved systolic performance. Although the natural history of obesity hypertension associated with compromised LV systolic function is not well defined, it appears that this characterizes that group of patients who ultimately develop congestive failure. Finally, I have included mention of some potentially deleterious circulatory and cardiac effects deriving from fasting or markedly restricted caloric regimens.

References

1. ALEXANDER JK: Obesity and the circulation. Mod Concepts Cardiovasc Dis 1963; 32: 799–803.
2. MESSERLI FH, CHRISTIE B, DECARVALHO JGR, ARISTIMUNO GG, SURAEZ DH, DRESLINSKI GR, FROHLICH ED: Obesity and essential hypertension: hemodynamics, intravascular volume, sodium excretion, and plasma renin activity. Arch Intern Med 1981; 141: 81–85.
3. ALEXANDER JK, AMAD KH, COLE VW: Observations on some clinical features of extreme obesity with particular reference to cardiorespiratory effects. Am J Med 1962; 32: 512–524.
4. DE DEVITIIS O, FAZIO S, PETITTO M, MADDALENA G, CONTALDO F, MANCINI M: Obesity and cardiac function. Circulation 1981; 64: 477–482.
5. MESSERLI FH, VENTURA HD, REISIN E, DRESLINSKI GR, DUNN FG, MACPHEE AA, FROHLICH ED: Borderline hypertension and obesity: two prehypertensive states with elevated cardiac output. Circulation 1982; 68: 55–60.
6. ALEXANDER JK: Obesity and cardiac performance. Am J Cardiol 1964; 14: 860–865.
7. MESSERLI FH, SUNDGAARD-RIISE K, REISIN ED, DRESLINSKI GR, VENTURA HO, OIGMEN W, FROHLICH ED, DUNN FG: Dimorphic cardiac adaptation to obesity and arterial hypertension. Ann Intern Med; 1983; 99: 757–761.
8. BACHMAN L, FREYSCHUSS U, HALLBERG D, MELCHER A: Cardiovascular function in extreme obesity. Acta Med Scand 1973; 193: 437–446.
9. AMAD KH, BRENNAN JC, ALEXANDER JK: The cardiac pathology of obesity. Circulation 1965; 32: 740–745.
10. ALEXANDER JK, WOODWARD CB, QUINONES MA, GASSCH WH: Heart failure from obesity. In: Mancini M, Lewis B, Cartaldo F, eds. Medical complications of obesity. London: Academic Press, 1978.
11. CUETO GARCIA L, LAREDO C, ARRIAGA J, GONZALEZ BJ: Echocardiographic findings in obesity. Rev Invest Clin (Mex) 1982; 34: 235–242.
12. ADLERSBERG D, COLER H, LAVAL J: Effect of weight reduction on course of arterial hypertension. J Mt Sinai Hosp 1946; 12: 984.
13. ASHLEY FW JR, KANNEL WB: Relation of weight changes in atherogenic traits: the Framingham Study. J Chron Dis 1974; 27: 103–114.
14. GREMINGER P, STUDER A, LUSCHER T, MUTTER B, GRIMM J, SEIGENTHALER W, VETTER W: Gewichtsreduktion und Blutdruck. Schweiz Med Wochenschr 1982; 112: 120–123.
15. ALEXANDER JK, PETERSON KL: Cardiovascular effects of weight reduction. Circulation 1972; 45: 310–318.
16. BACKMAN L, FREYSCHUSS U, HALLBERG D, MELCHER A: Reversibility of cardiovascular changes in extreme obesity. Effects of weight reduction through jejunoileostomy. Acta Med Scand 1979; 205: 367–373.
17. DRENICK EF: Starvation in the management of obesity. In: Wilson NL, ed. Obesity. London: Academic Press, 1978.
18. SIGLER MH: The mechanism of the natriuresis of fasting. J Clin Invest 1975; 55: 377–387.
19. YOUNG JB, LANDSBERG L: Weight loss and reduction in blood pressure. N Engl J Med 1978; 298: 1033.

20. JUNG RT, SHETTY PS, BARRAND M, CALLINGHAM BA, JAMES WP: Role of catecholamines in hypotensive response to dieting. Br Med J 1979; 1: 12–13.

21. DeHAVEN J, SHERWIN R, HENDLER R, FELIG P: Nitrogen and sodium balance and sympathetic-nervous-system activity in obese subjects treated with a low calorie protein or mixed diet. New Engl J Med 1980; 302: 477–482.

22. CUBBERLY PT, POLSTER SA, SCHULMAN CL: Lactic acidosis and death after treatment of obesity by fasting. New Engl J Med 1965; 272: 628–630.

23. SPENCER IOB: Death during therapeutic starvation for obesity. Lancet 1968; 1: 1288–1290.

24. GARNETT ES, BARNARD DL, FORD J, GOODBODY RA, WOODEHOUSE JA: Gross fragmentation of cardiac myofibrils after therapeutic starvation for obesity. Lancet 1969; 1: 914–916.

25. SANDHOFER F, DIENSTL F, BOLZANO K, SCHWINGSHACKL H: Severe cardiovascular complication associated with prolonged starvation. Br Med J 1973; 1: 462–463.

42

Exercise and the Heart in Hypertension

SAXON W. WHITE, M.D.

Compared to the figures for 1965 to 1967, there has been a 40% decline in mortality[1,2] due to ischemic heart disease for each sex and for all age groups in Australia and the United States, an event that has focused attention on the mechanisms of the phenomenon. A similar time course of decline in mortality for cerebrovascular disease in these countries has also been noted.[2] Nevertheless, cardiovascular disease remains by far the greatest killer in both countries, and in Australia the mortality rate for cerebrovascular disease is 40% to 55% greater than and the prevalence of hypertension is double that found in the United States.[2] To date, we still do not know whether the declining mortality is due to better patient management or to the subtle effects of changing community behavior. Nevertheless, the question continues to be raised as to whether attacking the "weaker" risk factor of lack of physical activity can in itself modify such risk factors as hypertension and thereby reduce cardiovascular mortality.

Epidemiologic Studies

In the 1970s, a number of articles with improved experimental design and data analysis relating physical inactivity to cardiovascular disease appeared. In the study of San Franciscan longshoremen[3] hypertension, prior heart disease, and cigarette smoking were identified as significant risk factors for coronary heart disease, the risk increasing three fold in the younger population for less active workers. If low energy output was combined with hypertension and smoking, there was a 20-fold increased risk; elimination of these combined factors, however, would have reduced the rate of fatal heart attack by 88% over 22 years! These outcomes were supported by other studies from Brand et al[4] who showed that coronary heart disease risk was inversely related to a work level of about twice resting oxygen uptake, an effect increased by an oxygen uptake at work of four fold above resting. It was postulated that the lower work effect may have been due to catecholamine hormone "detuning," and that the higher work effect probably represented additional physiologic training effects on cardiorespiratory function. Among others, the studies from Göteborg[5] of men born in 1913 and a large prevalence study involving 3,000 men by Cooper et al[6] also supported the thesis; in the latter study there was an inverse relationship between physical fitness and systolic blood pressure, an effect confirmed by Paffenbarger et al[7] in a study on a large group of Harvard alumni. By contrast, Sedgwick and co-workers[8] evaluated the effects of a physical fitness intervention program over 5 years on the classic risk factors in 370 sedentary men aged between 20 and 65 years and found that men who had substantially improved in fitness did not differ in risk factors (including arterial pressure levels) from men whose fitness had not changed or declined. Nevertheless, two recent studies reinforce the earlier data on the potential importance of exercise. Blair and coworkers[9] followed 4,820 men and 1,219 women aged 20 to 65 years over 1 to 12 years to estimate the independent contribution of physical fitness (maximal treadmill test) to the risk of becoming hypertensive, and found that persons with low levels of fitness had a relative risk of 1.52 compared with highly fit persons. Paffenbarger and colleagues[10] showed in 16,936 Harvard alumni that habitual post-college exercise is associated with low coronary heart disease risk. Sedentary alumni, even former highly trained athletes, have a high risk. They also showed, as have others,[11] that the exercise benefit is independent of hypertension and other risk factors. It was concluded that the exercise revolution may improve lifestyle, cardiovascular health, and longevity. An interesting and important principle emerging from these studies is that relatively low levels of exercise are required for protection against both coronary artery disease and hypertension.

The Exercise Response in the Normotensive State

Recently, the exercise response and what we know of its initiating and sustaining mechanisms have been comprehensively reviewed.[12] Systolic arterial pressure in men and women increases sharply during exercise (Fig. 1). The effect reflects a marked increase in myocardial contractility, and provides the energy for driving systolic flow through the dilated skeletal muscle bed. On the other hand, the diastolic pressure hardly changes. This effect reflects the balance between the increase in flow conductance in the exercising beds, and the decrease in the nonexercising beds (including skeletal muscle), and provides the driving pressure for coronary blood flow. There is also an increase in circulating catecholamines,[13] including epinephrine, which plays an integrative role by facilitating the availability of substrate for energy production (through the breakdown of glycogen to glucose in muscle and liver and the release of free fatty acids) and by enhancing cardiac performance.

Much interest has focused on neural controls during exercise. Although our understanding of the relative roles of "central command," and the secondary sensory inputs from skeletal muscle, arterial baro- and chemoreceptors and cardiac receptors during exercise responses is incomplete,[12,14] it is now apparent that the arterial baroreflex is functionally intact in relation to modifying changes in arterial pressure during exercise.[12,15] The gain of some components of the reflex, such as the neural controls regulating heart rate, are reduced more than others.[15] In effect, this means that the arterial

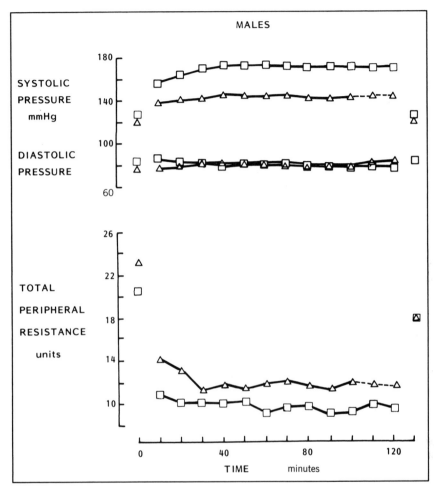

Figure 1. *Systolic and diastolic arterial pressure (measured using sphygmomanometry), and total peripheral resistance (cardiac output measured using impedance cardiography) changes in 2 groups each of 6 men, trained, VO_{2max} is 67.0 ± 1.98 ml · kg · min^{-1}, and untrained, VO_{2max} is 37.6 ± 2.15 ml · kg · min^{-1}. Each subject worked at 55% of his predetermined VO_{2max}. Mean resting systolic pressure for trained was 129 ± 4.4 mmHg, and for untrained it was 120 ± 2.5 mmHg. Note higher systolic pressures during exercise in trained groups, $p < 0.001$. The ages of the respective groups were 25.5 ± 1.69 (trained), and 25.8 ± 1.76 (untrained). □ = trained; △ = untrained. (Reprinted with permission from Brown.[16])*

baroreflex may normally restrain any untoward increases in arterial pressure during exercise.[12]

Not reviewed, however, were the exercise-evoked changes in sex steroids and other hormones. Recent studies on exercising normotensive men in our laboratory[16] showed an increase in serum estradiol (Fig. 2) and 17-hydroxyprogesterone, as well as in testosterone, androstenedione, and cortisol. Increases in female sex hormones in women in response to exercise have been previously documented,[17] but we were surprised initially to find them increased also in men. During incremental exercise, serum estrogen increases to levels comparable to those found in the female at rest in the luteal phase of the menstrual cycle. Since the hormone can determine the pattern of substrate utilization (for example, it causes carbohydrate sparing during endurance performance,[18]), it now turns out that any advantages proposed for the presence of the hormone in women may also apply to the physically active man. For example, data from von Eiff et al[19,20] suggest that estrogen plays a significant role in control of systolic arterial pressure levels in women at rest and during reactions to arithmetic and emotional stress. The presence of progesterone adds no further effect. Estrogen is also capable of stimulating increases in serum high density lipoproteins,[21] as does exercise,[22] and is widely accepted as playing a significant role by unknown mechanisms in the protection of women against ischemic heart disease, at least until the menopause. The significance of these findings to men and women in relation to physical activity and behavior, to the short- and long-term control of arterial pressure, and to the protection of both sexes against ischemic heart disease, awaits further elucidation.

Effects of Training on Arterial Pressure in the Normotensive State: Exercise training has clear-cut effects on the resting neural controls of normotensive people. There is increased vagal and decreased sympathetic activity directed to the sinoatrial node, which also undergoes a slowing of its intrinsic rate.[23,24] Recently, in a carefully controlled single blind, randomized cross-over study involving confined subjects, each subjected to four different levels of physical activity, resting arterial pressure was shown to be lowered in those exercising at least three times weekly.[25] This was due to a lowered total peripheral resistance, suggesting a decrease in resting sympathetic tone in the peripheral circulation. This was confirmed by the observed reduction in norepinephrine spillover rate at rest using tracer doses of ^{3}H norepinephrine. It is not known whether there is modification to underlying non-neural vascular tone. However, the data support and extend previous findings highly suggestive of a reduction in resting peripheral sympathetic tone induced by regular exercise and leading to a reduction in resting arterial pressure.[26–28]

Exercise training also has clear-cut effects on resting hormone levels in both sexes. The female athlete can become amenorrheic; the few highly trained female endurance performers recently studied in our laboratory[16] showed low resting estradiol levels at rest, confirming other reports of persistently low estradiol and prolactin levels.[29] In these women there is also altered thyroid function (subclinical hypothyroidism[30]) and reduced gona-

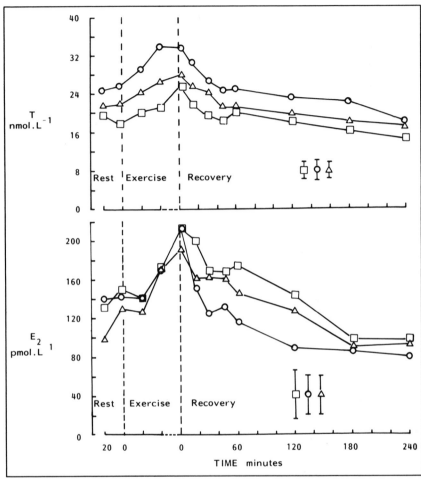

Figure 2. *Serum testosterone (T) and estradiol (E₂) concentrations in 6 highly trained, 6 trained, and 6 untrained men at rest, during 50 to 60 minutes of graded exercise to maximal effort working on a bicycle ergometer, and over a 240 minute recovery period. Vertical bars indicate ± 1 SED between 2 time intervals, calculated by analysis of variance. There were no significant differences in the responses between groups. Note, however, the delay in the E₂ increase relative to the T, which might be expected if T is aromatized to E₂ in peripheral tissues. VO₂max in highly trained was 67.0 ± 1.98 ml · kg · min⁻¹, in trained, VO₂max was 57.0 ± 0.97 ml · kg · min⁻¹, and in untrained, VO₂max was 37.6 ± 2.15 ml · kg · min⁻¹. □ = highly trained; ○ = trained; △ = untrained. (Reprinted with permission from Brown.[16])*

dotropin responses to gonadotropin releasing hormone stimulation. In resting male distance runners, reduced serum testosterone and prolactin concentrations have been reported,[31] and it is known that testosterone levels decrease after acute, prolonged exercise,[32] returning to preexercise levels within 24 hours. Similar effects were noted in men in our laboratory in relation to both testosterone and estradiol (Fig. 2), in whom after incremental exercise to maximal oxygen uptake the levels tended to decline to below preexercise levels. All these data taken together strongly suggest that as a result of repetitive physical activity, a reduction in resting arterial pressure is accompanied by changes in autonomic and endocrine function in favor of heightened vagal activity, and depression (or "detuning") of sympathoadrenal and pituitary-gonadal activity.

Exercise training also modifies the response to exercise. Recent studies in our laboratory (Fig. 1) have shown that male and female athletes who commence exercise with arterial pressures similar to their untrained counterparts increase the systolic pressures to significantly higher levels than those untrained when each subject works at 55% of maximal oxygen uptake, an effect that is much greater in males. On the other hand, the heart rate response remained systematically below those of the untrained subjects, as expected. Thus, the downward conditioning effect on heart rate noted at rest persisted during exercise, but the effect on arterial pressure did not. Presumably, the greater systolic pressure effects reflect an amplification effect of the trained heart.[33] Other laboratories report a normal or reduced catecholamine release during exercise in trained subjects,[34] so that the systolic pressure effect is unlikely to be due to a greater than normal orthosympathetic response. Our own data (Fig. 2) concerning sex and other steroid hormone responses show little difference in the responses between trained and untrained men, and little difference in the postexercise nadir. Thus, although there are quantitative differences in resting cardiovascular status and the activity of its control due to training, the quantitative response to exercise in trained men and women is near normal, except for the arterial pressure response. Qualitatively, the effects in both sexes are surprisingly similar. It is speculated that in more active men and women, the daily average concentrations of these hormones would be considerably higher than in their inactive counterparts, leading to negative feedback suppression of components of the neuroendocrine system; a similar argument could be advanced for the blood pressure control system.

Exercise in the Hypertensive State

In established essential hypertension at rest, it is evident that structural changes in the heart and arterial tree tend to sustain the high arterial pressure,[14] even though cardiac function may be compromised by a change in ventricular compliance secondary to the increase in connective tissue and myocardial hypertrophy.[35] In addition, there are adjustments to components of baroreflex function.[12,36] Thus, apart from the hyperkinetic state of the autonomic nervous system in young people with essential hypertension, the resting autonomic status in established hypertension appears relatively normal,[37] as is the renin-angiotensin system.[38] The reason given for increased circulating catecholamines[37] relates to the presence of left ventricular dysfunction. There are no data concerning the status of pituitary-gonadal function. During exercise, deficiencies in performance do become manifest, but whether this is due to structural change,[35] underlying cardiac ischemia,[39] altered control systems,[36] or to combinations of such effects is poorly understood. In some studies the cardiac output response for a given workload is less than normal,[1] in others it is greater,[39] with usually greater than normal total peripheral resistance effects. The increases in arterial pressure are variously reported; Lund-Johansen[37] reports an effort-dependent increase in arterial pressure systematically above the increase in normotensive controls. Others report a greater than normal increase at any given effort. Isometric exercise with its relatively greater increase in arterial pressure for a given exercise effort should be undertaken with caution; there is a greater risk of stroke during effort (lifting, straining, pushing) of this kind.[40]

Effects of Exercise Training in Hypertension: The effects of running and of weight training on resting arterial pressure in essential hypertension have been investigated, but in general these studies have also been poorly controlled. Hypertensive men and women training on treadmills, cycle ergometers, or playing games some three to five times per week for periods ranging from 4 to 12 weeks show, if anything, a small reduction in arterial pressure up to 17/7 mmHg,[41] usually accompanied by a training effect on heart rate. The best results have been obtained in mild to moderate hypertensive young people, suggesting an effect can be achieved, as in normotensive people, by training the neural control systems when they are possibly hyperactive,[26] and before major structural changes are manifested. Other data show that any beneficial effects on arterial pressure depend on the maintenance of the training program,[41] but the time course of the off-effect has not been defined in either hypertensive or normotensive people.

Conclusion

Evidence from both epidemiologic and laboratory studies suggests that repetitive physical activity lowers resting arterial pressure. Although the mechanism of this effect is not yet elucidated, there are data to suggest that in normotensive people at rest, the vagus nerve is more active, and there is a reduction in activity of the sympathoadrenal and pituitary-gonadal systems. All these effects would tend to reduce arterial pressure. During exercise in trained normotensive men and women, systolic arterial pressure may rise to higher levels than in their untrained counterparts, but from low resting baselines the autonomic and hormonal systems appear to respond normally. In uncomplicated essential hypertension at rest, data of this kind are even less complete; superimposed on profound structural alterations sympathoadrenal activity appears to be somewhat heightened rather than depressed, but during exercise the autonomic nervous system appears to respond normally. Repetitive physical activity will lower resting arterial pressure in hypertensive people, especially in the younger hypertensive. There is more consistent evidence[42] for heightened sympathoadrenal activity in an untrained person at rest. These considerations and the known effectiveness of sympatholytic antihypertensive therapy on hypertensive people at rest and during exercise, justify the speculation that relatively low-grade but regular aerobic exercise may in itself play a role in the prevention of hypertension and ischemic heart disease, and in the enhancement of sympatholytic drug effects in selected hypertensive patients. There would be a profound effect on cardiovascular mortality and morbidity if we could, by getting everyone to exercise, lower the population mean arterial pressure by 3 mmHg. This is apparent from the continuous relationship between risk and systemic arterial pressure.

Acknowledgments

The original work in this study was supported by a Grant-in-Aid from the Research Committee of the Faculty of Medicine, University of Newcastle, and by a University of Newcastle Postgraduate Scholarship. I am grateful to The Garvan Institute for Medical Research, Sydney (Dr. R. Vining and R. McGinley) for the radioimmunoassay measurements of serum hormones shown in Figure 2, and to Judith Wood, Janet Brice, and Kathy Pearson for help in preparing the manuscript.

References

1. Leeder SR, Gibberd RW, Dobson AJ, Lloyd DM: Declining mortality rates from ischaemic heart disease in Australia. Aust NZ J Med 1984; 14: 388–394.
2. MacMahon SW, Leeder SR: Blood pressure levels and mortality from cerebrovascular disease in Australia and the United States. Am J Epidemiology 1984; 120: 865–875.
3. Paffenbarger R, Hale WE, Brand RJ, Hyde RT: Work energy level, personal characteristics, and fatal heart attack: a birth cohort effect. Am J Epidemiol 1977; 105: 200–213.
4. Brand RJ, Paffenbarger R, Sholtz RI, Kampert JB: Job activity and fatal heart attacks studied by multiple logistic risk analysis. Circulation 1976; 54 (4): II–51.
5. Wilhelmsen L, Tibblin G, Aurell M, Bjure J, Ekstrøm-Jodal B, Grimby G: Physical activity, physical fitness and risk of myocardial infarction. Adv Cardiol 1976; 18: 217–230.
6. Cooper KH, Pollack ML, Martin RP, White SR, Linnerud AC, Jackson A: Physical fitness levels vs selected coronary risk factors. Cross-sectional study. JAMA 1976; 236: 166–169.

7. PAFFENBARGER R, WING AL, HYDE RT, JUNG DL: Physical activity and incidence of hypertension in college alumni. Am J Epidemiol 1983; 117: 245–257.

8. SEDGWICK AW, BROTHERHOOD JR, HARRIS-DAVIDSON A, TAFLIN RE, THOMAS DW: Long-term effects of physical training programme on risk factors for CAD in otherwise sedentary men. Br Med J 1980; 5 July, 7–10.

9. BLAIR SN, GOODYEAR N, GIBBONS LW, COOPER KH: Physical fitness and incidence of hypertension in healthy normotensive men and women. JAMA 1984; 252: 487–490.

10. PAFFENBARGER R, HYDE RT, WING AL, STEINMETZ CH: A natural history of athleticism and cardiovascular health. JAMA 1984; 252: 491–495.

11. KANNEL WB, SORLIE P, McNAMARA P: Relation of physical activity to risk of coronary heart disease: The Framingham Study. In: Larson OA, Malmborg RO, eds. Coronary heart disease and physical fitness. Copenhagen: Munksgaard, 1971; 256–260.

12. ROWELL LB: What signals govern the cardiovascular response to exercise? Med Sci Sports Exerc 1980; 12: 307–315.

13. FERGUSON RK, VLASSES PH, KOFFER H, CLEMENTI RA, KOPLIN JR, WILLCOX CM: Effect of captopril and propranolol, alone and in combination, on the responses to isometric and dynamic exercise in normotensive and hypertensive men. Pharmacotherapy 1983; 3: 125–130.

14. KORNER PI: The role of the heart in hypertension. In: Robertson JIS, ed. Handbook of hypertension, vol. 1. Clinical aspects of essential hypertension. Amsterdam: Elsevier, 1983; 97–132.

15. FARIS IB, JAMIESON GG, LUDBROOK J: Effect of exercise on gain of the carotid-sinus reflex in rabbits. Clin Sci 1982; 63: 115–119.

16. BROWN WB: Endurance exercise in man: metabolic, cardiorespiratory, and steroid hormone correlates in males and females. PhD Thesis. Newcastle, University of Newcastle, 1983.

17. JURKOWSKI JE, JONES NL, WALKER WC, YOUNGLAI EC, SUTTON JR: Ovarian hormonal responses to exercise. J Appl Physiol 1978; 44: 109–114.

18. GORSKI J, STANKIEWICZ B, BRYCKA R, KICZKA K: The effect of estradiol on carbohydrate utilization during prolonged exercise in rats. Acta Physiol Pol 1976; 27: 361–367.

19. VON EIFF AW, PIEKARSKI C: Stress reaction of normotensives and hypertensives and the influence of female sex hormones on blood pressure regulation. In: De Jong W, Provost AP, eds. Progress in brain research. Hypertension and brain mechanisms. Vol. 47. 1977; 289–299.

20. VON EIFF AW, PLOTZ EJ, BECK KJ, CZERNICK A: The effect of estrogens and progestin on blood pressure regulation in normotensive women. Am J Obstet Gynecol 1971; 109: 887–892.

21. MASAREI JRL, ARMSTRONG BK, SKINNER MW, RATAJCZAK T, HÄHNEL R, CROOKE D, CLARKE HT: HDL-cholesterol and sex-hormone status. Lancet 1980; 1: 208.

22. MILLER N, RAO S, LEWIS B, BJØRSUIK G, MYHRE K, MJØS OD: High-density lipoprotein and physical activity. Lancet 1979; 1: 111.

23. BOLTER CP, HUGHSON RL, CRITZ JB: Intrinsic rate and cholinergic sensitivity of

isolated atria from trained and sedentary rats. Proc Soc Exp Biol Med 1973; 144: 364–367.

24. SCHEUER J, PENPARGKUL S, BHAN AK: Experimental observations on the effects of physical training upon intrinsic cardiac physiology and biochemistry. Am J Cardiol 1974; 33: 744–751.

25. JENNINGS G, NELSON L, ESLER M: Effects of changes in physical activity on blood pressure and sympathetic tone. Xth Scientific Meeting, International Society of Hypertension, Interlaken, abstr. 13, 1984.

26. COOKSEY JD, REILLY P, BROWN S, BOMZE H, CRYER PE: Exercise training and plasma catecholamines in patients with ischemic heart disease. Am J Cardiol 1978; 42: 372–376.

27. DUNCAN JJ, HAGAN RD, UPTON J, FARR JE, OGLESBY ME: The effects of an aerobic exercise program on sympathetic neural activity and blood pressure in mild hypertensive patients. Circulation 1983; 68: 285.

28. EDWARDS MT, DIANA JN: Effect of exercise on pre-and postcapillary resistance in the spontaneously hypertensive rat. Am J Physiol 1978; 234: H439–H446.

29. BOYDEN TW, PAMENTER RW, GROSSO D, STANFORTH P, ROTKIS T, WILMORE JH: Prolactin responses, menstrual cycles and body composition of women runners. J Clin Endocrinol Metab 1982; 54: 711–714.

30. BOYDEN TW, PAMENTER RW, STANFORTH P, ROTKIS T, WILMORE JH: Evidence for mild thyroidal impairment in women undergoing endurance training. J Clin Endocrinol Metab 1982; 54: 53–56.

31. WHEELER GD, WALL SR, BELCASTRO AN, CUMMING DC: Reduced serum testosterone and prolactin levels in male distance runners. JAMA 1984; 252: 514–516.

32. MORVILLE R, PESQUIES PC, GUENNENEC CY, SERRURIER BD, GUIGNARD M: Plasma variations in testicular and adrenal androgens during prolonged physical exercise in man. Ann Endocrinol 1979; 40: 501–510.

33. EHSANI AA, HAGBERG JM, HICKSON RC: Rapid changes in left ventricular dimensions and mass in response to physical conditioning and deconditioning. Am J Cardiol 1978; 42: 52–56.

34. HARTLEY LH: Growth hormone and catecholamine response to exercise in relation to physical training. Med Sci Sports 1975; 7: 34–36.

35. KUNZ J, BRASELMAN H, GOTTSCHALK J, KREHER C, PIEPER K: The myocardial collagenous connective tissue in experimental cardiac hypertrophy induced by swimming exercise and hypertension. Exp Pathol 1981; 19: 206–218.

36. SUAREZ DH, MESSERLI FH, VENTURA HO, ARISTIMENO G, DRESLINSKI GR, FROHLICH ED: Baroreceptor stimulation and isometric exercise in normotensive and borderline hypertensive subjects. Clin Sci 1982; 62: 307–309.

37. LUND-JOHANSEN P: Physical activity and hypertension Scand J Soc Med 1982; 29 (suppl): 185–194.

38. AMERY A, FAGARD R, LIJNEN P, REYBROUCK J: Role of renin-angiotensin and of the adrenergic system in the blood pressure regulation at exercise in normotensive subjects and in hypertensive patients. Cardiology 1981; 68: 103–117.

39. WHITE SW, TRAUGOTT FM, QUAIL AW, SCRIVEN L, SMITH K, CHILVERS C: Heightened stroke volume response during moderate exercise in man with mild hy-

pertension and ischaemic heart disease. Xth Scientific Meeting, International Society Hypertension, abstr. 926, 1984.

40. FUKUDA Y: Epidemiology of the occurrence of cerebral stroke and heart attack—with particular reference to influence of hypertension control and living conditions. Kenkyukai, Japan: Rodoigaku, 1978.

41. CHRASTEK J, ADAMIROVA J, KRIZ V, et al: Testing the cardiorespiratory capacity and training in hypertensive disease stage II. Rev Czech Med 1974; 20: 58–75.

42. KLEIN AA, McCRORY WW, ENGLE MA, ROSENTHAL R, EHLERS KH: Sympathetic nervous system and exercise tolerance response in normotensive and hypertensive adolescents. J Am Coll Cardiol 1984; 3: 381–386.

43

Effects of Antihypertensive Therapy on Cardiac Function During Exercise

CLIVE ROSENDORFF, M.D., Ph.D., D.Sc.(Med.), F.R.C.P.
CARMEL GOODMAN, M.D., B.Ch. (LOND.)
ANNE COULL, B.Sc. Hons.

Although there has been increasing interest in the changes of cardiovascular function characterizing both early and established hypertension, less is known of the way in which antihypertensive drugs modify hemodynamics, especially during exercise.

In hypertension most patients with no functional cardiovascular impairment respond to modest exercise the same as normal subjects, but in the majority of WHO stage II and III patients,[1] both blood pressure and heart rate increase significantly higher than normal during exercise.[2-4] Normalization of these exaggerated, exercise induced, hemodynamic changes would be a desirable effect of any antihypertensive therapy. Another attribute of any antihypertensive drug would be the achievement of a more favorable ratio between myocardial oxygen supply and demand, thereby to ensure an adequate coronary blood flow during exercise.

Of all classes of antihypertensive agents, the most intensively studied have been beta-adrenergic drugs. These decrease heart rate, stroke volume (SV), and cardiac output (CO) at rest and during exercise, reduce systolic arterial pressure during exercise, and elevate the left ventricular (LV) end-diastolic pressure.[5-10] However, nearly all of these studies have been on the acute effects of beta-blocking drugs, assessed invasively. Of the other antihypertensive agents, few have been studied during dynamic exercise and with sustained therapy. These include thiazide diuretics,[11-13] methyldopa,[10,13] and captopril.[14,15]

In the present study we evaluate, using noninvasive methods, the effects of sustained (16 weeks) therapy of mild to moderate essential hypertension with hydrochlorothiazide, propranolol, methyldopa, and the angiotensin converting enzyme inhibitor enalapril on resting and exercise hemodynamics and myocardial perfusion.

Methods

Ambulatory patients of either sex, 25 to 65 years old, with essential hypertension and an untreated supine diastolic blood pressure of 95 to 120 mmHg (phase 5) were eligible for entry into the study. Exclusion criteria included patients with secondary or malignant hypertension, cardiac disease, previous myocardial infarction or cerebrovascular accident, diabetes, abnormal hematologic or biochemical parameters, and any other underlying disease that might have affected results.

Informed consent was obtained from 43 patients who entered the study. They were randomly assigned to one of four treatment groups: hydrochlorothiazide (n = 9), propranolol (n = 9), methyldopa (n = 9), and enalapril (n = 16). The study commenced with a 4-week washout period during which each patient received 2 placebo tablets daily, 1 in the morning and 1 in the evening. This dosage regimen was continued into the treatment period. The active treatment period consisted of 16 weeks of hydrochlorothiazide up to 100 mg/day, propranolol up to 400 mg/day, methyldopa up to 2 g/day or enalapril up to 40 mg/day, titrated every 2 weeks to achieve a supine diastolic blood pressure of less than 90 mmHg.

At the end of the placebo period, and again at the end of the treatment period, each patient had a full physical examination, chest radiographs, electrocardiograph, hematologic, and biochemical investigation and routine urinalysis. Toward the end of the placebo period, the patients had the first of the exercise sessions on a supine bicycle ergometer (Quinton Instruments). This exercise test served three functions: to familiarize the patients with the exercise apparatus, to confirm that no patients with exercise-inducible signs of disease were included, and to establish work load values for R_{50max} (see below).

This was done by beginning the bicycle exercise at 50 W and increasing by 25 W every three minutes until the patient could no longer continue exercising. The heart rate was measured at each work load. R_{50max} was calculated from the formula $R_{50max} = R_0 + (R_{max} - R_0)/2$ where R_0 and R_{max} were the patient's heart rate at rest and during maximal effort. All subsequent exercise tests were done at the work load that corresponded to R_{50max}.

Thereafter, four sets of exercise tests were performed at R_{50max}, two at the end of the placebo period and two at the end of the treatment period. The exercise tests were used to evaluate the effects of therapy on exercise-induced changes in heart rate and blood pressure responses, in myocardial blood flow and in LV function.

All tests were performed in the morning, and patients were instructed not to eat, drink, or smoke for 4 hours before the test. The heart rate was monitored before and during each exercise test by continuous electrocardiographic recording, and blood pressure was recorded before and at two-minute intervals during each exercise period using a manual sphygmomanometer. At the first of the two exercise tests, at least 2 days apart, performed at the end of the placebo period, myocardial perfusion was assessed by thallium-201 scintigraphy.[16] Once the exercising subject attained the R_{50max} heart rate, 1.5 to 2 mCi of thallium was injected intravenously via an antecubital vein. The subject then continued exercising for another 3 minutes at a constant workload corresponding to R_{50max}. At the completion of exercise, acquisitions were made in the anterior and left anterior oblique (LAO) 45°

positions. The myocardial images were recorded with a high-resolution scintillation camera (Searle Scintiview) with a high-resolution collimator. In each position 300,000 counts were collected over the relevant region of the myocardium with a 20% window set symmetrically around the x-ray peak. The time taken to reach 300,000 counts was recorded. A coronary flow index (CFI) was derived, which was defined as $10^4/t$, where t is time in seconds to 300,000 counts. With careful attention to retaining a constant counting geometry, the same acquisitions were repeated after 3 hours of rest and were taken as the resting value with which the exercise value was compared.[17] At the second of the two visits, the left ventricular ejection fraction (LVEF) was measured using the gated blood pool imaging technique.[18] Thirty minutes before the commencement of the exercise test, red blood cells were labeled in vivo by an intravenous injection of stannous pyrophosphate followed 20 minutes later by an intravenous injection of 20 mCi of technetium-99m (^{99m}Tc) pertechnetate. Studies were performed with a patient in the supine position under a mobile, single-crystal scintillation camera and images were recorded in the LAO 45° position in a continuous electrocardiographic-synchronized mode, with 24 frames per cardiac cycle. The scintillation camera data were collected for 4-minute periods immediately before commencing exercise, twice during 10 minutes of exercise at R_{50max}, and once during the recovery period.

All data were stored on a floppy disc and transferred to a dedicated computer. The LVEF was calculated as the difference between background-corrected end-diastolic and end-systolic counts, divided by end-diastolic counts, and was reported as the average of two separate determinations. The same procedures for measurement of myocardial perfusion and LVEF were performed again at the end of each of the treatment periods.

All data were acquired during rest and exercise during the placebo period and again during the treatment period, for each of the four modalities of treatment. The derived data for the pretreatment phases were compared using a paired difference *t*-statistic. Differences between the four treatment modalities were compared using Student's *t*-test between independent groups.

Results

Table I summarizes the blood pressure and heart rate responses to submaximal exercise off therapy and on each of the four modalities of treatment. All four drugs significantly decreased resting systolic and diastolic blood pressures, but, although all four drugs attenuated blood pressure responses to exercise, only hydrochlorothiazide (diastolic) and enalapril (systolic and diastolic) values achieved statistical significance at $p < 0.05$.

Therapy had no effect on the heart rate responses (Table I) to exercise, except in the case of propranolol, for which both resting and exercise heart rates were significantly lower than pretreatment levels, as well as being significantly lower than values in the other treatment groups.

TABLE I   Changes in Blood Pressure (mmHg) and Heart Rate

	Rest		Exercise	
	Before Therapy	After Therapy	Before Therapy	After Therapy
Blood pressure				
Hydrochlorozide				
Mean	183/113	158*/92[†]	216/129	205/111*
SEM	6.2/3.6	5.2/2.9	6.9/4.8	6.6/2.3
Propranolol				
Mean	181/112	156*/94*	219/126	191/110
SEM	9.0/5.1	7.9/4.5	13.3/5.4	5.7/3.9
Alpha-methyldopa				
Mean	163/107	154*/93*	207/121	192/115
SEM	7.8/4.1	5.5/4.6	7.4/4.7	4.8/3.9
Enalapril				
Mean	162/103	149*/92[†]	209/116	190*/110*
SEM	5.5/2.8	5.4/3.6	8.0/2.7	4.5/1.9
Heart rate				
Hydrochlorozide	72 ± 2.2	75 ± 3.3	119 ± 3.6	119 ± 4.9
Propranolol	71 ± 4.9	57 ± 4.6[†]	126 ± 10.0	108 ± 8.0[†]
alpha-Methyldopa	78 ± 5.1	70 ± 3.9	121 ± 4.3	117 ± 5.5
Enalapril	81 ± 3.0	74 ± 2.8	131 ± 3.6	125 ± 2.6

*$p < 0.05$.
[†]$p < 0.005$.

The LVEF (Fig. 1) was unchanged in patients treated with hydrochlorothiazide, from a mean of 58% before exercise to 57% during the first 10 minutes of exercise and 56% in the second 10 minutes of exercise, dropping to 51% in the recovery phase. In patients treated with propranolol, the LVEF decreased from a preexercise value of 55% to 50% during the first 10 minutes of the exercise period and to 49% during the second 10 minutes of exercise, and returned to 55% during the recovery phase. In the methyldopa group, LVEF increased from 52% before exercise to 55% in the first 10 minutes of exercise, returning to 44% during the recovery phase. In patients treated with enalapril, LVEF increased from a resting value of 47% to 55% during the first 10 minutes of exercise and returned to a recovery value of 53%.

There was no difference between the four groups in the resting CFI, both baseline and treated. Exercise values were higher in all groups, but again there was no significant difference between the four treatment group modalities in terms of CFI during exercise for baseline and therapy periods.

Rate-pressure product (RPP), calculated as the product of heart rate and systolic blood pressure, was significantly lower during rest and exercise in the propranolol-treated group ($p < 0.05$) and the enalapril-treated group ($p < 0.005$) compared with placebo. Propranolol caused a significantly larger attenuation of the RPP response to exercise than did hydrochlorothiazide ($p < 0.05$), methyldopa ($p < 0.05$), or enalapril ($p < 0.005$).

The CFI to RPP ratio, which is a useful index of the myocardial oxygen supply versus demand status, was not significantly different from pretherapy levels in any of the four treatment groups (Fig. 2), nor were there any significant differences between the four groups.

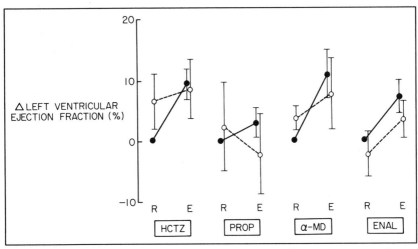

Figure 1. *Changes in left ventricular ejection fraction (LVEF) from the mean values of resting LVEF during the pretreatment phase (%). (Solid circles, 0 value). Means ± SEM are shown. Note that LVEF increases with exercise in all cases except the propranolol-treated group, in which there is a decrease. HCTZ = hydrochlorothiazide; PROP = propranolol; α-MD = methyldopa; ENAL = enalapril; R = resting; E = exercise; ●—● = pretreatment; ○—○ = after 14 to 16 weeks of therapy.*

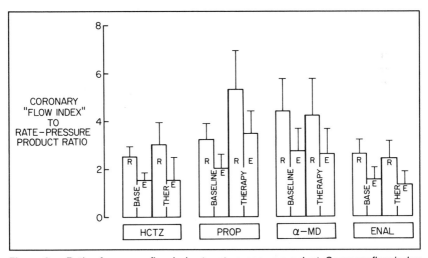

Figure 2. *Ratio of coronary flow index to rate-pressure product. Coronary flow index is defined as $10^4/t$, where t is time in seconds to acquire 300,000 counts during a thallium-201 scintiscan, and rate-pressure product is (heart rate × systolic blood pressure)/10^3. This ratio, which is an index of myocardial oxygen supply to demand, was not significantly altered by any of the four types of therapy. For abbreviations, see Figure 1.*

Comment

The attenuation of the blood pressure responses to exercise in the four treatment groups was virtually indistinguishable, although the enalapril-treated group was the only one in which this effect was statistically significant. However, there were clear differences between the propranolol-treated group and the other groups in the heart rate and ejection fraction responses to exercise. Both resting heart rate and the heart rate during exercise were significantly lower in the propranolol-treated group than before therapy, and the propranolol-treated group was the only one in which the ejection fraction clearly decreased with exercise and returned to normal values after exercise. The attenuated heart rate response to exercise with propranolol is in agreement with previous studies, in which beta blockers significantly inhibited exercise-induced tachycardia[5–8,10,19–21] and the relative lack of effect of hydrochlorothiazide, methyldopa, and enalapril on heart rate responses to exercise has been noted by others.[13,22–24] Also, the negative inotropic effect, suggested by the decrease in ejection fraction during exercise in the propranolol group has been well documented by other investigators.[8,21,25]

There is, however, an obvious reservation about equating changes in ejection fraction with changes in SV. If the effect of propranolol is to increase LV end-diastolic volume, a decrease in ejection fraction does not necessarily mean a decrease in SV. Put another way, a constant SV in the presence of an increased end-diastolic volume will be measured as a decrease in ejection fraction. Nevertheless, the data in the present study are, qualitatively at least, in accord with those obtained from invasive measurements of SV.[8,21,25] This, together with the large difference in exercise heart rate between the propranolol-treated and the other groups strongly suggests that, for any given level of exercise, the CO is lower in the propranolol-treated group than in other groups. Since the blood pressure responses to exercise were very similar among all groups, the corollary is that, for any given level of exercise, the peripheral resistance is higher in patients treated with propranolol than those on the other three forms of therapy. This may be an important factor in the limitation of exercise tolerance in patients on beta blockers.[7,26,27]

The exercise-induced increase in RPP, an index of myocardial oxygen consumption (MVO_2), was significantly attenuated by propranolol, due mainly to a decreased heart rate response to exercise. Propranolol was the most effective of the four drugs in attenuating the increased myocardial oxygen demand that normally occurs with exercise. These findings are in agreement with previous studies in which the major determinants of myocardial oxygen demand, namely, heart rate, afterload, and myocardial contractility, are significantly decreased by beta blockers during exercise.[8,28] Because changes in myocardial oxygen supply are largely dependent on myocardial oxygen demand,[29,30] we would have expected to find a lower myocardial perfusion corresponding to the lower RPP. However, CFI was no different in the propranolol-treated patients than the other groups. It was possible that there was no effect of propranolol, in the dose used, on coronary vascular resistance, or that the noninvasive thallium imaging technique failed to elicit subtle differences in myocardial perfusion between the propranolol and other groups. The CFI to RPP ratio, which is a useful index of the ratio of myocardial perfusion to MVO_2, that is, the supply to demand ratio, was unaffected by any of the four drugs, implying that all of the drugs tested were equally effective in maintaining a rate of myocardial perfusion appropriate to the oxygen demand.

Conclusion

The limitation of exercise tolerance often reported by patients on beta blockers, and described in various studies,[7,26,27] does not appear to be due, on the basis of our findings, to coronary insufficiency during exercise. It may be due to a limitation or a ceiling on heart rate and contractility, that is, the CO response to exercise, associated with a peripheral resistance that is inappropriately high for any particular level of exercise. It is well known that during moderate to severe exercise in the presence of beta blockers, the sympathetically mediated responses of the cardiovascular system are markedly attenuated.[5,31] Thus, CO responses to exercise may be depressed through antagonism of cardiac beta-adrenoreceptors, and the skeletal muscle blood supply may be impaired by blockade of beta$_2$-adrenoreceptors in vascular smooth muscle. Also, beta blockers affect fatty acid, glucose, and lactic acid metabolism and have a direct effect on beta receptors on the motor end-plate and skeletal muscle cells[32] to contribute to muscle fatigue.

Therefore, it is probably prudent not to prescribe beta blockers in young hypertensive patients undergoing moderate to severe exercise. However, ischemic heart disease should not be regarded as a contraindication to the use of beta blockers in hypertension, provided that there are no signs of cardiac failure or bradyarrhythmias.

References

1. World Health Organisation Report Series: Hypertension and coronary artery disease: classification and criteria for epidemilogical studies. Geneva: WHO, 1959.
2. WONG HO, KASSER IS, BRUCE R: Impaired maximal exercise performance with hypertensive cardiovascular disease. Circulation 1969; 39: 633–638.
3. SANNERSTADT R: Haemodynamic findings at rest and during exercise in mild arterial hypertension. Am J Med Sci 1969; 258: 70–79.
4. TAYLOR SH, DONALD KW, BISHOP JM: Circulatory studies in hypertensive patients at rest and during exercise. Clin Sci 1957; 16: 351–376.
5. EPSTEIN SE, ROBINSON BF, KAHLER RL, BRAUNWALD E: Effects of beta-adrenergic blockade on the cardiac response to maximal and submaximal exercise in man. J Clin Invest 1965; 44: 1745–1753.
6. MCKENNA DH, CORLISS RJ, SIALER S, ZARNSTORFF WC, CRUMPTON CW, ROWE

GG: Effect of propranolol on systemic and coronary hemodynamics at rest and during simulated exercise. Circ Res 1966; 19: 520–527.

7. ANDERSON SD, BYE PTP, PERRY CP, THEOBALD G, NYBERG G: Limitation of work performance in normal adult males in the presence of beta-adrenergic blockade. Aust NZ J Med 1979; 9: 515–529.

8. PORT S, COBB FR, JONES RH: Effects of propranolol on left ventricular function in normal men. Circulation 1980; 61: 358–366.

9. TAYLOR SH, SILKE B, LEE PS: Intravenous beta-blockade in coronary artery disease. N Engl J Med 1982; 306: 631–635.

10. MAGNANI B, AMBROSIONI E, COSTA FV, MALINI PL, MAGELLI C: Comparison of antihypertensive activity of atenolol and methyldopa at rest and during exercise. Int J Clin Pharmacol Ther Toxicol 1981; 19: 440–444.

11. KUMAR EB, NELSON GIC, SILKE B, AHUJA RC, OKOLI RC, TAYLOR SH: Circulatory dose-response effects of hydrochlorothiazide at rest and during dynamic exercise in essential hypertension. J Roy Coll Physicians Lond 1982; 16: 232–235.

12. VARNAUSKAS E, CRAMÉR G, MALMCRONA R, WERKÖ L: Effect of chlorothiazide on blood pressure and blood flow at rest and on exercise in patients with arterial hypertension. Clin Sci 1961; 20: 407–416.

13. LEE WR, FOX LM, SLOTKOFF LM: Effects of antihypertensive therapy on cardiovascular response to exercise. Am J Cardiol 1979; 44: 325–328.

14. FAGARD R, BULPITT C, LIJNEN P, AMERY A: Response of the systemic and pulmonary circulation to converting-enzyme inhibition (captopril) at rest and during exercise in hypertensive patients. Circulation 1982; 65: 33–39.

15. FAGARD R, LIJNEN P, VANHEES L, AMERY A: Hemodynamic response to converting enzyme inhibition at rest and exercise in humans. J Appl Physiol 1982; 53: 576–581.

16. STRAUSS HW, HARRISON K, LANGAN JK, LEBOWITZ E, PITT B: Thallium-201 for myocardial imaging. Relation of thallium-201 to regional myocardial perfusion. Circulation 1975; 51: 641–645.

17. POHOST GM, ZIR LM, MOORE RH, MCKUSICK KA, GUINEY TE, BELLER GA: Differentiation of transiently ischemic from infarcted myocardium by serial imaging after a single dose of thallium-201. Circulation 1977; 55: 294–302.

18. PITT B, STRAUS HW: Evaluation of ventricular function by radioisotope techniques. N Engl J Med 1977; 296: 1097–1099.

19. CRAWFORD MH, LINDENFELD J, O'ROURKE RA: Effects of oral propranolol on left ventricular size and performance during exercise and acute pressure loading. Circulation 1980; 61: 549–554.

20. SKLAR J, JOHNSTON GD, OVERLIE P, GERBER JG, BRAMMELL HL, GAL J, NIES AS: The effects of a cardioselective (metoprolol) and a nonselective (propranolol) beta-adrenergic blocker on the response to dynamic exercise in normal men. Circulation 1982; 65: 894–899.

21. LUND-JOHANSEN P: The effect of beta-blocker therapy on chronic hemodynamics. Prim Cardiol 1980; 1 (suppl): 20–24.

22. REID JL, MILLAR JA, CAMPBELL BC: Enalapril and autonomic reflexes and exercise performance. J Hypertens 1983; 1 (suppl 1): 129–134.

23. LUND-JOHANSEN P: Hemodynamic changes in long-term diuretic therapy of essential hypertension. Acta Med Scand 1970; 181: 509–518.

24. LUND-JOHANSEN P: Hemodynamic changes in long-term alpha-methyldopa therapy of essential hypertension. Acta Med Scand 1972; 192: 221–226.

25. GOMOLL AW, McKINNEY GR: Sotalol: cardiac and haemodynamic actions in the anaesthetized dog. In: Snart AG, ed. Advances in beta-adrenergic blocking therapy. London: Excerpta Medica, 1974; 6–22.

26. PEARSON SB, BANKS DC, PATRICK JM: The effect of beta-adrenergic blockade on factors affecting exercise tolerance in normal man. Br J Clin Pharmacol 1979; 8: 143–148.

27. KAIJSER L, KAISER P, KARLSSON J, RÖSSNER S: Beta-blockers and running. Am Heart J 1980; 100: 943–944.

28. HEYNDRICKX GR, PANNIER J-L, MUYLAERT P, MABILDE C, LEUSEN I: Alteration in myocardial oxygen balance during exercise after beta-adrenergic blockade in dogs. J Appl Physiol 1980; 49: 28–33.

29. KLOCKE FJ, ELLES AK: Control of coronary blood flow. Annu Rev Med 1980; 31: 489–508.

30. FEIGL ED: Coronary physiology. Physiol Rev 1983; 63: 1–205.

31. SHANKS RG: The properties of beta-adrenoreceptor antagonists. Postgrad Med J 1976; 52 (suppl 4): 14–20.

32. BOWMAN WC: Effect of adrenergic activators and inhibitors on the skeletal muscles. In: Szekeres L, ed. Adrenergic activators and inhibitors. Berlin: Springer-Verlag, 1980; pp 47–182.

44

How Does Antihypertensive Therapy Modify Other Risk Factors?

NORMAN M. KAPLAN, M.D.

A number of chapters have addressed specific effects of various antihypertensive drugs and nondrug therapies on overall and individual aspects of cardiac function. I have been asked to go beyond these more obvious and direct effects and to assess the ways in which antihypertensive therapy modifies risk factors for cardiovascular diseases other than the high blood pressure. In order to do so, I will use mainly the information from the Framingham Study, since it is the source of the best quantitative risk assessment data now available.[1]

The Risk Factors for Cardiovascular Disease

The Framingham Study identified these six factors to be of greatest utility for the prediction of subsequent coronary morbidity: systolic blood pressure, cigarette smoking, serum total cholesterol and high-density lipoprotein (HDL) cholesterol, glucose tolerance, and left ventricular hypertrophy (LVH) by electrocardiography (ECG).[1] The rather striking contributions of these risk factors in predicting the likelihood of the development of major cardiovascular disease in the next 8 years are shown in Figure 1, which is for 40-year-old men. Similar Framingham data are available for coronary disease and stroke for both men and women at various ages in the American Heart Association Risk Factor handbooks and in sliderule calculators provided by pharmaceutical companies.

These six factors do not cover all those that may be involved in adding risk for cardiovascular disease. Some others are listed in Table I. Those listed as minor are either relatively weak in their predictive strength or relatively infrequent in the population. Others, such as the proved protective effects of small amounts of alcohol or the likely protection offered by regular intake of small doses of aspirin, cannot be entered into the risk profile, since there are no quantitative data to assess the degree of risk reduction they may provide.

Of those risk factors used in the Framingham analyses, cigarette smoking should not be influenced by therapy and, although it may be used in the future, LVH by ECG has not yet been assessed repeatedly in enough studies to be considered. We are left then with solid data only about changes in lipids

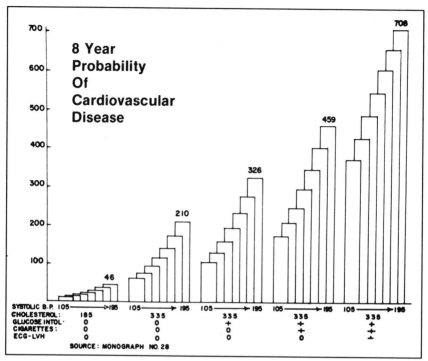

Figure 1. *The 8-year probability of cardiovascular disease, in 1,000 men of age 40 years, according to systolic blood pressures from 105 to 195 mmHg at specified levels of other risk factors, in the Framingham Study, monograph no. 28. (Used with permission from Kannel.)[1]*

and glucose tolerance of the various Framingham risk factors other than blood pressure. Therefore, I will mainly examine the evidence about the effects of antihypertensive therapy on lipids and glucose tolerance. Even though the evidence is less certain, I will also consider their effects on other probable risk factors.

The Effects of Therapy On Risk Factors

There are no definitive data on what the various treatments will do to cardiovascular risk when given to the same population. Unfortunately all of the currently available controlled therapeutic trials have used the diuretic-first stepped care approach. Therefore, until publication of the results from the ongoing Medical Research Council (MRC) of England's trial,[2] we cannot make any meaningful comparisons between different therapies. There have been numerous short-term comparisons between efforts of different agents on individual risk factors, but none on overall morbidity or mortality.

Lipids: As shown in the recent review of all published data by Weidmann et al,[3] diuretic therapy has almost always been shown to increase total

TABLE I   Known Risk Factors for Cardiovascular Disease

Major	Minor
Cigarette smoking	Obesity
Hypercholesterolemia	Physical inactivity
Hypertension	Diabetes and glucose intolerance
	Stress and personality type
	Excessive alcohol intake
	Estrogen intake

serum cholesterol and the low-density lipoprotein (LDL) and very low-density lipoprotein (VLDL) components, while having little or no effect on HDL cholesterol (Fig. 2).

In most studies using beta blockers alone, total cholesterol and LDL cholesterol are usually unchanged, but triglycerides almost always are increased and HDL cholesterol is lowered (Fig. 3). Although some have found these adverse effects to be less marked with more cardioselective agents,[4] the summation by Weidmann et al[3] of all published data found a mean decrease of 7% in HDL cholesterol with both selective and nonselective agents.[3] On the other hand, beta blockers with high intrinsic sympathomimetic activity caused only a 2% decrease in HDL cholesterol.

The amount of data on other agents is more limited, but an increasing number of studies have shown beneficial changes in total cholesterol, triglycerides, and HDL cholesterol with the alpha-blocker prazosin.[5]

Glucose Tolerance: Here again, the largest body of data is on diuretics and beta blockers, showing a definite tendency for glucose tolerance to worsen in some patients with diuretics. In the ongoing MRC trial, impaired glucose tolerance was observed about three times more frequently in those who received bendroflumethiazide compared with those who received a placebo, but no more frequently in those given propranolol.[6] The true incidence of glucose intolerance may have been higher, since testing was done only when fasting and random blood glucose levels exceeded 108 and 150 mg/dl, respectively.

In a much smaller group of patients followed much more closely over 14 years of continuous diuretic therapy, glucose tolerance tended to worsen progressively, returning toward normal within 7 months after withdrawal of therapy.[7]

The mechanism for diuretic-induced glucose intolerance is likely a reduced pancreatic beta-cell secretion of insulin in response to glucose, mediated via hypokalemia.[8] In the study by Helderman et al,[8] glucose tolerance, beta-cell sensitivity to glucose, and tissue sensitivity to insulin remained unchanged after 10 days of 100 mg hydrocholothiazide in subjects whose serum potassium was kept normal by the concomitant administration of 80 mEq of potassium per day. Glucose tolerance and pancreatic secretion of insulin were decreased in those given the diuretic alone and allowed to become hypokalemic.

Beta blockers alone may increase fasting and postprandial blood sugars a

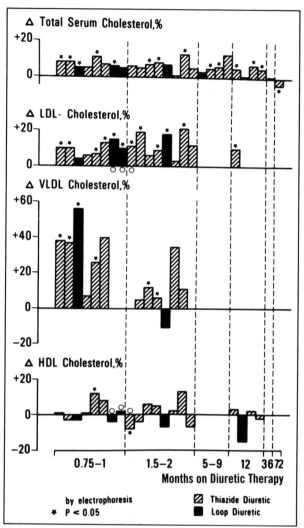

Figure 2. *An analysis of all published reports with a minimum of 12 subjects per study showing the percentage changes in serum lipoprotein cholesterol fractions as related to the duration of monotherapy with thiazide-type or certain loop diuretics. Loop diuretics are indicated by black columns. Asterisks denote statistically significant changes compared with pretreatment conditions, p < 0.05. (Reprinted with permission from Weidmann et al.[3])*

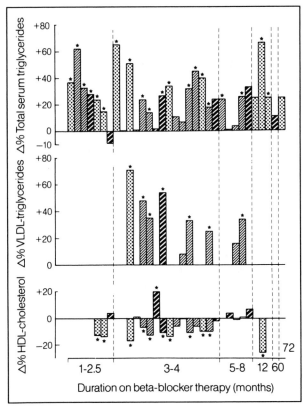

Figure 3. *An analysis of all published reports with a minimum of 12 subjects per study showing the percentage changes in serum total and VLDL triglycerides and HDL cholesterol as related to the duration of monotherapy with beta blockers. Asterisks denote statistically significant changes compared with placebo conditions, p = 0.05 or less. (Reprinted with permission from Weidmann et al.[3])*

small amount, but little overt glucose intolerance is usually observed with them or with other adrenergic inhibitors.

The potential harm of drug-induced glucose intolerance is less widely documented and appreciated than for hyperlipemia.[9] Nonetheless, the Whitehall study of 18,403 men found a significant increase of 10-year mortality rates from both coronary heart disease and stroke when the 2-hour blood glucose values were greater than 97 mg/dl.[10] The major portion of this increased risk for coronary disease and stroke could not be explained by the effects of age, blood pressure, or other known risk factors. Thus, glucose intolerance and, to a much more obvious degree, diabetes cause significant increases in cardiovascular risk.

Other Possible Risk Factors: Beyond hyperlipemia and glucose intolerance, a host of possible deleterious effects may accompany various antihypertensive agents. These have been most clearly recognized with the use of diuretics, perhaps because diuretics have been used in more patients for the longest times, but also because they may provoke more derangements in biochemical and metabolic functions.

Hypokalemia

Since hypokalemia has been covered elsewhere, I will only reiterate two points. First, diuretic-induced hypokalemia is common, appearing in as many as a third of patients given the equivalent of 50 mg of hydrochlorothiazide a day. Second, the frequency of ventricular ectopic activity (VEA) is increased in the presence of diuretic-induced hypokalemia.[6] Whether this increase and the subsequent development of ventricular fibrillation is responsible for the apparent lack of protection against coronary mortality in the therapeutic trials is uncertain, but it is certainly plausible. Furthermore, we should recall the higher coronary mortality rate, mostly from sudden death and likely from arrhythmias, noted among those who entered the MRFIT study with an abnormal ECG and who were then given more intensive therapy with 50 to 100 mg a day of either chlorthalidone or hydrochlorothiazide.[11] Hypokalemia was noted almost three times more frequently among those patients who were given high doses of diuretic.

Increased Circulating Catecholamines

Plasma catecholamine levels are usually increased in patients who take diuretics, beta blockers, or vasodilators, whereas they may be lower in those who take drugs that diminish adrenergic activity, such as reserpine, methyldopa, or clonidine.[12] Such elevated catecholamine levels may only limit the antihypertensive effectiveness of those drugs that cause them to increase, but they may also add to cardiovascular risks in other ways.

One way that elevated levels of catecholamine could add to risk is by increasing further the epinephrine-induced shifts of potassium out of the blood into cells, a shift that has been measured to be as much as 1.0 mEq/liter during the infusion of epinephrine.[13] Such shifts could increase the propensity for arrhythmias during stress, such as after an acute myocardial infarction. The connection between preexisting diuretic-induced hypokalemia and the elevations of plasma epinephrine from both diuretic therapy and the stress of coronary ischemia with the increased sudden deaths observed in the high-risk MRFIT patients cannot be proved, but, at the least, is plausible.

Other Considerations

We could speculate a good deal more about proved and probable ways that antihypertensive therapy may either improve or worsen other risk factors. Unfortunately, we have no properly collected hard data to quantitate these effects. A paper presented at the 1983 American Heart Association meeting compared the changes in four risk factors noted over 8 years among people in Framingham who either were started on antihypertensive drug therapy or were not.[14] The lowered blood pressure in those given therapy provided a significant decrease in overall predicted risk.

Such data still do not answer the basic question: can risks for premature cardiovascular disease be minimized to an even greater degree by the more cautious use of antihypertensive drug therapy?

As hopeful as these data from Framingham are, they do not provide the definitive evidence that one or another form of antihypertensive therapy can more significantly reduce the high level of coronary disease mortality in hypertensive patients. Such evidence will, it is hoped, come from the ongoing MRC trial. In the meantime, we should do all that is possible to minimize the known and possible risks of therapy.

References

1. KANNEL WB: An overview of the risk factors for cardiovascular disease. In: Kaplan NM, Stamler J, eds. Prevention of coronary heart disease: practical management of the risk factors. Philadelphia: W.B. Saunders, 1983; 1–19.

2. Report of Medical Research Council Working Party on Mild to Moderate Hypertension: Randomised controlled trial of treatment of mild hypertension: design and pilot trial. Br Med J 1977; 1: 1437–1440.

3. WEIDMANN P, GERBER A, MORDASINI R: Effects of antihypertensive therapy on serum lipoproteins. Hypertension 1983; 5 (suppl III): III-20–III-131.

4. DAY JL, METCALFE J, SIMPSON CN: Adrenergic mechanisms in control of plasma lipid concentrations. Br Med J 1982; 284: 1145–1148.

5. LOWENSTEIN J: The effects of prazosin on serum lipids in patients with essential hypertension. Am J Med 1984; 76 (suppl 2A): 79–84.

6. GREENBERG G, BRENNAN PJ, MIALL WE: Effects of diuretic and beta-blockers therapy in the Medical Research Council Trial. Am J Med 1984; 76 (suppl 2A): 45–51.

7. MURPHY MB, KOHNER E, LEWIS PJ, SCHUMER B, DOLLERY CT: Glucose intolerance in hypertensive patients treated with diuretics; a fourteen-year follow-up. Lancet 1982; 2: 1293–1295.

8. HELDERMAN JH, ELAHI D, ANDERSEN DK, RAIZES GS, TOBIN JD, SHOCKEN D, ANDRES R: Prevention of the glucose intolerance of thiazide diuretics by maintenance of body potassium. Diabetes 1983; 32: 106–111.

9. KAPLAN NM: Diabetes and glucose intolerance. In: Kaplan NM, Stamler J, eds. Prevention of coronary heart disease: practical management of the risk factors. Philadelphia: WB Saunders, 1983: 113–119.

10. FULLER JH, SHIPLEY MJ, ROSE G, JARRETT RJ, KEEN H: Mortality from coronary heart disease and stroke in relation to degree of glycaemia: the Whitehall study. Br Med J 1983; 287: 867–870.

11. Multiple Risk Factor Intervention Trial Research Group: Multiple risk factor inter-

vention trial: risk factor changes and mortality results. JAMA 1982; 248: 1465–1477.

12. POLAK G, REID JL, HAMILTON CA, JONES DH, DOLLERY CT: Sympathetic nervous function and renin activity in hypertensives on long term drug treatment with propranolol, methyldopa or bendrofluazide. Clin Experimental Hypertension 1978; 1: 1–9.

13. HEIDBREDER E, SCHAFFERHANS K, KIRSTEN R, HEIDLAND A: Effect of diuretics and calcium antagonists on circulatory parameters and plasma catecholamines during mental stress. Eur J Clin Pharmacol 1983; 23: 19–22.

14. SHEA S, COOK EF, KANNEL WB, GOLDMAN L: Effects of antihypertensive treatment on cardiovascular risk factors: data from the Framingham Heart Study [abstract]. Circulation 1983; 68 (suppl III): 1144.

45

Reduction of Sympathetic Tone and Myocardial Hypertrophy in Hypertensive Patients after Relaxation Therapy

VINCENT DEQUATTRO, M.D.
IGOR K. SHKHVATSABAYA, M.D.
ALEXEI P. YURENEV, M.D.
VIKTOR V. KHRAMELASHVILI, M.D.
ELENA V. PARFENOVA, M.D.
BORIS B. SALENKO, M.D.
VLADIMIR B. LEBEDEV, Ph.D.
ELENA G. DYAKONOVA, M.D
SVETLANA E. USTINOVA, M.D.
IRINA A. LICHITEL, M.D.
EDWARD BLANCHARD, Ph.D.
ROBERT BARNDT, M.D.
ANDRAS G. FOTI, Ph.D.

Relaxation therapy and biofeedback-enhanced relaxation techniques have lowered blood pressure of hypertensive patients, but generally their effects have been marginal or of short duration compared with the results of pharmacologic trials.[1] Furthermore, as attested to by the findings presented and referenced elsewhere in this book, various types of pharmacologic agents have reduced left ventricular (LV) mass in hypertensive patients.[2]

We visited the Myasnikof Heart Institute in Moscow in July, 1982, as a continuation of our joint interest with our Soviet colleagues in the sympathetic nervous system, stress, psychologic factors, and nonpharmacologic therapy of hypertension. We attempted to determine if relaxation techniques, as developed by our Soviet colleagues, could reduce blood pressure in Soviet patients with primary hypertension classified according to psychologic profiles. The different profiles were validated earlier in our laboratory or those of the Soviets. We attempted to determine if there were concomitant effects on sympathetic tone and blood pressure at rest and during mental stress and isometric and dynamic exercise. Furthermore, we were interested to know whether or not relaxation therapy could affect psychologic profiles and noninvasive assessments of cardiac function.

Patient Selection

At the onset, 20 patients with primary hypertension, ages 25 to 51 years, were admitted to the Myasnikov Institute of Clinical Cardiology after having been off medications for at least 3 weeks. Complete history and physical examination, including laboratory workup to exclude secondary hypertension, were performed on patients admitted to the Myasnikov Institute. Patients had blood pressures taken in the morning and evening daily. The patients underwent psychologic testing using scales previously employed in our laboratory, modified by Sullivan et al[3] from Speilberger. These were interpreted verbally for the patients by one of the Soviet psychologists in a group session. The patients were also classified according to Soviet psychologic scales, including those for neuroticism, clinical rating, and by the Mini-Mult, a shortened version of the Minnesota Multiphasic Personality Inventory (MMPI).[4] On a separate day, M-mode echo was performed[5] and measurements of cardiac function included septal thickness, posterior wall thickness, fiber shortening, and velocity of fiber shortening. Systolic time intervals and electroencephalographic records were also made.

Protocol

After 3 or 4 days of baseline assessments, the patients underwent a laboratory protocol as follows: nothing orally after midnight on the day of the test; patient was supine and first blood pressure taken immediately. A needle with heparinized tubing was placed in the antecubital vein for the purpose of withdrawing blood. After 30 minutes, blood pressure, pulse, and blood samples were obtained.

Relaxation Therapy Technique

The relaxation training sessions were conducted for 14 consecutive days by the same psychiatrist in a quiet room with comfortable high-backed, padded chairs. Two separate sessions were conducted at 11 and 12 o'clock daily, and the patients faced the front of the room and were asked to look at a large symbol ("Zen-like") whose dual purpose was to provide a point of concentration and also an image that could be recalled in the future away from the sessions. The purpose of the first session was for instruction and goals. The goal was for the patient to attain an altered state of consciousness in which he was at peace and harmony with his thoughts, body, and surroundings. Music and repetitive phraseology were used to allow this state of relaxation. Musical recordings early in the session were more soothing pieces to induce calm, whereas later they were replaced by more lively music to create arousal in preparation for the end of the session. The psychiatrist gradually diminished his own role in leading the group as they learned the technique. Repetition of internal self-statements, such as "I'm relaxed, I am calm" were used in the initial several minutes of the sessions. Muscle relaxation was employed, but statements expressing heaviness were avoided. Patients were trained to connect the symbol with the relaxation and were to recall the symbol to initiate their own self-practice. They did this for 5 to 10 minutes 3 times a day (self-hypnosis?). One measure of reaching the desired goal was the sense of relaxation of the facial muscles when the points of the image seemed to appear and disappear in a pulsating manner. The relaxation formula appeared to have elements of autogenic training and symbolism similar to those of Zen Buddhism and aspects of Pavlovian conditioning. A full analysis of the methodology is forthcoming from Dr. Salenko of the Myasnikof Institute.

Although the relaxation therapy was in the group format, individual consultation was available to the patient by the therapist between sessions. In addition, the patient was asked to practice relaxation three times during the day for a total of 20 to 30 minutes. The patients remained hospitalized during the 14 days of relaxation therapy, although some left the hospital on occasion for a period of 2 to 3 hours. At the completion of the relaxation therapy phase, the patients underwent testing as before and, in addition, underwent psychologic profile evaluation, echo, and systolic time interval assessment.

Assessments: Echo estimations of LV mass using an SKF Echoline I were made in the conventional fashion.[6] Systolic time intervals were assessed after 30 minutes supine rest and the ratio of preejection period (PEP) to left ventricular (LV) ejection time was calculated.[7] Plasma norepinephrine was measured using a radioenzymatic method.[8] Psychologic assessments were taken from both American[3] and Soviet scales.[4,5]

Results

Blood Pressure Changes in Established Versus Borderline Hypertensive Patients: Eleven patients had hypertension, that is, they had greater than 140 mmHg systolic blood pressure after five days hospitalization. Of these, six had reduced norepinephrine, four had increased norepinephrine, and one had no change in plasma norepinephrine after the relaxation therapy and at restudy. Of the reduced norepinephrine subgroup, four reduced their blood pressure with relaxation therapy, one had no change, and one increased his blood pressure by the 15th day. Of the group with increased norepinephrine levels, one had no change in blood pressure and three had a reduction in blood pressure with therapy. The one patient with no change also had no change in blood pressure after relaxation training. Thus, of the 11 patients who were clearly hypertensive, seven reduced their blood pressure and, of these, four had a reduction of norepinephrine and three had an increased norepinephrine after relaxation. The prevalence rate for having a blood pressure reduction in the range of 6% or more for the established hypertensive patients was 65%. Nine patients had at least a 6% reduction in systolic blood pressure, and the average reduction in these patients was 11%. Five patients had no change, one had a 6% increase in blood pressure, and the remaining four had less than a 4% reduction in blood pres-

TABLE I   **Characteristics of Patients with Systolic Blood Pressure Reduction of 6% or More after Relaxation Therapy**

Basal Blood Pressure (mmHg)	Blood Pressure (%)	Basal NE (μg/liter)	NE (%)
188/135	−24	287	+63
170/100	−12	498	−47
160/80	−12	282	+52
130/90	−15	253	−15
160/100	− 6	487	−36
150/105	− 7	449	−10
160/100	− 6	201	+16
150/90	− 7	299	−10
118/80	− 7	485	− 7
154 ± 7*	−11 ± 2*	360 ± 39*	.67 ± 12*
98 ± 6*			

*Means + SEM.

sure after 16 days relaxation treatment. Of the nine patients with good blood pressure response, one was normotensive and one was a borderline hypertensive (See Table I). The ambulatory blood pressure of the patients is given in Figure 1 for both before and after relaxation therapy.

The mean blood pressure of the patients before relaxation therapy taken while on the ward was 151 ± 4 systolic and 95 ± 2 diastolic. After 14 days of relaxation therapy, day blood pressures were reduced 13 mmHg (a mean of 9%) systolic and 4 mmHg diastolic with $p < 0.001$ and < 0.01, respectively. Nighttime systolic blood pressures were also reduced, by 5 mmHg, but without a diastolic blood pressure change. Change in nighttime pressures was significant ($p < 0.01$).

Plasma Norepinephrine Before and the Changes After Relaxation Therapy: Overall there was a 10% reduction of basal plasma norepinephrine after relaxation ($p < 0.01$). Of the seven patients with high basal norepinephrine, that is, greater than 450 ng/liter (1 SD above the mean) after 30 minutes supine rest, five reduced both their blood pressure and norepinephrine with relaxation training. Of the six with the highest norepinephrine, there was a mean reduction of norepinephrine of 25% and a reduction on blood pressure of 6%. Of the five patients with the lowest norepinephrine at the time of the basal study, there was a 14% reduction in blood pressure despite a 20% increase in norepinephrine after relaxation training. Of all the hypertensive patients, 10 reduced their basal norepinephrine at a range of 10% to 50%, with an average reduction of 32% ($p < 0.01$). However, nine patients had a less than 10% reduction in norepinephrine, with the range of 6% decrease to 65% increase, with an average change of a 15% increase.

Relaxation Therapy Sessions. Blood pressures of each patient were measured during two of the therapy sessions. The first session utilized relaxation therapy throughout, and the second session employed the biofeedback technique of a skin thermometer during the last half hour. Systolic blood pressures were reduced during the relaxation training session, both with and

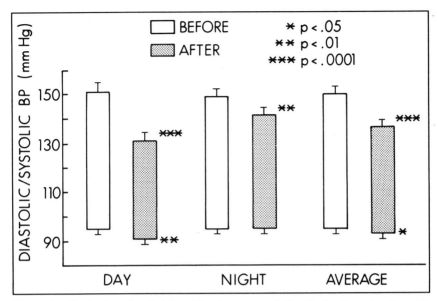

Figure 1. *Reduction of ambulatory blood pressure of all patients after relaxation trial.*

without the biofeedback. There was a significant reduction of systolic blood pressure during these sessions. Blood pressure tended to increase toward the end of the session during the rearousal process. There were no significant changes in skin temperature or there was a further reduction in systolic and diastolic blood pressure during the biofeedback therapy (Fig. 2).

Psychologic Evaluations: American Scales. Hypertensive patients in Moscow appeared to have less depression than the American counterparts that we studied previously. The mean scale of depression was 5.5 ± 1.0, less than that of the American hypertensive patients, 14.2 ± 1.4 ($p < 0.01$). However, there was a significant reduction in the depression rating after the 14th day of relaxation therapy, ($p < 0.01$). The Soviet patients had similar anxiety levels, but state and trait at 40 ± 1 and 46 ± 1, respectively, compared with the American patients studied previously. Furthermore, patients in Moscow had lower prevalence rates of "anger in," approximately 35%, compared with 76% for Californians.[3] There were no significant changes of the scales for anxiety, both state and trait, anger, or guilt after the relaxation training sessions.

Soviet Scales. Using the instruments developed in the USSR, 6 of the 20 patients were classified definitely neurotic and 5 definitely non-neurotic. The remaining 9 patients had characteristics somewhere in between. The average blood pressure of those who were definitely neurotic at the time of study of laboratory measurements was 137/88 mmHg, which was less than the non-neurotic group whose blood pressure was a mean of 159/104 mmHg ($p < 0.08$ and < 0.05), respectively. Of the neurotic group, three were hyper-

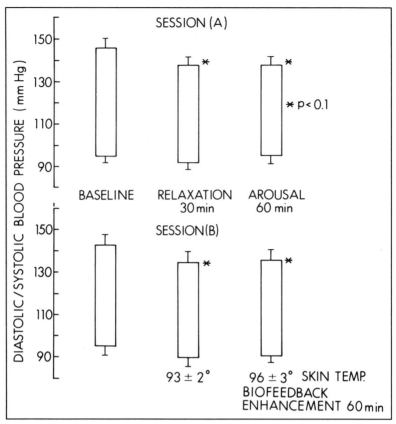

Figure 2. *Blood pressure changes during relaxation and arousal **(a)** or bio-feedback enhancement **(b)** of relaxation.*

tensives, two had borderline hypertension, and one was normotensive. However, in the non-neurotic group, all patients had established hypertension. There was an average systolic blood pressure reduction of 11% in this group after relaxation therapy compared with a reduction of only 3% in the neurotic group. The difference in the degree of blood pressure reduction after relaxation therapy was significant ($p < 0.02$). The norepinephrine levels were increased in the neurotic group, value of 447 ± 75 compared with 354 ± 46, but these differences were not significant. There was a greater reduction of norepinephrine after relaxation therapy (21%) in the neurotic patients compared with the 7% change in patients who were characterized as non-neurotic ($p < 0.05$; Fig. 3). Interestingly, when the American scale of depression was employed, the neurotic patients scored highest with a value of 8.5 ± 2.0; whereas, the non-neurotic patients had a 3.0 depression rating ($p < 0.03$). In our previous studies of 65 California patients,[2] there was a close correlation of depression with anxiety ($r = 0.67$, $p < 0.001$).

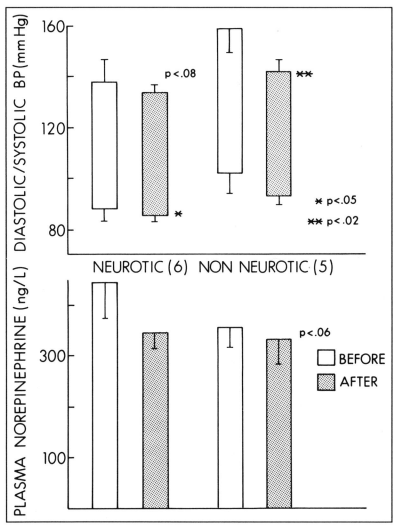

Figure 3. *Reduction of blood pressure and plasma NE in hypertensive subgroups after the relaxation trial.*

Echo Assessments of LV Mass and Systolic Time Intervals: Measurements were made of both septal (12.2 ± 0.2) and posterior wall (11.3 ± 0.7) thickness using standard techniques. There was a 5% reduction in septal thickness in the 19 patients after relaxation therapy (p < 0.08). Furthermore, the reduction was pronounced in non-neurotic patients, 15% (p < 0.07) and blood pressure responders (p < 0.01, Table II). There were no significant changes in posterior wall thickness. The systolic interval, PEP to LV ejection time ratio, was increased in the patients after relaxation therapy (0.27 ± 0.02

TABLE II   **Regression of Septal Hypertrophy and Reduction of Cardiac Autonomic Tone, After Relaxation Therapy**

Patients		All	Neurotic		Blood Pressure Responders	
			Yes	No	Yes	No
Septal Thickness (mm)	Before	12.2 ± .2	10.7 ± 1	14.6 ± 3	12.6 ± 2	12.6 ± 2
	After	12.0 ± .8*	10.8 ± 1	13.6 ± 1.4*	11.6 ± 1*	12.5 ± 2
No.	19		6	5	9	5
PEP	Before	0.27 ± 0.02	0.22 ± 0.02	0.33 ± 0.02	0.27 ± 0.02	0.29 ± 0.03
LVET	After	0.30 ± 0.01†	0.28 ± 0.02‡	0.32 ± 0.02	0.31 ± 0.01‡	0.29 ± 0.03

PEP = preejection period; LVET = left ventricular ejection time.
*p < 0.07.
†p < 0.05.
‡p < 0.01.

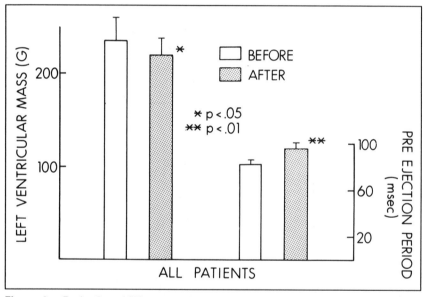

Figure 4. *Reduction of LV mass and cardiac sympathetic tone (as measured by an increase in PEP) in all patients after the relaxation trial.*

versus 0.30 ± 0.01; $p < 0.001$). The changes were even greater in the neurotic and blood pressure responder subgroups ($p < 0.01$, < 0.05, Table II).

Similar findings were present when LV mass index was calculated according to the standard formula.[8] When all patients were considered, there were small but significant reductions in LV mass ($p < 0.05$) and increases in the PEP, respectively ($p < 0.01$; Fig. 4). When these two factors were assessed in the patients according to subgroups, LV mass was reduced significantly after relaxation for both non-neurotic and blood pressure responders ($p < 0.05$).

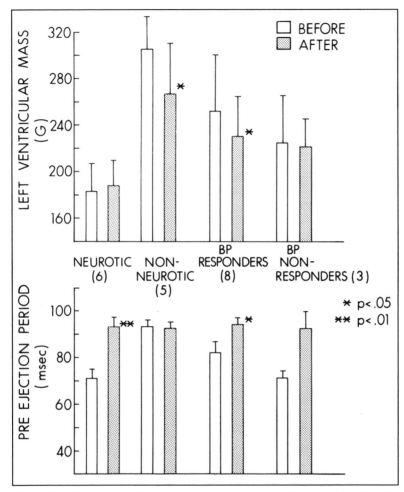

Figure 5. *Reduction of LV mass and cardiac sympathetic tone after relaxation in neurotic patients and blood pressure responders.*

Cardiac sympathetic tone was reduced significantly in the neurotic (p < 0.01) and blood pressure responder groups (p < 0.05; Fig. 5).

Comment

There were reductions of systolic blood pressure in the majority of hypertensive patients during the trial. This was observed both on the ward and in the laboratory. Furthermore, blood pressure reductions were seen during the relaxation therapy session, and one attempted biofeedback therapy seemed to lower blood pressure further during that session. It was surprising, indeed, to find that blood pressure reduction was greatest in patients with the lowest plasma norepinephrine and those who were classified as non-neurotic by the Soviet scale. It was also of interest to note that the majority of the patients reduced their plasma norepinephrine and that reduction of norepinephrine was most marked in neurotic patients as characterized by the Soviet scale.

The American scale may not have been a valid assessment of the psychologic characteristics of patients from the USSR. Patients in Moscow rated much lower in depression and slightly less in anxiety and anger than their American counterparts. However, there was a tendency for patients who scored the highest in the USSR scale for neuroticism to score high for depression by the American scale. It also seems important to note that systolic blood pressure, not diastolic blood pressure, was lowered during the basal state both in the laboratory and at the bedside.

There were significant reductions in septal thickness, LV mass, and cardiac correlates of sympathetic nerve tone after relaxation therapy. It is also possible that the institutionalization was responsible for all the observed changes. However, most patients were admitted to the hospital for three to five days before the entry examination and the relaxation therapy.

Patients characterized according to Soviet features of neuroticism tended to have more depression on the American scales and higher plasma norepinephrine, lower blood pressure after acclimatization, greater reduction of cardiac and peripheral neural tone after relaxation, and less change in ventricular mass after relaxation. On the other hand, reductions in LV mass after relaxation were in the order of 5% to 10% greater in blood pressure responders and non-neurotic patients. Thus, the changes in sympathetic tone and blood pressure appeared to be divergent as often as parallel.

Both excessive neural tone and afterload may be pathogenic in the myocardial hypertrophy of some patients with primary hypertension. It may be of great clinical importance, therefore, by either hemodynamic, neural, or psychologic attributes to predict which hypertensive patients with myocardial hypertrophy are likely to respond to pharmacologic or nonpharmacologic interventions that neutralize neural tone.

References

1. BLANCHARD EB, MILLER ST: Psychological treatment of cardiovascular disease. Arch Gen Psych 1977; 34: 1402–1413.
2. SHKHVATSABAYA I: Left ventricular hypertrophy in mild hypertension. In: Mild hypertension. London: Raven Press, 1982.
3. SULLIVAN P, SCHOENTGEN S, DEQUATTRO V, PROCCI W, LEVINE D, VAN DER MEULEN J, BORNHEIMER J: Anxiety, anger and neurogenic tone at rest and in stress in patients with primary hypertension. Hypertension 1981; 3 (suppl II): 119–123.
4. ZAITSEV VP: The Russian Version of the Mini-Mult. Psichologicheskiy Zhurnal (Rus.), 1981.

5. ZAITSEV VP: Psychological measurements. In: Handbook of cardiology (Rus.), Meditsina, Moscow, 1982.
6. WEISSLER AM, HARRIS WS, SCHOENFELD CD: Systolic time intervals in heart failure in man. Circulation 1968; 37: 149.
7. PEULER JD, JOHNSON GA: Simultaneous single isotope radioenzymatic assay of plasma norepinephrine, epinephrine and dopamine. Life Sci 1977; 21 (5): 625–636.
8. DEVEREUX RB, REICHEK N: Echocardiographic determination of left ventricular mass in man: anatomic validation of the method. Circulation 1977; 55: 613.

SUBJECT INDEX